Building Core
Competencies
in Pharmacy
Informatics

Notices

The authors, editors, and publisher have made every effort to ensure the accuracy and completeness of the information presented in this book. However, the authors, editors, and publisher cannot be held responsible for the continued currency of the information, any inadvertent errors or omissions, or the application of this information. Therefore, the authors, editors, and publisher shall have no liability to any person or entity with regard to claims, loss, or damage caused or alleged to be caused, directly or indirectly, by the use of information contained herein.

Readers should note that the informatics field is rapidly changing. Although this book underwent an expedited publication process, some of the content has likely changed since it was written. Readers are encouraged to visit www.pharmacy-informatics.com for the latest developments concerning informatics topics found in this book as well as other, related informatics topics.

The inclusion in this book of any product in respect to which patent or trademark rights may exist shall not be deemed, and is not intended as, a grant of or authority to exercise any right or privilege protected by such patent or trademark. All such rights or trademarks are vested in the patent or trademark owner, and no other person may exercise the same without express permission, authority, or license secured from such patent or trademark owner.

The inclusion of a brand name does not mean the authors, the editors, or the publisher has any particular knowledge that the brand listed has properties different from other brands of the same product, nor should its inclusion be interpreted as an endorsement by the authors, the editors, or the publisher. Similarly, the fact that a particular brand has not been included does not indicate the product has been judged to be in any way unsatisfactory or unacceptable. Further, no official support or endorsement of this book by any federal or state agency or pharmaceutical company is intended or inferred.

Building Core Competencies in Pharmacy Informatics

EDITORS

Brent I. Fox

Margaret R. Thrower

Bill G. Felkey

Center for Graduate Studies
West Coast University
Los Angeles, CA

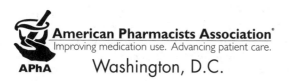

American Pharmacists Association
Improving medication use. Advancing patient care.
APhA   Washington, D.C.

Managing and Content Editor: Linda L. Young
Acquiring Editor: Sandra J. Cannon
Editorial Services: Potomac Indexing Services, LLC, Linda L. Young, and
Kathy E. Wolter
Book Design and Layout: Circle Graphics Inc.
Cover Design: Mariam Safi, APhA Creative Services

© 2010 by the American Pharmacists Association
APhA was founded in 1852 as the American Pharmaceutical Association.
Published by the American Pharmacists Association
2215 Constitution Avenue, NW
Washington, DC 20037
www.pharmacylibrary.com; www.pharmacist.com
All rights reserved.

To comment on this book via e-mail, send your message to the publisher at
aphabooks@aphanet.org.

Library of Congress Cataloging-in-Publication Data
Building core competencies in pharmacy informatics / editors, Brent I. Fox,
Margaret R. Thrower, and Bill G. Felkey.
    p. ; cm.
  Includes bibliographical references and index.
  ISBN 978-1-58212-144-4
  1. Pharmacy informatics. 2. Core competencies. I. Fox, Brent I. II. Thrower,
Margaret R. III. Felkey, Bill G. IV. American Pharmacists Association.
  [DNLM: 1. Medical Informatics Applications. 2. Pharmaceutical Services.
3. Professional Competence. QV 26.5 B932 2010]
  RS122.2.B85 2010
  615'.1023—dc22

                                                          2010023805

How to Order This Book
Online: www.pharmacist.com/shop_apha
By phone: 800-878-0729 (770-280-0085 from outside
the United States and Canada)
VISA®, MasterCard®, and American Express® cards accepted.

Dedication

To my parents, Larry and Debbie Fox: I am immensely grateful
for your love, support, and guidance.

To Greg Thrower, Anne Cancelosi, and Carol and Richard Ryman:
Thanks for your support, love, and always being there for me. To my
mentor and residency preceptor, Sheldon Holstad: Thanks for
the encouragement, the support, and believing in me
throughout the years.

To Judy: Your giving heart and beautiful smile make me appreciate
how lucky I have been to be with you through it all.

Contents

Foreword

Change is afoot in pharmacy, at a pace that is outstripping any other time in the history of the profession. Certain core aspects remain essential for practitioners, for example, pharmacotherapeutic expertise, critical thinking and communications skills, and compassion. However, there is undeniably a growing need for pharmacists to understand the role of informatics. Informatics is no longer just the domain of the computer-savvy pharmacist. It is increasingly part of everyday practice. This shift toward pharmacy informatics is due to internal factors as well as external factors, such as federal mandates requiring conversion of elements of the medication use process to an electronic format.

Being a pharmacist today may also be more challenging than at any time in history. There are more medications, more responsibilities, more expectations, and a seemingly unmanageable amount of information to process. However, learning about informatics is not just another item on a checklist to complete. When used properly, the principles of pharmacy informatics have the potential to reduce medication errors, streamline workflow, and enhance information management. Pharmacy informatics has even shown promise to help with the Holy Grail of reducing the burden of distributive functions so that pharmacists can have a greater focus on patient counseling—with the added benefit of clinical decision support tools. Gaining a firm understanding of the fundamentals of informatics is the first step in achieving this promise. *Building Core Competencies in Pharmacy Informatics* helps with that step and beyond. For example, this book provides a well-structured introduction to the implementation and challenges unique to the electronic medical record, electronic health record, and personal health record. Anyone who does not know the differences between those three and the impact each could have on medication reconciliation requirements will want to read this book. *Building Core Competencies in Pharmacy Informatics* also takes seemingly abstract issues such as interoperability and employs actual examples, such as the aftermath of Katrina, to make them very real. Although this book covers all of the fundamentals such as electronic prescribing, computerized provider order entry, electronic medical records, etc., it also goes beyond the basics. It explores topics of growing importance such as the pharmacist's role in the patient-centered medical home. Similarly, the participatory medicine model and Health 2.0 are discussed by one of the pioneers of pharmacy informatics.

I was happy to see a book written by leading clinicians with expertise in informatics, rather than information technology theorists who lack the necessary practice component. *Building Core Competencies in Pharmacy Informatics* is not only technically sound, it is also written in a very accessible style and allows the "voice" of the authors to come through. If you listen closely you can hear their enthusiasm, which comes only from living the subject as part of their day-to-day practice. The editors and chapter authors are optimistic about informatics but share a pragmatic perspective. They recognize that informatics is not a solution; rather it is an approach used as a means to the end of improving patient outcomes. Readers will benefit from this balanced approach, which is not always seen in this type of text.

The authors use the same tools and techniques as those of effective educators. They have created chapters composed of relevant topics and clearly defined purposes tailored to pharmacists. They also convey the information effectively and provide opportunities to put ideas into action with suggested activities. In doing so, the book is not limited to just informing readers about the ways in which informatics is affecting pharmacy—it delivers insight on how to manage that change. *Building Core Competencies in Pharmacy Informatics*, published by the American Pharmacists Association, is an invaluable tool to prepare you for practice today and for the change of tomorrow.

Kevin A. Clauson, PharmD
Associate Professor, Pharmacy Practice
College of Pharmacy
Adjunct Associate Professor, Biomedical Informatics
College of Osteopathic Medicine
Nova Southeastern University

About the Authors

Note: *The numbers in parentheses denote the chapter(s) written by the author.*

Frederick Albright, MS, PhD (4)
Director for Graduate Studies and Research Assistant Professor,
Department of Pharmacotherapy, and Research Assistant Professor,
Pharmacotherapy Outcomes Research Center, University of Utah
College of Pharmacy, Salt Lake City, Utah

Bradford N. Barker, BSEE (26)
President, NetConsult, Inc., Dalton, Georgia

Jennifer J. Boehne, PharmD (2)
Pharmacy Informatics & Outcomes Research Fellow, Division of General
Internal Medicine and Primary Care, Brigham and Women's Hospital,
Boston, Massachusetts

Michael J. Brownlee, PharmD, MS (25)
Director of Pharmacy, Oregon Health & Science University,
Portland, Oregon

P. Neil Edillo, PharmD, BCPS, CPHIMS (25)
Clinical Informatics Pharmacist, Oregon Health & Science University,
Portland, Oregon

Bill G. Felkey, MS (19, 24, 28)
Professor Emeritus, Department of Pharmacy Care Systems, Auburn University Harrison School of Pharmacy, Auburn, Alabama

Helen L. Figge, PharmD, MBA, CSSBB, CLSSS (22)
Vice President, Allscripts; and Board Member, HIMSS New York, Clifton Park, New York

Allen J. Flynn, PharmD, CPHIMS, CHS (18)
Medication Lead, Clinical Design Team, University of Michigan Health System, Ann Arbor, Michigan

Christopher R. Fortier, PharmD (27)
Manager, Pharmacy Support Services, and Clinical Assistant Professor, Medical University of South Carolina Medical Center, Charleston, South Carolina

Brent I. Fox, PharmD, PhD (1, 5, 6, 8)
Assistant Professor, Department of Pharmacy Care Systems, Auburn University Harrison School of Pharmacy, Auburn, Alabama

Karl F. Gumpper, BS Pharm, BCPS, FASHP (3)
Director, Section of Pharmacy Informatics & Technology, American Society of Health-System Pharmacists, Bethesda, Maryland

Christian Hartman, PharmD, MBA (20)
Medication Safety Officer, UMass Memorial Medical Center, Worcester, Massachusetts; and President and Director at Large, American Society of Medication Safety Officers, Horsham, Pennsylvania

Joan E. Kapusnik-Uner, PharmD, FASHP, FCSHP (7)
Manager Disease Decision Support, First DataBank, San Francisco, California; and Associate Clinical Professor, Department of Clinical Pharmacy, University of California San Francisco

William A. Lockwood, III, BA, MA (17)
Senior Editor, *ComputerTalk for the Pharmacist*; and Assistant Executive Director, American Society for Automation in Pharmacy, Blue Bell, Pennsylvania

Kevin Marvin, RPh, MS, FASHP (10)
Consultant, Medication Systems Informatics, Burlington, Vermont

Sandi H. Mitchell, BS Pharm, MSIS (27)
Senior Consultant, maxIT Healthcare, Westfield, Indiana

Shobha Phansalkar, RPh, PhD (11)
Instructor in Medicine, Brigham and Women's Hospital and Harvard
Medical School; and Senior Medical Informatician, Partners Healthcare,
Boston, Massachusetts

Steve Pickette, PharmD, BCPS (21)
Director, System Pharmacy Clinical Services, Providence Health &
Services, Renton, Washington

Terry L. Seaton, PharmD, BCPS, FCCP (Introductory Chapter)
Professor and Associate Director, Division of Pharmacy Practice, St.
Louis College of Pharmacy, St. Louis, Missouri

Andrew C. Seger, PharmD (2)
Senior Research Pharmacist, Division of General Internal Medicine and
Primary Care, Brigham and Women's Hospital; and Clinical Quality and
Information Systems Analysis, Partners HealthCare Systems, Inc.,
Boston, Massachusetts

Valerie Castellani Sheehan, PharmD (13, 14)
Clinical Program Development Coordinator, McKesson Pharmacy
Optimization, McKesson Corporation, Golden Valley, Minnesota

Mark H. Siska, RPh, MBA/TM (12)
Assistant Director, Informatics & Technology Pharmacy Services, Mayo
Clinic, Rochester, Minnesota

Margaret R. Thrower, BS, PharmD, BCPS (9, 15, 23)
Clinical Advisor, McKesson Pharmacy Optimization, McKesson
Corporation, Golden Valley, Minnesota

Dennis A. Tribble, PharmD (16)
Chief Pharmacy Officer, Baxa Corporation, Englewood, Colorado

Charles W. Westergard, BSPharm, MBA (21)
Vice President, Clinical Affairs, Pharmacy OneSource, Inc., Bellevue,
Washington

Setting the Stage: Consensus-Based Development of Pharmacy Informatics Competencies

Terry L. Seaton

T he new millennium has ushered in an enhanced interest in the application of technology and automation in health care. The resultant growth in emphasis on informatics has exposed a significant lack of an organized approach to education and training in this field. An adequate workforce to meet the current and future informatics needs in health care cannot be sustained without formally addressing key developmental issues.

Although the discipline known as medical informatics has been reasonably well established for decades, most physicians practicing medical informatics have largely been "self-trained." Nursing informatics specialists, who developed their field shortly after physicians developed medical informatics, have had a long history of a more structured approach to their professional development. Despite the extensive incorporation of computer applications in the pharmacy profession, pharmacy informatics has been the slowest of the major clinical informatics specialties to adopt an approach to formalized informatics training.

The original publication of a set of recommendations on education of medical and health informatics, by the International Medical Informatics Association (IMIA) in 2000, represented the first attempt to establish formal standards and expectations. These recommendations have recently been updated.[1] The intended audience for those recommendations included both clinicians who use informatics tools to support their daily practice and information technologists who practice health informatics.

Quickly following the original IMIA recommendations, in 2003, the Institute of Medicine (IOM) identified five core competencies to reform education within the health professions.[2] Among those educational objectives was a declaration to utilize informatics. Special emphasis was to be placed on using information technology to manage knowledge, reduce medical errors, support clinical decision making, and facilitate communication.

The IOM's recommendations then received the attention of both health professionals and the bodies that accredit educational programs for health professions. In 2006, the Accreditation Council for Pharmacy Education (ACPE) released a draft of the revised *Standards and Guidelines for the Professional Program in Pharmacy Leading to the Doctor of Pharmacy Degree*. The draft version was released to allow open comment from stakeholders. The finalized standards, which became effective in July of 2007, included a new expectation that entry-level Doctor of Pharmacy (PharmD) graduates "demonstrate expertise in informatics."[3]

Although the inclusion of informatics in ACPE's accreditation standards represents a significant step, the standards do not provide extensive details that pharmacy educators can use to inform curricular revision. A footnote simply states, "Competencies in informatics include basic terminology (data, information, knowledge, hardware, software, networks, information systems, information systems management); reasons for systematic processing of data, information and knowledge in health care; and the benefits and current constraints in using information and communication technology in health care."[3]

Recognizing the need for expansion on the informatics requirement in ACPE's standards, a group of experts in the area of pharmacy informatics began a process to develop a set of pharmacy informatics competencies in the fall of 2005. Coordinating their efforts through the Pharmacoinformatics Working Group leadership team of the American Medical Informatics Association (AMIA; www.amia.org/working-group/pharmacoinformatics), these experts identified an extensive list of possible competencies in pharmacy informatics. Suggestions were based on the previously published IMIA recommendations, American Society of Health-System Pharmacists' (ASHP's) goals and objectives for postgraduate year 2 pharmacy informatics residencies, and ideas developed through personal experience of the experts. This list was refined and revised many times, continuing into the fall of 2006, into an eventual draft of approximately 110 competency statements.

The next step in the process was to use a modified Delphi technique to develop consensus regarding the highest priority competencies that eventually would be recommended to be taught and assessed as part of an entry-level PharmD curriculum. To allow more pharmacy informatics experts to verify the competency statements, the St. Louis College of Pharmacy housed a Web-based portal. Individuals affiliated with ASHP's Section of Pharmacy Informatics and Technology, the Technology in Pharmacy Education and Learning Special Interest Group of the American Association of Colleges of Pharmacy (AACP), AMIA, and several other knowledgeable individuals were invited to review the statements.

During the spring of 2007, these pharmacy informaticians were invited to log on to the Web site and independently rate their level of agreement for each of the 110 competency statements as to whether the statement should be included in a final list. Raters could choose whole numbers ranging from "0" (disagree) to "9" (agree). The first round of ratings lasted approximately 3 weeks, and experts were allowed to rate the statements only once (limited by Internet Protocol address). A total of 19 experts formally rated the competency statements in the first round (Table 1). Participants reported their length of pharmacy informatics experience as being greater than 10 years (32%), 5 to 10 years (26%), 2 to 5 years (26%), and 0 to 2 years (16%).

The second round of competency statement ranking took place during the AACP annual meeting in the summer of 2007. From the original draft of 110 prioritized competency statements, participants attending an educational session titled "Developing Student Competencies in Informatics" were invited to provide their input and validate the previous ratings. Participation was voluntary and facilitated by the use of a

TABLE 1

Characteristics of Participants Involved in Round 1 and Round 2
Ratings of Competency Statements*

Characteristic	Round 1 (%)	Round 2 (%)
Total number of raters	19	94
AACP TiPEL SIG	11 (58)	31 (33)
ASHP SOPIT	10 (53)	4 (4)
AMIA PIWG	4 (21)	3 (3)
Faculty/preceptor	16 (84)	75 (80)
Resident	1 (5)	2 (2)
Informatician	2 (11)	3 (3)
Director/manager	2 (11)	2 (2)

AACP = American Association of Colleges of Pharmacy; AMIA = American Medical Informatics
Association; ASHP = American Society of Health-System Pharmacists; PIG = Pharmacoinformatics
Working Group; SOPIT = Section of Pharmacy Informatics and Technology; TiPEL SIG = Technology in
Pharmacy Education and Learning Special Interest Group.
*Participants may have more than one professional affiliation.

handheld anonymous audience response system. The system allowed each rater to enter a single response per competency statement. Because of time constraints, not all of the original 110 statements could be validated in the second round. Therefore, a total of 30 competency statements were selected to be rated by the symposium participants using the same "0" to "9" scale used in the initial phase of competency statement development. The top 10 highest rated statements (based on mean rating in round 1), the bottom 10 lowest rated statements, and 10 statements randomly selected from the middle 90 statements were used. This process was used so that the extremes of the round 1 rankings could be validated. In theory, there should be significant separation between the highest and lowest statements from round 1.

Baseline demographics were again obtained from the raters (Table 1). Although a total of 103 seminar attendees rated at least one of the competency statements, correlation statistics were based only on the 94 participants who rated ≥75% of the items. Most of the attendees (56%) did not belong to an informatics group of a professional organization. There was good correlation ($r = 0.88$) between the items rated during rounds 1 and 2. After analysis, the items were then grouped into five domains (Table 2) and the wording was finalized. This final list of competencies is used throughout this book as described in subsequent text.

TABLE 2
Informatics Competency Statements*

Entry-level Doctor of Pharmacy graduates should be able to use information technology to:

1. Store, retrieve, and analyze health information.
   a. Discuss the benefits and limitations of systematically processing data, information, and knowledge in health care.
   b. Discuss the impact of data quality on health outcomes.
   c. Describe the structure and key elements of an electronic health record.
   d. Describe measures used to ensure the privacy, security, and confidentiality of health information.
   e. Discuss legal and ethical issues pertaining to health information.
   f. Discuss standards for interoperability related to medications, diagnoses, communication, and electronic data interchange.
   g. Discuss key issues affecting human-computer interaction.
   h. Differentiate between spreadsheets, databases, and user interfaces.

2. Optimize the medication prescribing/ordering process.
   a. Describe the structure and key elements of computerized provider order entry and electronic prescribing processes.
   b. Describe the impact of provider order entry and electronic prescribing on health care outcomes.

3. Aid in clinical decision making.
   a. Demonstrate efficient and responsible use of clinical decision support tools to solve patient-related problems.
   b. Apply principles of evidence-based medicine to the medication use process.
   c. Discuss the development of electronic decision support tools and their strengths and limitations.
   d. Discuss the impact of alerts on workflow and health care outcomes.
   e. Identify common clinical decision support tools.

4. Automate the medication delivery process.
   a. Discuss technologies used to automate the medication delivery process.
   b. Discuss the value of bar-coded and radiofrequency identification for medication distribution and administration.

5. Facilitate pharmacy management.
   a. Describe the role of information systems in health care management.
   b. Collaborate with other health care professionals to optimize informatics projects.
   c. Apply project and change-management principles and methods to informatics projects.
   d. Document and report health care quality benchmarks.

*These statements assume preexisting basic computer knowledge and skills on which to build further informatics-related competencies.

The development of educational competencies is often an iterative process that is continually refined and improved as experience with and knowledge of a domain grows. Although medical informatics has existed in Europe since the 1960s and first appeared in the United States in the following decade, the field of pharmacy informatics is very much in its infancy. The competency development process described here was grounded in an internationally developed group of consensus standards for health and medical informatics education. The resulting competencies represent collective recommendations regarding the core informatics knowledge that all U.S. pharmacists should obtain.

The competencies do not represent the knowledge required to develop expertise that would allow someone to establish a pharmacy informatics practice. Instead, the competencies are intended to expand on ACPE's call for informatics education across all PharmD programs. The competencies should serve as the foundation of pharmacy informatics education in all PharmD programs.

In the context of this book, the competencies serve as the guide for the content found in each unit. The beginning of each unit includes appropriate competencies from the list in Table 2. Each chapter within a unit begins with actionable objectives, drawn from the unit competencies. Some competencies are used more often than others. Activities that readers can perform to expand on the content found in the chapter are placed at the end of each chapter. The incorporation and linkage of competencies, objectives, and activities are intended to establish working knowledge in readers of the consensus-based competencies that were developed in the process described previously. Boldface words in the chapters, excluding text subheads, represent terms that are defined in the glossary. Understanding these terms will aid readers in mastering the competencies.

The first three units provide foundational information that is necessary to understand the concepts, technologies, and responsibilities found in subsequent units. Units IV through VIII are organized around the medication use process (as explained in Chapter 1) to demonstrate the various pharmacy informatics tools that are found in each step of the process. The final unit employs a systems view to address various topics that influence the role, opportunities, and contextual factors that impact use of pharmacy informatics as a tool to support pharmacy practice.

References

1. Mantas J, Ammenwerth E, Demiris G, et al., IMIA Recommendations on Education Task Force. Recommendations of the International Medical Informatics Association (IMIA) on education in health and medical informatics. First revision. *Methods Inf Med.* 2010; 49(2):105–20.
2. Institute of Medicine. Health Professions Education: a Bridge to Quality. Available at: http://www.iom.edu/Reports/2003/Health-Professions-Education-A-Bridge-to-Quality.aspx. Accessed March 26, 2010.
3. Accreditation Council for Pharmacy Education. Accreditation standards and guidelines for the professional program in pharmacy leading to the doctor of pharmacy degree. Available at: http://www.acpe-accredit.org/standards/default.asp. Accessed October 23, 2009.

Foundations of Pharmacy Informatics

UNIT COMPETENCIES

- Discuss key issues affecting human-computer interaction.
- Describe the structure and key elements of computerized provider order entry and electronic prescribing processes.
- Describe the impact of provider order entry and electronic prescribing on health care outcomes.
- Discuss the development of electronic decision support tools and their strengths and limitations.
- Discuss technologies used to automate the medication delivery process.
- Describe the role of information systems in health care management.

UNIT DESCRIPTION

Chapters in this unit address foundational concepts and environmental factors related to pharmacy informatics. This discussion includes core informatics definitions and relationships that all pharmacists should know and understand. Additional topics include the relationship between medication safety and informatics, which provide an "advanced organizer" to the remainder of the book. The unit concludes with an examination of driving factors of informatics, as well as barriers to widespread adoption of informatics.

Informatics and the Medication Use Process

Brent I. Fox

OBJECTIVES

1. Articulate definitions and relationships of key informatics terms.
2. Articulate the goals of biomedical and health informatics.
3. Describe the Institute of Medicine's five core competencies for health care professions education.
4. Enable readers to appreciate the driving forces behind pharmacy informatics educational requirements.
5. Describe the differences and examples of the two broad categories of information used in the clinical informatics domains.
6. Distinguish between a pharmacist who uses informatics in practice and a pharmacy informatician.
7. Describe the pharmacist informatician's roles and responsibilities in biomedical and health informatics.
8. Describe the foundational knowledge and skills required of pharmacy informaticians.
9. Describe the medication use process and each step within the process, including the pharmacist's responsibilities in each step.

This chapter introduces two topics: informatics and the medication use process. Informatics plays a critical, enabling role in a safe and efficacious medication use process. "Setting the Stage: Consensus-Based Development of Pharmacy Informatics Competencies" describes the development of informatics competencies for Doctor of Pharmacy programs accredited by the Accreditation Council for Pharmacy Education and how those competencies relate to the organization of this book. This chapter provides a foundational introduction to informatics, information technology (IT), other key concepts and terms, and related topics. The latter part of this chapter describes the organization of this book, with a focus on the medication use process as the framework for how the book is organized. The majority of the other chapters in this text address specific applications of pharmacy informatics' supporting role in the medication use process.

Historical Foundations and Contemporary Definitions

The term *medical informatics* first appeared in the 1960s in France. The first informatics programs appeared in the United States in the 1970s.[1] Today, the National Library of Medicine defines **medical informatics** as "the field of information science concerned with the analysis, use and dissemination of medical data and information through the application of computers to various aspects of health care and medicine."[2] Simply stated, **informatics** is the use of computers to manage data and information. Figure 1–1 illustrates that informatics exists at the intersection of people, information, and technology.[3] Throughout this chapter and book, authors will expand on these components of informatics.

Although the foundational definition of informatics is simple, in today's health care environment, many are likely to encounter confusion and a lack of clarity surrounding informatics. This chapter describes the most widely accepted terminology and structure for informatics, which is also the editors' preferred method for describing the field. Confusion about informatics has been attributed to what has been described as an "adjective problem" within informatics. The adjective problem arises from the addition of words—such as *pharmacy, dentistry, nursing,* and others—in front of informatics to narrow its focus. The most comprehensive term ***biomedical and health informatics*** describes the "optimal use of information, often aided by the use of technol-

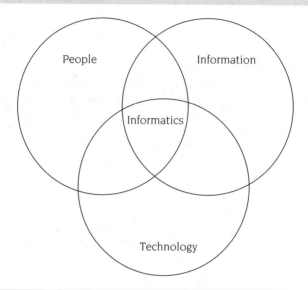

FIGURE 1–1

Core components of informatics.

Source: Information extracted from Reference 3.

ogy, to improve individual health, health care, public health, and biomedical research."[3] The terms may be used separately (i.e., *biomedical informatics* and *health informatics*) in place of the comprehensive term.

The term *medical informatics* is also often used. In the strictest sense, medical informatics describes the application of informatics in health care settings (which closely matches the National Library of Medicine's definition) and is a subordinate component of biomedical and health informatics. Other key definitions include the following[3]:

- **Bioinformatics:** Application of informatics to cellular and molecular biology.
- **Public health informatics:** Application of informatics in areas of public health (surveillance, reporting, and health promotion).
- **Consumer health informatics:** Application of informatics to support the patient's health activities.
- **[Other clinical field] informatics:** Application of informatics to specific health care disciplines.

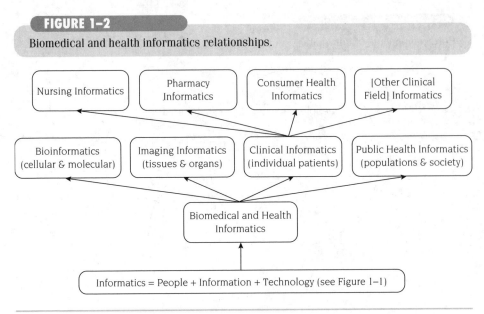

FIGURE 1-2

Biomedical and health informatics relationships.

Source: Adapted from References 3 and 4.

Figure 1–2 depicts the relationships between these terms.[3,4] The figure illustrates that people, information, and technology provide the foundation of biomedical and health informatics. Bioinformatics and clinical, imaging, and public health informatics are subordinate components of biomedical and health informatics; these components exist on the same tier. Recall that medical informatics represents the application of informatics in health care settings to the care of individual patients. *Medical informatics* is often used interchangeably with *clinical informatics*. Pharmacy informatics and nursing informatics, for example, represent informatics applied to these specific health care disciplines and are types of clinical informatics. Consumer health informatics exists on the same tier as the informatics applied to pharmacy, nursing, and other clinical fields.[3] Table 1–1 contains additional definitions with which readers should become familiar.[3,5,6] These terms will be encountered throughout this text and in pharmacy practice.

The Case for Informatics: National Perspectives

In 1996, the Institute of Medicine (IOM) launched a series of reports (books) that examined the state of health care delivery in the United States. The first book identified and defined the problem, which was quite startling: Medical

TABLE 1-1

Core Informatics Terms and Their Definitions

Term	Definition
Information technology (IT)	Activities and tools used to locate, manipulate, store, and disseminate information.
Information and communication technology	Term often used to indicate IT with a focus on communication and networking.
Health information technology (HIT)	Use of information and communication technology in health care settings.
Health information management (HIM)	Discipline historically focusing on medical record management (in a paper environment); as medical records transition to digital, HIM has begun to overlap with informatics.
Imaging informatics	Broad term indicating the application of informatics to the management of images in health care.
Research informatics	Broad term indicating the application of informatics to health and biomedical research.
Informatician (informaticist)	Practitioners of informatics; they focus more on information than technology.
Clinical informatician	Clinically trained individuals whose expertise is applied at the intersection of IT and health care; focus is on successful adoption and use of HIT.

Source: References 3, 5, and 6.

errors lead to thousands of deaths each year in hospitalized patients, with estimates ranging from 44,000 to 98,000. The problem, however, was not found to originate with the people providing care; instead, the problem resided in the systems of care that lead to the occurrence of errors.[7] In an effort to improve the safety and quality of health care, subsequent books looked at the challenge of increasing the quality of health care delivery[8] and the role of the government (as a purchaser, provider, and regulator of health care) in influencing the private sector.[9] The fourth book brings us to the topic of informatics.

The IOM series of books had significant impact on health professions education, including the field of pharmacy and the domain of informatics. In the series, a clear progression was made: The first two books define the patient safety and medical error problem, identify factors influencing the problem, and identify methods to solve the problem. The third book (which focused on health care quality) called for an interdisciplinary summit to determine the reform necessary to shift health professions education to a focus on safety and quality. The fourth book reports on the findings of the summit.

The summit, which included 150 participants from a variety of health-related disciplines, focused on the reality that health professions education did not adequately address the current and desired future state of health care delivery; health care professionals were not being educated in a manner that equipped them to adequately address the challenges they would face in practice. These challenges included:

- A health care system that was significantly segmented, leading to poor communication and continuity of care.
- A focus on acute care although the largest area of need is chronic care.
- An inability to efficiently and appropriately use the growing scientific knowledge base.
- Inadequate rate of adoption of IT.
- Inadequate involvement of the patient as a decision maker in the patient's care.
- An impending workforce shortage and discontentment among current health care workers.

The combination of all of these challenges indicated a need for substantial change in how health care was delivered in this country. This redesign of health care delivery could not occur without the efforts of the health care professionals within the delivery system. Unfortunately, the report concluded that health care professionals were not being educated in a manner that would equip them with the knowledge and skills to perform the necessary redesign. This signaled a need to change the content of health professions education.[10]

On the basis of the described challenges, the summit developed recommendations for the changes that should occur in health professions education. Specifically, the summit identified five core competencies. These competencies were intended to equip health care professionals with the knowledge and skills necessary to effectively navigate today's health care system while focusing on the requisite redesign that must occur to address the described challenges. The five core competencies are as follows[10]:

1. Provide patient-centered care: Focus on patients' needs, desires, and values by placing them at the center of their care; emphasize wellness and prevention.
2. Work in interdisciplinary teams: Providers should collaborate on patient care to ensure continuity.
3. Employ evidence-based practice: Augment clinical experience with the best available research.
4. Apply quality improvement: Apply safety principles to the process of care; measure quality and improve processes and systems where appropriate.
5. Utilize informatics: Use IT to communicate, manage knowledge, and support clinical decision making.

The publishing of these core competencies established a benchmark for health professions education. Some of the recommendations require a change (the necessary redesign) in the philosophy of health care delivery (establishing the patient as the driver of care), whereas others focus on the systems of care (interdisciplinary teams and quality improvement). The requirement to utilize informatics emphasizes the importance of health care providers' ability to use timely, relevant, and authoritative information that is critical to providing quality patient care. In fact, Leape et al. found that 78% of errors leading to adverse drug events (ADEs) and potential ADEs in a hospital setting were caused by seven system failures, and that all could have been improved through the use of better information systems.[11]

Does this suggest that informatics is intended to replace the judgment or knowledge of pharmacists and other health care professionals? Absolutely not. Informatics is a tool to support decision making by health care professionals. It extends the capabilities of pharmacists by equipping them with actionable knowledge to promote better patient care decisions. A theorem has been proposed to represent the relationships within informatics (Figure 1–3). The premise of the theorem is that a person working in conjunction with an information source is able to achieve greater results than if the person works alone. Several tenets of the theorem are important. First, the information source must provide information beyond what the person already possesses. Second, the person (pharmacist) and the information source work collaboratively to achieve a desired outcome. Although represented by a plus sign, the magnitude of the outcome is not numerically additive; instead, it is influenced by the interaction of the

FIGURE 1-3

A proposed theorem of informatics.

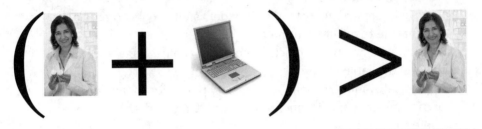

Source: Adapted from C. Friedman's description of the fundamental theorem of biomedical informatics in Reference 12.

person with the information source (as designated by the parentheses). Finally, the theorem does not suggest that the information source alone is able to achieve greater results than the pharmacist alone.[12]

Readers will see throughout this book that informatics tools are applied at the point of decision making. However, informatics activities also occur "upstream," where information is generated, collected, organized, and shared among systems to eventually be applied at the point of decision making. The key concept to recognize is that informatics supplements (or extends) the pharmacist's ability to provide patient care but does not replace the pharmacist as the medication use expert.

The Case for Pharmacy Informatics Education and Training

The Accreditation Council for Pharmacy Education (ACPE) is the national organization that defines the educational standards for pharmacy programs seeking accreditation. As described in the discussion of the development of competency standards, ACPE's current standards and guidelines (adopted in 2006 and became effective July 2007) identify informatics as a requirement for Doctor of Pharmacy programs. (See "Setting the Stage: Consensus-Based Development of Pharmacy Informatics Competencies" for discussion of the current state of the informatics requirement and how the requirement relates to the competencies in this book.) ACPE's standards are established through an extensive process that includes expert opinion, a multifaceted open comment process, and a thorough review of the literature. For the current standards, this process lasted 3 years.

The standards are designed to equip graduates with the knowledge and skills to enter pharmacy practice. Accordingly, the standards reflect the current and anticipated future state of pharmacy practice. As such, current pharmacists can also benefit from foundational informatics education. For student pharmacists and pharmacists alike, the goal of this book is to equip readers with fundamental pharmacy informatics concepts, skills, and information, as defined in the discussion of the development of the competencies and developed according to ACPE's Standards 2007. All pharmacists will be impacted by information systems in virtually every aspect of practice. Patient records, medication usage information, insurance information, laboratory tests and results, and medication administration histories are just a few of the categories of information that are managed in electronic environments. Pharmacists must be able to input, access, share, critically evaluate, and use information in these systems to support their patient care efforts, regardless of practice setting. This book was written for these patient care efforts that every pharmacist performs.

For readers who desire a career in pharmacy informatics, the foundational information in this book will serve as a core component of the education necessary to develop expertise in pharmacy informatics. This book, however, is not intended to develop pharmacy informatics experts who are ready to step into a pharmacy informatics position after closing the book. Expertise in informatics is often developed through years of practical experience. Table 1–2 lists additional informatics resources, including professional associations and journals. The list is not exhaustive but does include the majority of the most well-known informatics resources.

Pharmacy Informatics Applied to Pharmacy Practice

As described in previous text, all pharmacists rely on informatics to support their practice. Regardless of the setting, pharmacy practice (like the practice of most other health care providers) is an information-based science. Pharmacists spend much of their time gathering, synthesizing, and acting on information. There are two broad categories of information used in the clinical informatics domains (Figure 1–2), including pharmacy informatics: patient-specific and knowledge-based information.[13]

TABLE 1–2

Additional Informatics Resources

Resource	Web Site	Description
AHRQ Health IT Bibliography	www.bit.ly/1MstFh	Web site providing a collection of resources, selected by experts, on the topics of health care and HIT.
American Health Information Management Association	www.ahima.org	National association focusing on best practices and standards for health information management.
American Medical Informatics Association	www.amia.org	National association focusing on all aspects of biomedical and health informatics. Pharmacoinformatics Working Group focuses on the intersection of technology and medication management.
American Society of Health-System Pharmacists	www.ashp.org/informatics	National association for pharmacists who practice in institutional settings. Develops standards and accredits pharmacy informatics residencies. Section of Pharmacy Informatics and Technology (SOPIT) focuses on informatics issues. SOPIT publishes the Informatics Interchange column in the association's journal.
Health Informatics World Wide	www.hiww.org	Web site providing a regularly updated index of the most relevant links to Web sites on biomedical and health informatics.
Health Information Management Journal	www.himaa.org.au/HIMJ/journal.html	The refereed journal of the Health Information Management Association.
International Journal of Medical Informatics	www.ijmijournal.com	Official journal of the European Federation for Medical Informatics.
International Medical Informatics Association	www.imia.org	International association focusing on the application of information science and technology in the fields of health care and research in biomedical and health informatics.
Journal of the American Medical Informatics Association	www.jamia.org	Official journal of the American Medical Informatics Association.

AHRQ = Agency for Healthcare Research and Quality; HIT = health information technology.
Source: Author.

Patient-specific information is created and applied in the process of caring for individual patients.[13] It can include medication and medical histories, laboratory test results, and other information that is unique to the specific patient. In the not-so-distant past, the overwhelming majority of patient-specific information was created and housed in health care facilities, including pharmacies, hospitals, and clinics. Today, the growth of consumer health informatics has created an environment in which patients are generating and managing health-related information outside of the traditional four walls of health care facilities. The consumer health informatics field is a rapidly growing domain within biomedical and health informatics. This field is anticipated to continue to grow because it is consistent with the IOM's core competency of patient-centered care.

Knowledge-based information forms the scientific basis of health care.[13] It includes the understanding of how drugs work in the body; referential information (about medications, disease processes, procedures, etc.); clinical practice guidelines; and many other domains of health and medical knowledge that are found in health professions textbooks and journals. Pharmacists and other providers combine knowledge-based and patient-specific information to make patient care decisions. The growing challenge facing today's provider is integrating an overwhelming amount of knowledge-based information with widely scattered patient-specific information to obtain a complete and accurate picture of the patient's condition. Informatics addresses this challenge by using IT to manage information.

Chapters in this book address many of the informatics technologies with which pharmacists interact in their practice activities. These technologies include computerized provider order entry (CPOE) and electronic prescriptions (e-prescriptions), which are used to generate medication (and other types of) orders. Other technologies include pharmacy information management systems (PIMS), which are the administrative and clinical systems that support the pharmacist's daily medication management activities. Spurred by the federal government, adoption of electronic medical records (EMRs) and electronic health records (EHRs) is growing—and is a definitive area that needs pharmacist involvement. Other topics in this book with which pharmacists should be prepared to contribute include clinical surveillance systems and project management.

Clinical decision support systems (CDSS) are probably some of the most well-studied and visible informatics tools. These systems use patient-specific information and knowledge-based information to identify potentially critical situations or errors in care. Notifications are presented to providers who then make decisions on the basis of the notification.[13] CDSS are found throughout health care, especially within pharmacy systems and prescribing systems. In pharmacy, the best known CDSS is drug-drug interaction checking modules within PIMS. CDSS is discussed in several chapters in this book.

Pharmacy Informatics and HIT

Our pharmacy colleagues (those in practice and student pharmacists) have commented that the distinction between informatics and health information technology (HIT) is sometimes confusing. Are PIMS, EMRs, CDSS, and so on examples of informatics or HIT? The easiest way to conceptualize the difference is that the communication and information technologies comprising HIT provide the backbone that enables the information management found in informatics. Or, as shown in Figure 1–1, HIT occupies the circle labeled "Technology." In conjunction with people (clinicians and informaticians) and the actual information of interest, HIT completes the informatics domain. The three components together comprise informatics; it does not exist without all three pieces.

With regard to the people component in Figure 1–1, where does pharmacy informatics fit? What is its role? **Pharmacy informatics** has been defined as "the use and integration of data, information, knowledge, technology, and automation in the medication use process for the purpose of improving health outcomes."[14] Although this definition is not a mirror image of the informatics definitions above, the core elements are still found. Pharmacy informatics focuses on the use of information (including data and knowledge; see Chapter 6 for further discussion) and technology (including automation; described in several other chapters) to specifically address the medication use process.

Pharmacists' expertise is in the optimal use of medications to improve patient outcomes. The goal of pharmacy informatics is to enable the attainment of optimal patient outcomes through the use of HIT to manage medication-related information. As described previously, all pharmacists rely on informatics tools to support their practice. These tools provide the patient-specific and knowledge-based information that supports decision making across all levels and locations of care. These tools are so pervasive throughout practice that some have suggested that pharmacists who do not have basic computer skills are at a disadvantage in their practice.[15] Clearly, there is no model of future pharmacy practice that does not employ informatics as an enabler of improved patient outcomes. Although pharmacy informatics supports all pharmacists, not all pharmacists work directly with HIT as their primary mode of practice.

Pharmacy Informaticians

Although the intent of this book is not to prepare readers to be pharmacy informaticians, the topic deserves a brief discussion. Pharmacists whose practice is devoted to the development, implementation, management, and support of HIT systems are pharmacy informaticians. Much of the work with these systems addresses how they best fit into the daily workflow of pharmacy and other health care disciplines. Because of this focus on fitting the user's workflow, pharmacy informaticians must have a practical, working knowledge of pharmacy practice. This firsthand knowledge of the practice environment is a prerequisite to determining the best way to integrate HIT into the environment. This practical knowledge of pharmacy practice is gained through completion of a professional pharmacy (Doctor of Pharmacy) program, often includes residency training, and is frequently augmented by several years of practice.

Pharmacy informaticians fit in the broader category of clinical informaticians and are clinically trained individuals whose expertise focuses on successful adoption and use of HIT (Table 1–1). Chapters 3 and 8 detail current initiatives to increase HIT adoption on a national level. Chapter 3 addresses the role of accreditation, quality, and patient safety organizations as drivers of HIT adoption. Chapter 8 addresses the role of the federal government as a driver of interoperability, which is a prerequisite of successful HIT adoption. Nationwide adoption of HIT will depend heavily on a sufficient and appropriate workforce. Various publications have characterized the needs for the IT, HIT, and informatician workforces. Unfortunately, this interchangeable use of the terms IT, HIT, and *informatician* when describing workforce needs can create confusion regarding what types and numbers of workers are needed. For example, an individual trained in traditional IT does not have the same knowledge and skill set as an informatician, and vice versa. Accordingly, the IT person will focus on technical aspects of HIT, whereas the informatician focuses on fitting HIT into clinical workflow.

Despite this confusion and the relatively recent emergence of pharmacy informatics, the profession should have a solid understanding of the role of pharmacy informaticians. Pharmacy informatician responsibilities have been grouped into four broad categories[14]:

1. Participation in all aspects of informatics that support the medication use process.
2. Leadership that focuses on informatics to enable safe medication use.
3. Education at the local and national levels to prepare pharmacists for informatics in practice.
4. Research into various technical, workflow, outcomes, and related considerations.

These responsibilities reflect the varying roles of pharmacy informaticians in today's health care system. As preparation for these roles, a foundational set of knowledge and skills has been suggested for pharmacy informatician training programs[15]:

- Knowledge and understanding of (1) pharmacy practice, (2) automation technology, (3) basic software and database design, (4) basic data management tools, and (5) informatics standards and initiatives.
- Skills in (1) project management, (2) change management, (3) critical analysis, (4) communication, (5) program logic, (6) risk analysis, and (7) acquisition/request for proposal process.

The challenge before us is to use informatics, supported by HIT, as the building block for exchange of health information (see Chapter 8 for more information on this topic) in our efforts to improve the efficiency, safety, and quality of health care delivery. A report issued in 2004 by the Department of Health and Human Services identified four goals for the use of HIT[16]:

1. Inform clinical practice by bringing electronic health records to the point of care.
2. Interconnect clinicians to allow information to follow the patient from one location of care to another.

3. Personalize care by using HIT to engage patients to be more involved in their own care and to reach previously underserved patients.
4. Improve population health by enhancing public health monitoring, improving the process of monitoring health care quality, and accelerating the dissemination of new knowledge into clinical practice

Every informatician's daily practice is devoted to achieving these four goals. The majority of readers will be "customers" of an informatician as they develop, implement, manage, and support the HIT used each day in their practice.

The Medication Use Process and Pharmacy Informatics

The definition of pharmacy informatics presented previously depicts the medication use process as the "location" where pharmacy informatics exists in the health care system. In reality, all pharmacists focus their efforts on safe and effective medication use within the context of the medication use process. The medication use process is a system comprising a group of interconnected parts that work together to achieve a common goal. The goal of the medication use process is safe and effective medication therapy, ultimately leading to positive patient outcomes. The "interconnected parts" of the medication use process include the people, systems, procedures, and policies that manage medications and medication-related information in the care of patients. The most commonly cited depiction of the medication use process is presented in Figure 1–4.[17]

The figure demonstrates that the medication use process is cyclical in nature, beginning with an assessment of the need for medication therapy. As with the other steps in the process, the discussion will not focus on the clinical activities performed at each step but instead address informatics tools used at each step. When assessing the need for medication therapy, prescribers rely on patient-specific information such as diagnosis, laboratory values, previous response to medications and other treatments, and subjective information from the patient. Prescribers use electronic patient records, electronic prescribing systems,

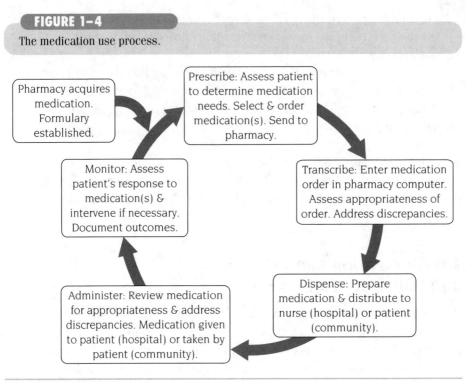

FIGURE 1-4

The medication use process.

Source: Adapted from Reference 17.

and clinical decision support tools in this step. These topics are addressed in Unit IV.

Prescribed medications are transferred (manually or electronically) to the pharmacy, where transcription occurs. Recent reports have called for a new term to replace *transcription*. Use of this new term, *perfection*, is intended to better capture the cognitive processes that pharmacists perform when presented with medication orders.[18] The editors acknowledge the need for a term that more appropriately reflects pharmacists' cognitive activities at this step. In keeping with the currently accepted terminology, however, this book will use *transcription* to reflect this step. In addition to assessing medication orders for drug-related problems at this step, pharmacists also transform the order into a dispensable form that can be safely and correctly interpreted at the administration step of the process.[18] In this step, pharmacists use pharmacy computer systems, evidence-based medicine tools, and CDSS to perform their cognitive and administrative functions. These topics are addressed in Unit V.

Medications are then dispensed and distributed to patients. The actual activities in this step depend on the setting: institutional or community pharmacy. Despite the differences in these settings, many similarities are found across the two settings. Medications are acquired from a supplier (wholesaler, central warehouse, or other distributor) and are stocked in the pharmacy according to historical, anticipated, and real-time needs of the setting. This acquisition step actually occurs repeatedly throughout the process but is addressed with the dispensing step because of the conceptual link between acquiring and dispensing. The medications are prepared—according to the transcribed order—in a variety of dosage forms, with the focus on safety and accuracy. In addition to safely and accurately dispensing the transcribed order, an important focus of today's pharmacy is to efficiently dispense medications and document the related activities. Unit VI addresses the informatics tools used in this step.

The administration step also varies considerably across institutional and community pharmacy settings. Nurses administer medications in institutional settings, whereas the patient (or the caregiver) is usually responsible for administration in the community setting. A key component of administration is to ensure the five rights of medication administration: right patient, right medication, right route, right dose, and right time. To ensure these rights, nurses perform numerous safety checks utilizing a variety of informatics tools. Although nurses are primarily responsible for medication administration, pharmacists have considerable involvement with the informatics tools that nurses use to ensure the patient's rights. In the community setting, often very little is known about the accuracy with which patients take (administer) their medications. However, a growing area of research is investigating the use of tools that help ensure patients appropriately take their medications. In both settings, the last step of administration is to document what was done. Unit VII addresses the informatics tools used in this step.

Once the patient has taken the medication and this action has been documented, the next step is to monitor the patient to determine the impact of the intervention and to document outcomes. Again, this step differs across the two settings. Monitoring and documentation within the hospital is performed by nurses at the patient's bedside. Increasingly, pharmacists are able to monitor patients using electronic tools that pull data from various components of the hospital computer system. Monitoring and documentation in the community setting are performed by the patient, the pharmacist, and the primary physician(s). As with administration, the ability to monitor and document medication therapy impact in the community setting is much more difficult than in institutional settings. However, new tools and models of care are being implemented to improve community-based monitoring and documentation. A growing area of emphasis for pharmacists in all settings is documentation of interventions that are performed to improve medication-related outcomes. These topics are addressed in Unit VIII.

The knowledge gained from monitoring a patient's response to medications (and the associated documentation) is the starting point for a new trip through the medication use process. As mentioned above, medication acquisition occurs throughout the process, even though the primary discussion of this topic is presented in Unit VI. This illustrates an important point: it is often difficult to definitively say that certain activities occur only at a single point in the process. Another example is pharmacists' documentation of interventions, which is depicted in Unit VIII as occurring during the monitoring step. The reality is that pharmacists continually assess medication therapy to determine the safety and efficacy of outcomes. Interventions that are made to improve medication therapy are performed whenever they should be. This can include during prescribing, dispensing, or any step in the process. Intervention documentation is performed accordingly. So, although the informatics tools and activities of pharmacists are categorized as fitting into discrete steps of the medication use process, readers should recognize that the tools and activities exist across all steps of the process.

Units II and III are not mentioned in the discussion of the medication use process. These units provide foundational information that is essential to understanding the tools and activities discussed in the other units. Units II and III are core components of this book because they provide information that readers must understand to apply the information found in the other units. Just as pharmacists must understand a medication's mechanism of action to know how the medication brings about change in the patient's condition, Units II and III provide the necessary information to understand how the tools discussed in the other units work.

Finally, Unit IX, the concluding section of the book, addresses topics related to informatics, including privacy and security of electronic information as well as project management skills for pharmacists involved with informatics projects. This unit also includes a chapter on future challenges and changes for pharmacy informatics. Several other chapters address other contextual topics related to pharmacy informatics.

Conclusion

The overarching goal for all health care professionals is safe and effective patient-centered care that is delivered efficiently and in a timely manner. Pharmacy informatics is a subset of the larger biomedical and health informatics field. The field of informatics is more about information and people than it is about technology. Over the last decade, a growing emphasis has emerged that identifies informatics as a primary driver for a safer health care system. Accordingly, pharmacy informatics has gained increased attention within professional and educational realms as a core skill and knowledge area for all pharmacists. Pharmacy informatics is a discipline that ultimately strives to enable safer and more efficacious medication therapy through optimal use of information and HIT to enable better patient care decisions. Pharmacy informatics tools are found throughout the medication use process, which is the structural framework for this book.

LEARNING ACTIVITIES

1. Consider a scenario in which you are filling a new prescription for a patient in a hospital pharmacy setting. Identify five pieces of information you would like to know about the patient to help you assess the safety and efficacy of the medication. For each piece of information, categorize it as referential or patient specific. Where is each piece of information found? How would you access the information if it is not normally found in the pharmacy computer system?
2. Consider the same scenario above, except now you are filling the new prescription for a patient in a community pharmacy setting. Answer the same questions in #1.

3. Before reading ahead in this book, use your own experiences in pharmacy to identify as many informatics tools as you can for each step of the medication use process.
4. Obtain Reference 10 and read Chapter 3, which describes the core competencies for health care professionals. The reference is available electronically through the National Academies Press Web site (www.nap.edu) or through most university libraries. What opportunities do you see for pharmacists? What challenges do you see for pharmacists? What contributions can pharmacists make by developing knowledge and skills in these competencies?

References

1. Vanderbilt University Department of Biomedical Informatics. What is biomedical informatics? December 13, 2002. Available at: http://www.mc.vanderbilt.edu/dbmi/informatics.html. Accessed October 11, 2009.
2. National Library of Medicine. Collection development manual: medical informatics. January 7, 2004. Available at: http://www.nlm.nih.gov/tsd/acquisitions/cdm/subjects58.html. Accessed October 11, 2009.
3. Hersh W. A stimulus to define informatics and health information technology. BMC Med Inform DCIS Mak. 2009;9(1):24.
4. Shortliffe E, Blois GO. The computer meets medicine and biology: emergence of a discipline. In: Shortliffe E, Cimino JJ, eds. *Biomedical Informatics: Computer Applications in Health Care and Biomedicine.* 3rd ed. New York, NY: Springer; 2006:29–35.
5. Fox BI. What is informatics? In: *Health Care Informatics: A Skills-Based Resource.* Washington, DC: American Pharmacists Association; 2006:1–24.
6. U.S. Department of Health and Human Services, Health Resources and Services Administration. Health information technology. Available at: http://www.hrsa.gov/healthit. Accessed October 26, 2009.
7. Kohn LT, Corrigan JM, Donaldson MS, eds. *To Err Is Human: Building a Safer Health System.* Washington, DC: National Academies of Science; 2000:1–5.
8. Committee on Quality of Health Care in America. *Crossing the Quality Chasm: A New Health System for the 21st Century.* Washington, DC: National Academies of Science; 2001.
9. Corrigan JM, Eden J, Smith BM, eds. *Leadership by Example: Coordinating Government Roles in Improving Health Care Quality.* Washington, DC: National Academies of Science; 2002.
10. Greiner AC, Knebel E, eds. *Health Professions Education: A Bridge to Quality.* Washington, DC: National Academies of Science; 2003:1–46.
11. Leape LL, Bates DW, Cullen DJ, et al. Systems-analysis of adverse drug events. JAMA. 1995;274(1):35–43.
12. Friedman C. A "fundamental theorem" of biomedical informatics. J Am Med Inform Assoc. 2009;16:169–70.

13. Hersh W. Medical informatics—improving health care through information. JAMA. 2002; 288:1955–8.
14. American Society of Health-System Pharmacists. ASHP statement on the pharmacist's role in informatics. *Am J Health Syst Pharm.* 2007;64(2):200–3.
15. Tribble DA, Poikonen J, Blair J, Briley DC. Whither pharmacy informatics. *Am J Health Syst Pharm.* 2009;66(9):813–5.
16. Brailer D. *The Decade of Health Information Technology: Delivering Consumer-Centric and Information-Rich Health Care.* Washington, DC: Department of Health and Human Services; 2004.
17. United States Pharmacopeia. The medication use process. 2004. Available at: http://www.usp.org/pdf/EN/patientSafety/medicationUseProcess.pdf. Accessed November 6, 2009.
18. Poikonen J. A new term for transcribing. *Am J Health Syst Pharm.* 2008;65(19):1801–2.

Medication Safety and Pharmacy Informatics

Jennifer J. Boehne and Andrew C. Seger

OBJECTIVES

1. Understand basic terminology associated with medication safety.
2. Describe the medication use process and various types of health information technologies that are available to promote medication safety.
3. Identify the advantages and disadvantages associated with various types of health information technology.
4. Develop an understanding of the limitations of clinical systems as they relate to medication safety.

The Institute of Medicine (IOM) brought medication safety into the forefront of both health care providers and media when it published the 1999 report *To Err Is Human: Building a Safer Health System*. The IOM estimated that 44,000 to 98,000 Americans die in hospitals each year because of adverse events.[1] It is important to note that adverse drug events (ADEs) are not limited to hospital settings; they frequently occur in a patient's home, nursing homes, and other settings. In addition to looking at the number of medical errors, the report takes a closer look at who is involved in errors, what the root causes are, and how pharmacists can go about making the health care system safer. Table 2–1 provides important terms related to medication safety and informatics that will be encountered in this and other chapters.

TABLE 2–1

Key Medication Safety and Informatics Terms

Term	Definition
Medication error	Any event that is considered preventable and can potentially lead to a drug being consumed or used in a way that was not originally intended. Medication errors can occur at any point in the medication use process. Medication errors are not limited to health care facilities; they can occur while the medication is in the control of a health care provider, a patient, or a caregiver.
Near miss	A situation in which the error was detected before it affected and/or reached the patient.
Adverse drug event (ADE)	Harm to a patient due to the administration of a drug. An ADE may be preventable (related to any error in the medication use process) or non-preventable.
Potential adverse drug event	An event in which an error occurred but did not cause injury (e.g., the error was detected before it reached the patient, or the patient received a wrong dose but was not harmed).
Side effect	Known reaction to a medication.
Error of commission	Occurs as a result of an action taken (e.g., an incorrect drug, dose, or timing of a dose).
Error of omission	Occurs as a result of an action not taken (e.g., a missed dose, failure to adjust doses according to laboratory results, missed prophylaxis, or inappropriate therapy selection).
Failure mode effects analysis (FMEA)	A method of assessing risk of occurrence of an error by identifying problems involving products or processes. FMEA involves a systematic analysis of possible problems and factors associated with them before the errors occur.
Root cause analysis (RCA)	An investigation technique that systematically seeks to understand the underlying causes of an error by looking at all the systems involved. RCA is predicated on the belief that problems are best solved by attempting to correct or eliminate root causes, as opposed to merely addressing the immediately obvious symptoms.

Source: Author.

By far the largest category of adverse events noted in the IOM report was due to medication errors, representing 19% of adverse events.[1] Other research studies have found even higher rates of ADEs in the hospital setting.[2,3] Traditional voluntary reporting systems typically underreport ADEs.[4] Classen et al. reviewed more than 36,000 hospital admissions over an 18-month period. They verified 731 ADEs in 648 patients using an automated detection system. Yet, only 92 of these 731 ADEs were reported by the traditional voluntary reporting systems.[2] Figure 2–1 is a graphic depiction of medication errors, ADEs, and potential ADEs.

Bates et al. looked at more than 4000 hospital admissions over a 6-month period and found 6.5 ADEs and 5.5 potential ADEs per 100 patients. Twenty-eight percent of the ADEs were judged preventable. Errors resulting in preventable ADEs occurred most often at the stages of prescribing (56%) followed by administration (34%), transcription (6%), and dispensing (4%). Errors were much more likely to be intercepted if the error occurred earlier in the medication use process: 48% at the prescribing stage versus 0% at the administration stage.[3] It is imperative that pharmacists

FIGURE 2–1

Relationship among medication errors, adverse drug events, and potential adverse drug events.

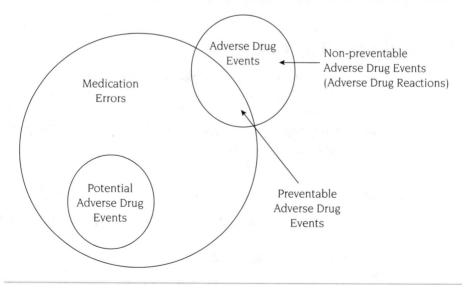

Source: Information extracted from Reference 4.

identify ADEs at the prescribing stage, thereby preventing them from being initiated.

The IOM released a second report in 2006 titled *Preventing Medication Errors*. This report determined that roughly 25% of ADEs are preventable. Although there is wide variation in the actual rates, medication errors are both surprisingly common and extremely costly to the health care system. IOM recommends using error prevention strategies including electronic prescribing (e-prescribing) with clinical decision support systems to prevent medication errors in hospital, long-term care, and ambulatory care settings.[5] A closer look at medication safety across health care institutions is needed, not only because of pressure from accrediting bodies, but also because it is the right thing to do for patients.[6] (Units IV through VIII comprise chapters that address informatics tools at each step in the medication use process.)

This chapter serves as an "advanced organizer" to help illustrate the connection between medication safety and informatics. Various health information technologies are discussed in the context of where they are employed in the medication use process. As indicated previously, research has found that the prescribing stage is a key source of medication errors. Accordingly, much effort has been extended and studied to impact the error rate at this step. It follows that much of what is discussed below focuses on this stage of the medication use process.

Medication Use Process

The medication use process is introduced in Chapter 1 (see Figure 1–4). The process is broken down into five stages: prescribing, transcribing, dispensing, administering, and monitoring. This chapter takes a closer look at each of these five stages and discusses how various types of technology can help improve medication safety.

Prescribing

Health information technology (HIT) tools used during prescribing include:

- Computerized provider order entry (CPOE).
- E-prescribing.
- Clinical decision support systems (CDSS).

Computerized Provider Order Entry and Clinical Decision Support Systems

Prescribing has traditionally been initiated by physicians, although a number of other health care practitioners including physician assistants, nurse practitioners, and even pharmacists are allowed to prescribe in certain circumstances. It is important to understand who is prescribing because it may impact the workflow process. Mid-level practitioners generally operate with pre-established clinical pathways in place to ensure consistent treatment of patients. In addition, if someone other than a physician writes the prescription, local regulations may require that the order or prescription be reviewed by the supervising physician prior to moving forward in the medication use process.

The traditional prescribing process is inherently error-prone and involves issues such as illegible hand writing, unclear abbreviations, the absence/presence of leading/trailing zeros, and confusing, vague, or incomplete directions. Electronic medical records (EMRs) and CPOE address many of these types of traditional issues by providing a structured format for ordering medications at the point of entry, in addition to making the prescription legible and standardizing medication nomenclature. CPOE allows the use of a standardized ordering process that requires the prescriber to provide information on the five basic patient rights: right patient, right drug, right dose, right route, and right time. CPOE also allows the use of a standardized ordering process that assists the prescriber in certain tasks that may prevent errors in care from occurring downstream. CPOE systems may also include clinical pathways to assist the clinician in following evidence-based guidelines and to promote safe mediation ordering.[7]

CDSS can be utilized to enhance medication safety in other areas. Once a medication is selected, CDSS can provide various levels of support to ensure that the medication is appropriate and dosed appropriately for the patient. The use of default dosing (the most common dose for the medication) and default frequency (the most common frequency for the medication) provides basic tools for the safe use of medication. In addition, the use of other CDSS (such as dosing for medications on the basis of renal function) can also enhance safer prescribing.

CPOE and CDSS can enhance medication safety through the following methods:

- Key patient identifiers should be visible at the top of the screen, including patient name, date of birth, and medical record number. In addition, the patient's height, weight, and allergies are also often displayed. Most systems also have a summary or snapshot screen that allows viewing of the patient's conditions/problems, medications, and allergies. Some systems have a placeholder where a picture of the patient may be displayed.

- Medications should be displayed and searchable by both generic and brand names. Drug information icons are available that link directly into a vendor's drug information monograph. In addition, systems frequently use tall-man lettering to differentiate sound-alike/look-alike drugs. Clinical decision support functionality can be added to identify known drug allergies, drug-drug interactions, therapeutic duplication, or opportunities for formulary substitution.[8]

- Medications can be defaulted to the most frequently prescribed dose. Clinical decision support can be added to ensure that the correct dose is selected on the basis of the patient's age (pediatric and geriatric dosing), weight, creatinine clearance (renal dosing), liver function (hepatic dosing), or body mass index. It is important to note that although harm typically is thought to occur because of toxicity issues, it is also possible for a patient to receive a less-than-effective dose.

- Medications can be defaulted to the most frequently prescribed route. In addition, inappropriate routes can be locked out so they cannot be ordered (e.g., intrathecal vincristine). Abbreviations for routes should always be spelled out to avoid confusion.

- Administration time should be spelled out to avoid confusion (e.g., QD versus once daily). Medications that are prescribed "as needed" should also include the reason for use. CPOE systems can offer a pick list of potential reasons for these medications as well as a free-text field for non-labeled uses.

Many types of CDSS are available within both pharmacy order entry systems and computerized order entry systems. CDSS functionality is often grouped into basic and advanced features. The majority of systems have basic forms of clinical decision support to alert the provider about known drug allergies, therapeutic duplication, or opportunities for formulary substitution. Advanced features such as drug-drug interactions, minimum-maximum-frequency dose checking, pediatric dosing, geriatric dosing, renal dosing, hepatic dosing, drug-disease contraindications, and drug-pregnancy contraindications may not be available in all systems or may apply only to a limited set of medications.

Although CDSS run in the background and are not readily visible, they require a substantial amount of reference information, which is maintained in tables in one or more databases. The information for these tables may be provided by a drug information provider (i.e., First Data Bank, Medi-Span, or Multum), developed and maintained by a health care system, or provided by a hybrid system of the two sources. It is important to note that just because a feature is available in a system, it may not be turned on or it may be only partially available depending on how it is configured. The success of CDSS is highly dependent on the time and effort that a health system puts into the implementation.[9] Although some do not consider order sets to be a form of CDSS, they may be seen as such because an order set would allow the clinician to select multiple medications (in addition to other types of orders such as general care orders) with a single keystroke via a template that has been vetted through a medical or surgical service.

e-Prescribing

In the past, e-prescribing systems relied on the pharmacy having a designated printer or fax machine on the receiving end. Numerous vendors now offer both stand-alone and integrated e-prescribing solutions that are integrated with the pharmacy system. Some issues still need to be worked out, but the goal of the e-prescribing system is to have information presented to the health care provider at the point of entry of the prescription order to ensure that all of the essential information is available and transmitted to the pharmacy. Ideally, this information would be integrated and flow into the pharmacy software system, eliminating the need for transcribing and phone calls to clarify orders.

Like CPOE programs, e-prescribing software helps ensure that the ordered medication contains the required elements for a complete prescription, and the software has basic CDSS to look for drug allergies, therapeutic duplication, or opportunities for formulary substitution. In addition, most systems alert the physician if there is a major drug-drug interaction and can help providers comply with treatment guidelines and "best practice" recommendations. The use of e-prescribing systems has the additional benefit of being interfaced with systems that verify coverage and identify formulary restrictions or medications that need a prior authorization to be filled. However, the process for creating a parallel prior authorization system is hampered by the varying requirements of the multitudes of insurance providers and the variability of the clinical information needed to process differing classes of medication.[10, 11]

Limitations for Use of HIT Tools during Prescribing

Potential issues that might hinder the safe utilization of CPOE and e-prescribing are varied and many. Information about a patient's conditions/problems, medications, and allergies is useful only if it is accurately maintained in the computer system. This also applies to basic information such as the patient's height and weight. Pharmacists and other health care providers must be diligent to ensure that this information is up to date and accurately reflects the patient's current clinical state.

Other issues include incorrect patient or medication selection. It is possible for the health care provider to select the incorrect patient; this frequently happens when too many patient records are open at the same time. It is also possible for the health care provider to select the incorrect medication; this frequently occurs when two medications have a similar spelling and the wrong drug is inadvertently selected.

In addition, there may be a mismatch in the signature section (SIG) and the additional instructions; this frequently occurs when the health care provider adds additional instructions as free text that conflicts with the structured SIG information. This conflict results in the pharmacist calling the physician to request clarification. Pharmacists may also receive calls when a health care provider needs assistance to enter a complex order for which the instructions change over time (i.e., titrate up, titrate down, etc.).

The ability for two-way messaging within these systems is also currently limited. If the pharmacist detects a potentially inappropriate dose, telephoning the prescribing provider is still one of the main ways to adjudicate the issue. If a prescriber decides to send a cancellation notice (e-prescribing) for a particular prescription, the pharmacy's system may not have a mechanism to notify the prescriber's system that the cancellation was received. This can lead to excessive medication use and potential patient harm.

In addition, some issues related to the systems need to be examined closely. Although most systems have a CDSS functionality imbedded in the product, it is sometimes difficult for the clinical user to understand the system's settings. For example, consider drug-drug interactions (DDIs), which are frequently a CDSS feature. Prescribers often assume that (or simply do not know if) DDI systems are active. This leads clinicians to believe that DDI systems are actively checking for interactions, when in fact the systems may not have been set to issue a DDI alert. In these situations, the CDSS interface does not have a way to inform prescribers that the DDI alert is turned off. Finally, because CPOE and e-prescribing systems are not fully standardized, health care providers who practice in more than one location may need to learn multiple systems to prescribe.

DDI alerting systems have been shown to have low rates for prediction of adverse events.[12] Although the process of tiering can improve clinicians' acceptance of these types of alerts, the process of adapting DDI alerting to improve the positive predictive value of alerts requires programmers, analysts, and pharmacists to evaluate these changes.[13] Many commercial vendors do not provide this extra-value feature, and it would ultimately add to the cost of implementing and maintaining the system.

e-Prescribing also has financial implications; however, they are not directly related to medication safety. Some see the additional transmission costs currently imposed on the pharmacy as an onerous requirement of e-prescribing systems. Others see a trade-off between the additional transmission charge and a decreased amount of time spent on the telephone with support staff clarifying orders. This trade-off has allowed some pharmacies to repurpose their staff to do tasks that were previously not tenable. Another major issue is that e-prescribing systems currently cannot be used to transmit prescriptions for federally controlled substances. It has been estimated that one of six prescriptions are for controlled substances, creating the need for two disparate systems for prescribers. At the time this chapter was written, the Drug Enforcement Administration was finalizing regulations to allow e-prescribing of controlled substances. Health care providers need a single process for prescribers to order medication to improve medication safety and fully realize the workflow efficiencies that the technology allows.

Transcribing

HIT tools used in transcribing include:

- CPOE.
- e-Prescribing.

The process of transcribing paper-based orders/prescriptions into the pharmacy system is eliminated when CPOE is implemented. If there is no interface between the CPOE and pharmacy systems, a computer-generated printout of medication orders is transmitted to the pharmacy processing area for entry into the pharmacy system. If there is an interface, the order may go directly into the patient's profile for assessment and processing by the pharmacist. The pharmacist's role transforms from deciphering the paper-based prescription/order and entering it into the pharmacy system to ensuring that the order was entered correctly and can be dispensed and charged for appropriately. Pharmacists may have to modify package size or quantity dispensed, or make substitutions according to the formulary and current inventory. Pharmacists also will often see additional alerts when they review orders and will have to use their clinical judgment to determine whether to intervene.

Limitations for Use of HIT Tools during Transcribing

If CPOE and pharmacy systems are not fully integrated, orders may have to be reentered into the pharmacy system, which reintroduces the chance of an error occurring. In addition, because of the complex nature of CPOE in various settings, such as oncology, neonatal, pediatrics, intensive care units, and obstetrics, and so on, some areas of the hospital may not be fully functional for CPOE, so dual systems will be in place. Health care providers who practice in these locations may need to learn multiple systems or use traditional paper-based orders to prescribe.

Dispensing

HIT tools (Unit VI) used at dispensing include:

- Bar code verification (during the picking process).
- Automated dispensing cabinet (ADC) scanning (during the filling and/or removal process).
- Syringe filler (bar code verification during the loading process).
- Total parenteral nutrition compounders (bar code verification during the loading process).
- Robotics (bar code verification during the loading process and automated pick process).

The dispensing process has traditionally been assigned to the workflow of both the pharmacist and pharmacy staff. Although the word *dispensing* implies a transfer of a medication from one person to another, it can also involve reviewing the order for completeness and accuracy, and resolving discrepancies before preparing the medication. CPOE can assist in eliminating transcription errors between the ordering and dispensing processes. In addition, there are a variety of pharmacy automation tools that use bar codes during the drug selection process to ensure that the correct drug, strength, and dosage form were dispensed before the medication is distributed to the patient.

Limitations for Use of HIT Tools during Dispensing

To ensure that clinical pharmacy systems function properly, pharmacists must maintain medication databases. These databases often need to be mapped to communicate with existing homegrown and commercial systems. In addition, legacy coding may be associated with billing systems and may need to be harmonized. Another potential major hurdle is the lack of standardized bar codes on medications (on receipt not all drugs will have useable barcodes and will need to be bar coded again). In addition, standard linear bar codes cannot accommodate information such as lot number and expiration dates that is essential in dealing with medication recalls. These limitations affect both the safety and efficiency of the medication use system.

Administration

HIT tools (Unit VII) used during administration include:

- Point-of-care/bedside bar coding.
- Electronic medication administration record (eMAR).
- Intelligent infusion ("smart") pumps.

The majority of medications are administered by nurses, but it is important to note that physicians, respiratory therapists, radiologists, and other health care providers also administer medications. In addition, in the ambulatory care setting, the patient often administers the medication. Although the patient is always the ultimate recipient of the medication, there may be others, such as patient care aides or other members of the patient's family, who are involved in medication administration. Prior to administering the medication, it is essential that the five basic patient rights (right patient, right dose, right medication, right route, and right time) are followed. In addition, the patient should be evaluated before administration to ensure that the medication is safe and effective for the condition(s) being treated.

The use of point-of-care bar-coding systems has been increasing over the past few years. The purpose of these systems is to ensure that the five basic patient rights are followed. Implementation of these systems has been hampered by a couple of major issues. First, many products in the marketplace that are utilized in the inpatient care setting do not contain bar codes. Second, products that are compounded for local use (i.e., intravenous antibiotics) need special bar codes that are not supported by the basic linear bar-coding format. Although some systems have upgraded to a two-dimensional bar code format to allow inclusion of this information, bar coding remains a costly endeavor.

eMARs are sometimes implemented alongside point-of-care/bedside bar-coding systems. These systems replace the paper records that are currently used to document medication administration. The paper-based systems can be handwritten or generated at a particular point of the day via a computer system, but changes in medications are handwritten, thus increasing the potential for an error in medication administration. The use of eMAR systems eliminates this manual process, and a change in a medication is updated in real time in the patient's record as soon as the order is approved by the pharmacist.

Smart pumps are infusion pumps that contain software to help eliminate pump programming errors that would result in a patient receiving an inappropriate dose of a medication. A smart pump allows hospitals to preprogram the pump's standard concentrations and upper and lower dose limits into a drug library. The pump will alert the nurse if the programmed information is outside of safe (soft) limits and will prevent administration of doses that are considered extremely unsafe (hard limits). The software is usually designed so that it can be specific to each type of unit. In studies utilizing these pumps, there has been less-than-optimal performance from a safety point of view; however, this may be due to the many systems interacting with them, both human and technological.[14,15]

Limitations for Use of HIT Tools during Administration

Although clinical systems are used as additional safety tools to assist with medication administration, the person administering the medication may see the systems as a barrier to the timeliness of all care provided to all of the person's patients. Some providers have developed workarounds to speed delivery of care. An example is a provider who may have copied bar codes onto a separate piece of paper and utilizes these codes if the bar code on the packaged product cannot be readily scanned. This problem may be an issue with the packaging or the scanning technique. In either case, the effectiveness of the bar-coding system may be decreased. When implementing any new system, the system developer must understand how the end users will use the CDSS. This applies not only to bar-coding systems but to all technology-based systems.

The maintenance of drug libraries for smart pumps is an arduous process. It requires either the physical connection of a computer to each pump or a wireless system to update the pump library. Radio frequency identification (RFID) is often used in these situations. RFID systems are costly because they require a wireless infrastructure to be in place. Independent of the mechanism for connecting the pump to a computer, the pump must be turned on, and the update has to be input manually and accepted to take effect. Drug libraries often vary from unit to unit. If a patient moves to a different unit, the new unit's drug library may list different medications, which potentially could cause problems. In addition, although a single pump may have multiple unit libraries, the user still has to select the appropriate drug library. Pumps also are moved throughout the hospital and may end up in a different physical location, potentially causing problems with the applicability of the medication library to patients in the unit where the pump is located.

Monitoring (Unit VIII)

HIT tools used for monitoring include:

- ADE surveillance.
- Antibiotic/drug surveillance.
- Rules engines.

Monitoring involves a variety of issues that include a patient's allergy information, current and historic medication information, current and historic medical conditions, laboratory results, radiologic findings, and physical assessment. Monitoring often was overlooked in the past because these information components often were scattered in both paper and electronic formats. The primary goal of monitoring is to assess whether the patient should continue to take the medication, and to report and document the results. The medication should be both safe and effective for the patient. Electronic medical records should ideally provide laboratory results as well as a patient's vital statistics and other pertinent data to allow the pharmacist and other health care providers to monitor both efficacy and safety of medication use. This information should be readily available, and the system should have the capability to alert providers of critical low and high values based on standardized values.

Pharmacists often need to report and document results in a note. Many systems have templates that can be developed to ensure that this documentation is standardized. These systems also can be linked with laboratory systems to pull across the most current laboratory values, reducing the chance of incorrect information being utilized in the decision-making process.

ADE surveillance tools (also known as ADE monitors) can be simple or complex. These tools use electronic data and predetermined rules to identify when an ADE may have occurred or is about to occur. These tools function by comparing the electronic data (from pharmacy, laboratory, or admission/discharge/transfer) to known indicators of a potential medication-related problem (the rules). Some ADE monitors contain as few as six rules, and some contain upwards of 100 rules. The monitors may contain only medication information (administration of naloxone), only laboratory data (serum potassium > 6.5 mEq/L), or a combination of both (receiving an angiotensin-converting enzyme inhibitor and serum potassium > 6.0 mEq). The use of these systems can also be modified on a patient by patient basis so that a clinician can intervene earlier in a patient's care to potentially prevent harm.

A more complex tool is surveillance related to antibiotic use. Culture and sensitivity data, along with historical information, can be ported into an ordering system to potentially prevent inappropriate prescribing of antibiotics. These systems are much more sophisticated and require many years to develop and maintain. This type of surveillance system is less ubiquitous because of its cost and complexity.

Rules engines are similar in structure to ADE surveillance systems. For example, a rule for patients receiving insulin would require documented delivery of the patient's meal to the room prior to the patient receiving meal time insulin. Although this rule does not ensure that the patient consumes the meal, it may reduce the incidence of hypoglycemia. Another example is monitoring the effectiveness of specific medications. If a patient has been receiving warfarin for 4 days and the patient's international normalized ratio (INR) is only 1.2, there might be an issue with the dose or some other issue that the clinician should investigate. These systems are more difficult to implement than ADE surveillance systems but less difficult than antibiotic surveillance tools.

Limitations for Use of HIT Tools for Monitoring

Implementing monitoring systems (and all alerting systems) creates the potential of increased volumes of alerts, which may cause alert fatigue. It is important that the alerts be pertinent to the patient's care to decrease alert fatigue. An example would be issuance of an alert about a drop in platelets to 98,000 cells/μL for a patient who recently received a chemotherapy medication. Although this information may be important, administration of the chemotherapy medication may make this alert seem superfluous to the clinician. In addition, one must be diligent about recording dates and times of laboratory results and assessment information, especially during review of progress notes because the information sometimes is cut and pasted into the note instead of being automatically inserted by the system.

Other Medication-Related Systems

Medication Reconciliation

Medication reconciliation is required by the Joint Commission (TJC) as part of its National Patient Safety Goals. Medication reconciliation is the process of comparing a patient's historical and current medications to determine the accurate, current medication list. This process should occur at all transitions of care: from the community to institutional settings, within an institution, and upon returning to the community from an institution. Although not currently being used as part of the scoring system for TJC review, medication reconciliation is an important part of medication safety.[16] This process is sometimes done on paper; however, some hospitals perform this process electronically.

Figure 2–2 shows a screen shot of a sample electronic form. The form is for a test patient and the process has not been completed (although the form is highlighted as completed). The development of this particular form requires considerable effort and coordination among many groups. The data must be normalized because it is coming from many outside sources, including community pharmacies, pharmacy benefit management companies, and other locations of care.

Medication Incident Reporting

Medication incident reporting may provide useful information to help identify "weak spots" in the medication use system. Proper documentation

FIGURE 2–2

Sample software application for medication reconciliation.

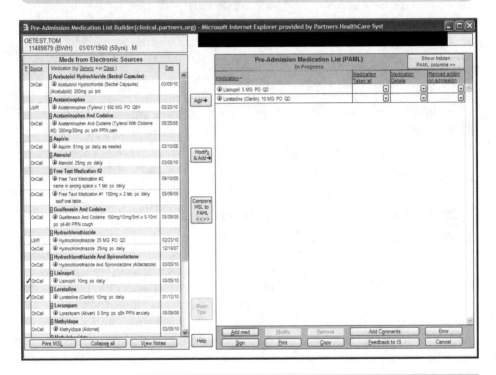

Source: Author.

of medication errors and adverse events can be analyzed to help improve workflow and minimize the chance of their recurrence. Rantucci et al. provide a useful summary of the different programs for reporting medication errors in the United States.[17] Although these types of systems are helpful, it is important to understand that because they are voluntary systems (the reporter is not required to report), they are potentially underpowered to detect all or even a fraction of the harm that patients experience secondary to medication use. Although they are one tool in pharmacists' toolbox, medication incident reporting systems do not provide a full understanding of medication issues. Their use should occur in conjunction with other tools described previously to create as vivid a picture as possible of medication issues.

Limitations for Use of Health Information Technology

Although many of the described technologies enhance the safety of the medication use process, it is essential to understand that there are limitations to the application of technology to medication systems. An example is how drug allergy alerting systems function. Only active ingredients are currently coded into the alerting system. A solid oral dose form may contain the excipient FD&C Yellow Number 5 (tartrazine). If a patient is allergic to this excipient, the drug allergy alerting system will not produce an alert and the patient may experience an allergic reaction if the oral dosage form is ingested. The same could be said for patients who are allergic to latex products. Good clinical decision making by health care providers is essential to preventing these types of adverse events. This is why computers will never fully replace human interaction in the medication use process.

As a second example, CPOE and e-prescribing systems may attempt to structure the directions-for-use portion of the medication order. The expression of clinical practice varies by region, practitioner, and patient, and even by the medication used. It is difficult to design a system that considers all of the variability and produces a seamless user experience. Ambulatory populations being prescribed liquid oral medications is an example. Pharmacists generally express volume in terms of units such as teaspoonfuls and tablespoonfuls. Although these measurements can be converted to "mL" (and there has been an increase in the number of prescribers using "mL" as a volume designation in recent years), system designers have to understand these conversions. Thus, the ability to develop standardized SIGs has fallen prey to the different terminology that clinicians use to describe to others how medications should be used by and for the patient.

Another example is the pull-down lists that some CPOE and e-prescribing systems utilize for medication selection. The medications oxybutynin and oxycodone may be adjacent to each other in a pull-down list. This potentially could lead to the incorrect selection of a medication and then lead to patient harm. This case demonstrates the tension between system developers who possess the skills to develop a working system and the potential that, as they develop the system, human-machine interface errors may be embedded in the design.

In a similar light, it is difficult to fine-tune the "volume" of an alerting system. Because programmers generally view the world in a binary mode (as an "on" or "off" function), applying this paradigm to clinical care might not be tenable. An analogy would be a radio that has only two volume settings: no volume or full volume. A potential way to provide an alternative solution would be to provide a patient-specific editor for each alert. For example, if reordering a medication, the clinician would not receive an alert unless the value changed in a range defined by the clinician. This way the system potentially can become "smarter" and potentially decrease the number of alerts reaching the clinician.

In terms of drug-drug interaction design, most systems are specific only for the active ingredients and do not consider other medication-specific factors that may play a role in determining if a patient is exposed to a true drug-drug interaction. Some systems alert on the combination of prochlorperazine and potassium supplements. The dynamics of this interaction is that if a patient receives a potassium supplement orally, the prochlorperazine will slow down the motility of the stomach and put the patient at risk for developing an ulcer because of the irritating nature of the potassium supplement. However, for patients receiving intravenous potassium, an alert should not be generated for this combination. Currently, some systems do not make the distinction between orally and intravenously administered potassium products and will "over alert" prescribers.

Although clinical systems can prevent potential harm to our patients, they are limited in their ability to prevent some types of administration errors. An example is errors related to the administration of medication via the incorrect route. It is possible for a patient to have an oral liquid form of an antibiotic administered through an IV line. Additionally, although a medication can have a patient-specific bar code attached to the product, the bar code will not prevent the wrong patient from being administered the medication or a patient from receiving the incorrect medication or strength of medication. It is still possible even with these clinical systems in place for the patient to receive the medication in an unsafe way.

Conclusion

Medication safety is a growing focus of health care providers, institutions, payers, and patients. Medications represent the largest portion of errors in the IOM reports and, as such, deserve the attention of health care providers. (See Table 2–2 for a listing of resources related to medication safety.) Much of the focus of medication safety efforts is to leverage HIT tools to improve

TABLE 2-2

Medication Safety Resources

Group	Web Site(s)	Description
Agency for Healthcare Research and Quality: Medical Errors and Patient Safety	www.ahrq.gov/qual/errorsix.htm	Primary federal agency concerned with quality and safety issues. The agency provides a collection of links to documents, reports, legislation, and other useful information for health professionals and consumers.
American Society of Health-System Pharmacists (ASHP)	www.ashp.org	National professional association that represents pharmacists who work in health care systems. ASHP provides a variety of health care resources, including:
	www.ashp.org/Import/practiceandpolicy/PracticeResourceCenters/PatientSafety.aspx	Resource Center on Patient Safety: Focuses on issues surrounding the safe use of medications in hospitals. Includes links to news, issue briefs, and reporting of medication errors.
	www.ashp.org/qii	Quality Improvement Initiative: Quality improvement resources to support pharmacist leadership and engagement in health care quality initiatives that improve patient outcomes and reward performance excellence.
Food and Drug Administration (FDA)	www.fda.gov	Federal agency responsible for the safety, efficacy, and security of human and veterinary drugs, biological products, medical devices, the nation's food supply, cosmetics, and products that emit radiation. FDA provides a number of Web sites regarding safety issues, including:
	www.fda.gov/Safety/MedWatch/SafetyInformation/default.htm	MedWatch: medical product safety information including searchable databases, information, and forms for submitting adverse events.

(continued)

TABLE 2–2

Medication Safety Resources (*Continued*)

Group	Web Site(s)	Description
	www.accessdata.fda.gov/ scripts/cdrh/cfdocs/psn/ index.cfm	Patient Safety News: newsletter with video clips.
Institute for Clinical Systems Improvement	www.icsi.org	Member organization that focuses on safety, quality improvement, and evidence-based medicine.
Institute for Healthcare Improvement (IHI)	www.ihi.org	Nonprofit organization driving the improvement of health by advancing the quality and value of health care. Offers the IHI Open School for Health Professionals, which offers a certificate in patient safety. Includes courses, cases, and resources on patient safety.
Institute for Safe Medication Practices	www.ismp.org	Nonprofit organization that provides resources and tools for education and prevention of medication errors.
Institute of Medicine (IOM) Reports	www.nap.edu/catalog.php? record_id=12610	Nonprofit organization that provides information on health care such as these reports from the committees of the IOM Quality of Care Initiative, available online.
The Joint Commission	www.jointcommission.org/ PatientSafety/National PatientSafetyGoals	Nonprofit organization that accredits health care organizations and programs, and provides resources for accreditation and quality and safety, including the 2010 National Patient Safety Goals.
National Patient Safety Foundation	www.npsf.org	Nonprofit organization that sponsors education programs, conferences, a speakers bureau, research programs, and other resources.

Source: Author.

the safety of the medication use process. This chapter briefly described several such technologies. These and other technologies are discussed in additional chapters in this book. This chapter also identified challenges and pitfalls to the use of HIT to address medication safety. The descriptions of potential issues related to the use of clinical systems in the medication use process should not be interpreted as barriers to installation and implementation of these systems. These systems will evolve over time and eventually will be enhanced to provide safer care. The overall goal to decrease risk to patients as they utilize medications to improve their health is one that pharmacists should strive for and adopt as rapidly as possible.

LEARNING ACTIVITIES

1. Review medication incident reports for your education or practice location. Discuss ways in which the incidents could have been prevented. Could they have been prevented by the use of technology, or was technology a factor?
2. Take part in a root cause analysis (RCA) or failure mode effect analysis (FMEA) of a medication, or perhaps a general safety incident.
3. Diagram the medication use process at your education or practice location from the time a medication is delivered to the pharmacy to the time it is administered to the patient. As part of moving toward a multidisciplinary team practice, understand the impact that processes in the pharmacy play in creating potential errors in other practices (i.e., medicine, nursing, and surgery). Discuss the similarities and differences in the process on the basis of whether the medication is available on the floor or in an ADC, or is sent up from the pharmacy.

References

1. Kohn LT, Corrigan JM, Donaldson MS, eds. *To Err Is Human: Building a Safer Health System.* Washington, DC: National Academies of Science; 2000:1–5.
2. Classen DC, Pestotnik SL, Evans RS, et al. Computerized surveillance of adverse drug events in hospital patients. JAMA. 199;266(20):2847–51.
3. Bates DW, Cullen DJ, Laird N, et al. Incidence of adverse drug events and potential adverse drug events. Implications for prevention. ADE Prevention Study Group. JAMA. 1995;274(1):29–34.

4. Gandhi TK, Seger DL, Bates DW. Identifying drug safety issues: from research to practice. *Int J Qual Health Care.* 2000;12(1):69–76.

5. Institute of Medicine. *Preventing Medication Errors.* Washington, DC: National Academies of Science; 2007. Available at: http://books.nap.edu/openbook.php?record_id=11623#. Accessed October 12, 2009.

6. The Joint Commission. 2010 National Patient Safety Goals. Available at: http://www. jointcommission.org/PatientSafety/NationalPatientSafetyGoals. Accessed October 12, 2009.

7. Cohen MR. *Medication Errors.* Washington, DC: American Pharmacists Association; 2007.

8. Greenes RA, ed. *Clinical Decision Support: The Road Ahead.* New York, NY: Elsevier Inc.; 2007.

9. Osheroff JA, Pifer EA, Teich JM, et al. *Improving Outcomes with Clinical Decision Support: An Implementer's Guide.* Chicago, IL: Healthcare Information and Management Systems Society; 2005.

10. HIMSS E-Prescribing Wiki. Available at: http://himsseprescribingwiki.pbworks.com. Accessed October 6, 2009.

11. Fincham JE. *E-Prescribing: The Electronic Transformation of Medicine.* Sudbury, MA: Jones and Bartlett; 2009.

12. Weingart SN, Simchowitz B, Padolsky H, et al. An empirical model to estimate the potential impact of medication safety alerts on patient safety, health care utilization and cost in ambulatory care. *Arch Intern Med.* 2009;169(16):1465–73.

13. Paterno MD, Maviglia SM, Gorman PN, et al. Tiering drug-drug interaction alerts by severity increases compliance rates. JAMA. 2009;16(1):40–6.

14. Rothschild JM, Keohane CA, Cook EF, et al. A controlled trial of smart infusion pumps to improve medication safety in critically ill patients. *Crit Care Med.* 2005;33(3):533–40.

15. Nuckols TK, Bower AG, Paddock SM, et al. Programmable infusion pumps in ICUs: an analysis of corresponding adverse drug events. *J Gen Intern Med.* 2008;23(Suppl 1):41–5.

16. Joint Commission Perspectives. Approved: will not score medication reconciliation in 2009. March 2009. Available at: http://www.jcrinc.com/common/PDFs/fpdfs/pubs/pdfs/ JCReqs/JCP-03-09-S1.pdf. Accessed October 26, 2009.

17. Rantucci MJ, Stewart C, Stewart I. *Focus on Safe Medication Practices.* Baltimore, MD: Lippincott Williams & Wilkins; 2009.

Health Information Technology Adoption: Drivers, Enablers, and Barriers

Karl F. Gumpper

OBJECTIVES

1. Discuss the role of accreditation and certification organizations in the adoption of health information technology (HIT) in hospitals and health systems.
2. Discuss the role of quality and patient safety organizations in enabling practitioners to adopt HIT.
3. Determine barriers to successful HIT adoption.
4. Describe the role of pharmacy organizations in HIT adoption.

Health information technology (HIT) is found throughout all aspects of pharmacy practice and health care. This chapter addresses several of the factors influencing adoption of HIT. Specifically,

---

The term *computerized provider order entry* is used throughout this book. However, this chapter follows the Joint Commission's preferred terminology of *computerized prescriber order entry.*

the chapter addresses organizations and other groups that influence hospital adoption of HIT through certification and other means. (Factors influencing practitioner-level adoption of HIT are an important and growing area of research, but this subject is beyond the scope of this chapter.) In today's health care environment, the primary focus on HIT adoption is in health systems, where the cost of care is higher. This focus on acute care is not intended to minimize the importance of ambulatory or outpatient care. Indeed, initiatives are underway to drive HIT adoption in community pharmacy environments. However, because there is a more focused and concerted effort in the acute care environment, the majority of this chapter will address initiatives in this setting.

Accreditation and Certification Organizations

The Joint Commission

The Joint Commission (TJC) is an independent, nonprofit organization that accredits and certifies more than 17,000 health care organizations and programs in the United States. TJC accreditation and certification is recognized nationwide as a symbol of quality that reflects an organization's commitment to meeting certain performance standards.[1] TJC provides accreditation services for the following types of organizations:

- General, psychiatric, children's, and rehabilitation hospitals
- Critical access hospitals
- Medical equipment services, hospice services, and other home care organizations
- Nursing homes and other long-term care facilities
- Behavioral health care organizations and addiction services
- Rehabilitation centers, group practices, office-based surgeries, and other ambulatory care providers
- Independent or freestanding laboratories

Many organizations seek accreditation for multiple reasons to validate that they provide quality, safe, and effective care to their patients. This validation may be voluntary or may be a component of a legal or regulatory requirement (Table 3–1).[2] TJC does not require health care organizations to adopt technology to meet the standards. Accreditation can be obtained by a health care organization's demonstration of the policy and procedures in caring for patients. If the process requires paper documentation and the

TABLE 3-1

Benefits of Joint Commission Accreditation

Benefit	Description
Helps organize and strengthen patient safety efforts.	Patient safety and quality-of-care issues are at the forefront of Joint Commission standards and initiatives.
Strengthens community confidence in the quality and safety of care, treatment, and services.	Achieving accreditation makes a strong statement to the community about an organization's efforts to provide the highest-quality services.
Provides a competitive edge in the marketplace.	Accreditation may provide a marketing advantage in a competitive health care environment and improve the ability to secure new business.
Improves risk management and risk reduction.	Joint Commission standards focus on state-of-the-art strategies for performance improvement that help health care organizations continuously improve the safety and quality of care, which can reduce the risk of error or low-quality care.
May reduce liability insurance costs.	By enhancing risk management efforts, accreditation may improve access to and reduce the cost of liability insurance coverage.
Provides education on good practices to improve business operations.	Joint Commission Resources, the Joint Commission's nonprofit affiliate, provides continuing support and education to accredited organizations, including good practices and other enhancements.
Provides professional advice and counsel, enhancing staff education.	Joint Commission surveyors are experienced health care professionals trained to provide expert advice and education during the on-site survey.
Provides a customized, intensive review.	Joint Commission surveyors come from a variety of health care industries and are assigned to organizations that match their background. The standards are also specific to each accreditation program, so each survey is relevant to the organization's industry.
Enhances staff recruitment and development.	Joint Commission accreditation can attract qualified personnel who prefer to serve in an accredited organization. Accredited organizations also provide additional opportunities for staff to develop their skills and knowledge.
Provides deeming authority for Medicare certification.	Some accredited health care organizations qualify for Medicare and Medicaid certification without undergoing a separate government quality inspection, which eases the burdens of duplicative federal and state regulatory agency surveys.

(continued)

TABLE 3-1

Benefits of Joint Commission Accreditation (*Continued*)

Benefit	Description
Recognized by insurers and other third parties.	In some markets, accreditation is becoming a prerequisite to eligibility for insurance reimbursement and for participation in managed care plans or contract bidding.
Provides a framework for organizational structure and management.	Accreditation involves not only preparing for a survey but also maintaining a high level of quality and compliance with the latest standards. Joint Commission accreditation provides guidance for an organization's quality improvement efforts.
May fulfill regulatory requirements in select states.	Laws may require certain health care providers to acquire accreditation for their organization. Those organizations already accredited by the Joint Commission may be compliant and need not undergo any additional surveys or inspections.

Source: Adapted from Reference 2.

organization meets the requirements and completes the documentation according to organizational policy, TJC will accredit the organization. Many organizations seek the assistance of computerization and technological solutions to ensure that the documentation is completed routinely and completely. Within the health care environment, tremendous amounts of data are produced during a patient's clinic visit, an acute hospital admission, or filling of a prescription. The assistance of computerization and technology often adds efficiencies in managing these data.

Organizations are required to continuously monitor their performance and report back to TJC on these performance measures as part of the survey process. TJC's ORYX initiative integrates outcomes and other performance measurement data into the accreditation process. ORYX measurement requirements are intended to support TJC-accredited organizations in their quality improvement efforts. Performance measures are essential to the credibility of any modern evaluation activity for health care organizations. These measures supplement and help guide the standards-based survey process by providing a more targeted basis for the regular accreditation survey, continuous monitoring of actual performance, and the guiding and stimulating of continuous improvement in health care organizations. Some accredited organizations are required to submit performance measurement data on a specified minimum number of measure sets or non-core measures, as appropriate, to TJC. Data collected or submitted to TJC are reviewed during the on-site survey.

TJC and the Centers for Medicare and Medicaid Services (CMS) work together to align the National Hospital Quality Measures. These measures are integral to improving the quality of care provided to hospital patients and bring value to stakeholders by focusing on the actual results of care. National Hospital Quality Measures and other core measure data were integrated into the priority focus process that TJC uses to help focus on-site survey evaluation activities. The public availability of performance measurement data permits user comparisons of hospital performance at the state and national levels. These data can be accessed at TJC's Quality Check Web site (www.qualitycheck.org). Because large amounts of data are required for collection and interpretation, organizations must have a systematic process for obtaining quarterly reports and providing them to TJC.

Within its standards, TJC has incorporated specific requirements for organizations to demonstrate compliance with technology and computerization. The standards do not contain a specific chapter that completely outlines these requirements to ensure organizational compliance. The chapter "Information Management" requires that the organization address planning for the management of information and preventing loss of electronic data. In addition, components in the chapter "Organizational Leadership" address a patient safety program and often include technology solutions. Published for TJC-accredited organizations and interested health care professionals, *Sentinel Event Alert* identifies specific sentinel events, describes their common underlying causes, and suggests steps to prevent occurrences in the future. Accredited organizations should consider information in an alert when designing or redesigning relevant processes; they should also consider implementing relevant suggestions or reasonable alternatives. An alert published in December 2008 describes suggestions for health care organizations to consider when implementing new technologies[3,4]:

1. Examine workflow processes and procedures for risks and inefficiencies, and resolve these issues prior to any technology implementation. Involving representatives of all disciplines—whether they are clinical, clerical, or technical—will help in the examination and resolution of these issues.

2. Actively involve clinicians and staff who will ultimately use or be affected by the technology, along with information technology (IT) staff with strong clinical experience in the planning, selection, design, reassessment, and ongoing quality improvement of technology solutions, including the system selection process. Involve a pharmacist in the planning and implementation of any technology that involves medication.

3. Assess your organization's technology needs beforehand (e.g., supporting infrastructure; communication of admissions, discharges, transfers, etc.). Investigate how best to meet those needs by requiring IT staff to interact with users outside their facility to learn about real-world capabilities of potential systems, including those of various vendors; to conduct field trips; and to look at integrated systems (to minimize reliance on interfaces between various vendor systems).

4. During the introduction of new technology, continuously monitor for problems and address any issues as quickly as possible, particularly problems obscured by workarounds or incomplete error reporting. During the early post-live phase, consider implementing an emergent issues desk staffed with project experts and champions to help rapidly resolve critical problems. Use interdisciplinary brainstorming methods for improving system quality and giving feedback to vendors.

5. Establish a training program for all types of clinicians and operations staff who will be using the technology, and provide frequent refresher courses. Training should be appropriately designed for local staff. Focus training on how the technology will benefit patients and staff (i.e., less inefficiency, fewer delays, and less repeated work). Do not allow long delays between orientation and system implementation.

6. Develop and communicate policies that delineate staff authorized and responsible for technology implementation, use, oversight, and safety review.

7. Prior to taking a technology live, ensure that all standardized order sets and guidelines are developed, tested on paper, and approved by the pharmacy and therapeutics committee (or institutional equivalent).

8. Develop a graduated system of safety alerts in the new technology that helps clinicians determine urgency and relevancy. Carefully

review skipped or rejected alerts as important insight into clinical practice. Decide which alerts need to be hard stops when using the technology, and provide appropriate supporting documentation.

9. Develop a system that mitigates potential harmful computerized prescriber order entry (CPOE) drug orders by requiring departmental or pharmacy review and sign-off on orders that are created outside the usual parameters. Use the pharmacy and therapeutics committee (or institutional equivalent) for oversight and approval of all electronic order sets and clinical decision support alerts. Ensure proper nomenclature and printed label design, eliminate dangerous abbreviations and dose designations, and ensure nurses' acceptance of the medication administration record.

10. To improve safety, provide an environment that protects staff involved in data entry from undue distractions when using the technology.

11. After implementation, continually reassess and enhance safety effectiveness and error detection capability, including the use of error-tracking tools and the evaluation of near-miss events. Maximize the potential of the technology to maximize the safety benefits.

12. After implementation, continually monitor and report technology-related errors and near misses or close calls through manual or automated surveillance techniques. Pursue system errors and multiple causations through the root cause analysis process or other forms of failure mode analysis. Consider reporting significant issues to well-recognized external reporting systems.

13. Reevaluate the applicability of security and confidentiality protocols as more medical devices interface with the IT network. Reassess compliance with the Health Insurance Portability and Accountability Act on a periodic basis to ensure that addition of medical devices to the IT network and the growing responsibilities of the IT department have not introduced new security and compliance risks.

The purpose of TJC's **National Patient Safety Goals** (NPSGs) is to promote specific improvements in patient safety. The requirements highlight problematic areas in health care as well as describe evidence and expert-based solutions to these problems. The requirements focus on system-wide solutions, wherever possible. Although TJC does not require a technology solution to meet the requirements, many organizations often adopt technologies for that purpose. Goals and requirements are guided and prioritized by the Sentinel Event Advisory Group. Each year, this group works with TJC to undertake a systematic review of the medical literature and available health care databases to identify potential new goals and requirements. The updated goals and their requirements are published annually by midyear after extensive vetting, public commentary, and approval phases.[5] Table 3–2 lists these goals and includes some possible technology solutions that could assist health care organizations to meet the requirements. As technology evolves and is refined, other solutions may assist the provider in ensuring appropriate and safe care of the patient.

TJC's 2008 report, "Health Care at the Crossroads: Guiding Principles for the Development of the Hospital of the Future," describes how IT plays a major role in improving health care quality and safety, and can help to support the migration of hospital-based care into the community and even the home. The technological transformation of health care also invites redefinition of the hospital, according to the report. To address technology in the hospital of the future, the expert roundtable suggests the following[6]:

- Define the business need and provide sustainable funding to support the widespread adoption of HIT.
- Redesign business and care processes in tandem with HIT adoption.
- Use digital technology to support patient-centered hospital care and extend that care beyond the hospital walls.
- Establish reliable authorities to provide technology assessment and technology investment guidance for hospitals.
- Adopt technologies that are labor-saving and integrative across the hospital.

TJC is a strong driver of IT adoption in most of the health care organizations that it accredits or certifies. The use of technology and computerization allows for reliable documentation to demonstrate compliance with the standards. As previously mentioned in this chapter, TJC does not *require* organizations to utilize technology in the provision of care to patients, but the voluntary use of technology must be implemented and utilized in a safe and efficacious manner.

TABLE 3-2

National Patient Safety Goals for Hospitals 2010

Goal	Sub-Goal	Title	Possible Technology Solution(s)
NPSG 1— Patient Identification	NPSG.01.01.01	Two Patient Identifiers	Bar code or RFID technologies, biometrics.
	NPSG.01.03.01	Transfusion Administration Safety	Bar code or RFID technologies, biometrics.
NPSG 2— Communication among Caregivers	NPSG.02.03.01	Critical Tests, Results, and Values	Wireless communication devices, real-time alerts and integration to electronic medical records.
NPSG 3— Medication Safety	NPSG.03.04.01	Labeling in Procedural Areas	Bar code technology.
	NPSG.03.05.01	Anticoagulation Therapy	CPOE, CDS, smart pump technology, real-time clinical surveillance programs.
NPSG 7— Health Care-Associated Infections	NPSG.07.01.01	Hand Hygiene	Real-time alerts and integration to electronic medical records.
	NPSG.07.03.01	Multiple Drug-Resistant Organisms	Real-time clinical surveillance programs, real-time alerts and integration to electronic medical records, CPOE, CDS.
	NPSG.07.04.01	Central Line-Associated Bloodstream Infection	Real-time clinical surveillance programs, real-time alerts and integration to electronic medical records, CPOE, CDS.
	NPSG.07.05.01	Surgical Site Infection	Real-time clinical surveillance programs, real-time alerts and integration to electronic medical records, CPOE, CDS.
NPSG 8— Medication	NPSG.08.01.01	Reconciliation Upon Arrival	Electronic health record, CPOE, CDS, reconciliation electronic prescribing.
	NPSG.08.02.01	Reconciliation Upon Transfer	Electronic health record, CPOE, CDS, electronic prescribing.
	NPSG.08.03.01	Reconciliation Upon Departure	Electronic health record, CPOE, CDS, electronic prescribing.

(continued)

TABLE 3-2
National Patient Safety Goals for Hospitals 2010 (*Continued*)

Goal	Sub-Goal	Title	Possible Technology Solution(s)
	NPSG.08.04.01	Modified Medication Reconciliation: medications are used minimally or prescribed for a short duration	Electronic health record, CPOE, CDS, electronic prescribing.
NPSG 15— Focused Risk Assessment (Suicide; Home Fires)	NPSG.15.01.01	Suicide Risk Reduction	Real-time alerts and integration to electronic medical records.
Universal Protocol	UP.01.01.01	Conduct a Preprocedure Verification Process	Electronic health record, real-time alerts and integration to electronic medical records.
	UP.01.02.01	Mark the Procedure Site	
	UP.01.03.01	A Time-Out Is Performed before the Procedure	

CPOE = computerized provider order entry; CDS = clinical decision support; NPSG = National Patient Safety Goal; RFID = radio frequency identification.
Source: Adapted from Reference 5.

Det Norske Veritas

Det Norske Veritas (DNV) is an independent foundation with the purpose of safeguarding life, property, and the environment. DNV's history goes back to 1864, when the foundation was established in Norway to inspect and evaluate the technical condition of Norwegian merchant vessels. DNV is the first and only CMS-approved accreditation service that surveys annually and integrates the International Organization for Standardization's ISO 9001 quality methods with Medicare Conditions of Participation. This approach turns accreditation into a strategic business advantage—by creating new standards of excellence from the skills, experience, and ingenuity that already exist in a hospital. The underlying NIAHO (National Integrated Accreditation for Health Organizations) accreditation requirements are tightly coupled with the Medicare Conditions of Participation. DNV accreditation introduces ISO 9001 quality methods into the hospital setting, resulting in self-sustaining improvement.[7–9]

ISO 9000 is a family of standards for quality management systems that is maintained by the International Organization for Standardization and administered by accreditation and certification bodies. The ISO rules are updated as the requirements motivate changes over time. A company or organization that has been independently audited and certified to be in conformance with ISO 9001, one of the standards included in ISO 9000, may publicly state that it is "ISO 9001 certified" or "ISO 9001 registered." Certification to an ISO 9001 standard does not guarantee any quality of end products and services; rather, it certifies that formalized business processes are being applied.[10]

The accreditation requirements of DNV are similar to those of TJC but are closely tied to a quality management system. The continuous feedback and reporting are important to demonstrate adherence to these requirements. As more health care organizations consider and adopt DNV accreditation, a higher emphasis on the use of technology and provision of the necessary reports will be required.

Quality Organizations

National Quality Forum

The National Quality Forum (NQF) is a nonprofit organization that aims to improve the quality of health care for all Americans through fulfillment of its three-part mission:

- Setting national priorities and goals for performance improvement.
- Endorsing national consensus standards for measuring and publicly reporting on performance.
- Promoting the attainment of national goals through education and outreach programs.

NQF's membership includes a wide variety of health care stakeholders, including consumer organizations, public and private purchasers, physicians, nurses, hospitals, accrediting and certifying bodies, supporting industries, and health care research and quality improvement organizations. The breadth and diversity of its membership allow NQF to be well positioned to maintain a constant drumbeat for health care quality. NQF's unique structure enables private- and public-sector stakeholders to work together to craft and implement cross-cutting solutions to drive continuous quality improvement in the American health care system.[11]

NQF believes that HIT is an essential foundation for the improvement of health care safety and quality. The federal government's recent funding to promote adoption of HIT will spur health care quality efforts by improving the ability to collect and share information. There is evidence that the adoption of HIT by clinicians reduces medical errors by increasing access to information, thereby improving response times, eliminating repetitive testing, and providing tools to facilitate evidence-based care. The NQF is interested in the adoption of HIT tools such as electronic prescribing, interoperable electronic health records, and quality registries to improve patient safety and the quality of health care.[12]

NQF has convened two expert panels to discuss the use of HIT and the sharing of quality data sets to improve overall patient care. The report of the first NQF Health Information Technology Expert Panel (HITEP-I) provides important building blocks for this effort. HITEP's report also identifies the common data quality types needed for quality measurement and a new method to assess data quality that should help the movement toward a more rational approach to measuring development and endorsement. Finally, this report presents key recommendations to help provide a common road map for addressing gaps and for moving forward. The technical and organizational approach described in the report should help define the common data quality types needed for electronic health record (EHR) quality measurement and assist in the transition of quality measurement to EHRs.[13]

The second Health Information Technology Expert Panel (HITEP-II) continues the work of HITEP-I, which identified 84 high-priority quality measures, their associated common data types, and a framework to evaluate the quality of electronic information required by performance measures through EHRs. Specifically, HITEP-II and its two workgroups have focused on recommendations for a standardized quality data set and more meaningful quality measurement through improved clinical data flows within and across care settings.[14] The findings of HITEP-II are available at www.qualityforum.org/projects/hitep2.aspx.

The original set of NQF-endorsed safe practices released in 2003, and updated in 2006, was defined to be universally applied in all clinical care settings to reduce the risk of error and harm for patients. The current 2009 updated report adds to the evolution of these practices and acknowledges their ongoing value to the health care community. This revised set of NQF-endorsed safe practices has been updated with current evidence and expanded implementation approaches, and it provides additional measures for assessing implementation of the practices. Each practice is specific and ready for implementation and has been shown to be effective in improving health care safety. Systematic, universal implementation of these practices can lead to appreciable and sustainable improvements for health care safety.[15]

One of the safe practices specifically addresses technology, Safe Practice 16: Safe Adoption of Computerized Prescriber Order Entry: "Implement a computerized prescriber order entry (CPOE) system built upon the requisite foundation of re-engineered evidence-based care, an assurance of healthcare organization staff and independent practitioner readiness, and an integrated information technology infrastructure." The safe practice standard provides guidance to health care organizations to better define their CPOE project and what should be included in the implementation. The practice setting; implementation strategy; opportunities for patient and family involvement; measurements (outcome, process, structure, and patient-centered); and new areas for research are stated within the consensus document (Table 3–3).[15]

Leapfrog Group

The Leapfrog Group is a voluntary program aimed at mobilizing employer purchasing power to alert America's health industry that big leaps in health care safety, quality, and customer value will be recognized and rewarded. Among other initiatives, Leapfrog works with its employer members to encourage transparency and easy access to health care information, as well as rewards for hospitals that have a proven record of high quality care. To fully meet the Leapfrog Hospital Recognition Program (LHRP) quality measures, hospitals must[16]:

1. Ensure that physicians enter at least 75% of medication orders via a computer system that includes prescribing-error prevention software.
2. Demonstrate, via a test, that their inpatient CPOE system can alert physicians to at least 50% of common, serious prescribing errors.

TABLE 3–3

National Quality Forum Safe Practice 16: Safe Adoption of Computerized Prescriber Order Entry

Safe Practice Statement

Implement a computerized prescriber order entry (CPOE) system built on the requisite foundation of reengineered evidence-based care, an assurance of health care organization staff and independent practitioner readiness, and an integrated information technology infrastructure.

Additional Specifications

Providers enter orders using an integrated, electronic information management system that is based on a documented implementation plan that includes or provides for the following:

■ Risks and hazards assessment to identify the performance gaps to be closed, including lack of standardization of care; high-risk points in medication management systems such as at point-of-order entry and upon administration of medications; and the introduction of disruptive innovations.

■ Prospective reengineering of care processes and workflow.

■ Readiness of integrated clinical information systems that include, at a minimum, the following information and management systems:

  ● Admit, discharge, and transfer

  ● Laboratory with electronic microbiology output

  ● Pharmacy

  ● Orders

  ● Electronic medication administration record (including patient, staff, and medication identification)

  ● Clinical data repository with clinical decision support capability

  ● Scheduling

  ● Radiology

  ● Clinical documentation

■ Readiness of hospital governance, staff, and independent practitioners, including board governance, senior administrative management, frontline caregivers, and independent practitioners.

■ The following CPOE specifications, which:

  ● Facilitate the medication reconciliation process.

  ● Are part of an electronic health record information system or an existing clinical information system that is bidirectionally and tightly interfaced with, at a minimum, the pharmacy, the clinical documentation department (including medication administration record), and laboratory systems, to facilitate review of all orders by all providers.

  ● Are linked to prescribing error prevention software with effective clinical decision support capability.

  ● Require prescribers to document the reasons for any override of an error prevention notice.

TABLE 3–3

National Quality Forum Safe Practice 16: Safe Adoption of Computerized Prescriber Order Entry (*Continued*)

- Enable and facilitate the timely display and review of all new orders by a pharmacist before administration of the first dose of medication, except when a delay would cause harm to a patient.
- Facilitate the review and/or display of all pertinent clinical information about the patient, including allergies, height and weight, medications, imaging, laboratory results, and a problem list, all in one place.
- Categorize medications into therapeutic classes or categories (e.g., penicillin and its derivatives) to facilitate the checking of medications within classes and retain this information over time.
- Have the capability to check the medication ordered as part of effective clinical decision support for dose range, dosing, frequency, route of administration, allergies, drug-drug interactions, dose adjustment based on laboratory results, excessive cumulative dosing, and therapeutic duplication.

Applicable Clinical Care Settings

This practice is applicable to Centers for Medicare and Medicaid Services care settings, including hospital inpatient service.

Sample Implementation Approaches

- CPOE may be adopted with a staged approach once integrated information systems are in place to support safe and effective CPOE systems. At least 75% of all inpatient medication orders should be entered directly by a licensed prescriber:
  - Stage 1: CPOE is in place on at least one ward/unit in the hospital.
  - Stage 2: CPOE is in place on three or more wards/units in the hospital.
  - Stage 3: CPOE is in place on more than 50% of the wards in the hospital.
  - Stage 4: Full compliance with at least 75% of all medications entered through the CPOE system by the prescriber.
- The system is tested against the Leapfrog Group Inpatient CPOE Testing Standards. These standards were developed to provide organizations that are implementing CPOE with appropriate decision support about alerting levels; these alerting levels need to be carefully set to avoid over alerting and under alerting.
- Strategies of progressive organizations: Certain progressive organizations have leveraged the integration of health information technologies and CPOE to optimize imaging, laboratory, and other areas of diagnostic testing. Some organizations are leveraging clinical decision support to maximize performance improvement, quality, and patient safety.

Opportunities for Patient and Family Involvement

- When appropriate, and within privacy standards, allow patients access to their health care information.
- Encourage patients to ask questions about their health care information and how they can best utilize their information to make informed health care decisions.

(continued)

TABLE 3-3

National Quality Forum Safe Practice 16: Safe Adoption of Computerized Prescriber Order Entry (*Continued*)

Outcome, Process, Structure, and Patient-Centered Measures

These performance measures are suggested for consideration to support internal health care organization quality improvement efforts, and all measures may not necessarily address external reporting needs.

- Outcome measures include reduced harm such as adverse drug events, death, disability (permanent or temporary), or preventable harm requiring further treatment; increased staff efficiency and throughput; return on investment calculations; reductions in medication; space and paper management cost; transcription cost savings; and reduced billing cycle costs with revenue cycle improvement.

- Process measures include medication errors; turnaround time for order to administration; compliance with the Joint Commission core measure requirements; medication management system performance metrics; compliance with local clinical protocols; and performance against Leapfrog CPOE testing standards and other performance metrics.

- Structure measures include verification of oversight or operational structures and documentation of readiness plans, including care reengineering and workflow design.

- Patient-centered measures: There are no published or validated patient-centered measures for CPOE.

Settings of Care Considerations

- Rural health care settings: It is recognized that small and rural health care settings are resource constrained. Clearly, achievement of widespread implementation of CPOE in rural health care settings may require special financial and technical assistance. However, it is not apparent from studies that limited application of CPOE or discrete aspects of CPOE (presumably at lower cost) will provide significant safety benefits. Indeed, studies suggest that CPOE, when implemented in rural hospitals, should conform to the specifications included in this practice without exception.

- Children's health care settings: All requirements of the practice are applicable to children's health care settings, with the understanding that there are special considerations for pediatrics, including that of availability of proven pediatric decision support electronic tools.

- Specialty health care settings: All requirements of the practice are applicable to specialty health care settings. The development of specialized standardized order sets for chemotherapy provides a good example that other specialty health care settings can follow.

New Horizons and Areas for Research

The area of clinical decision support and appropriateness offers a ripe avenue of investigation to further enhance the impact of CPOE on patient safety and quality of care. CPOE has emphasized medication safety; however, its ultimate impact may be through improved medical decision making and standardization of care. Further investigation is warranted for the study of implementation approaches involving the use of electronic medical records and CPOE, the short-term impact of risks to patients involved with rapid implementation, and the long-term risks of impact on gains in safety.

TABLE 3–3

National Quality Forum Safe Practice 16: Safe Adoption of Computerized Prescriber Order Entry (*Continued*)

Other Relevant Safe Practices

Safe practice 1: Leadership structures and systems.

Safe practice 3: Teamwork training and skill building.

Safe practice 4: Identification and mitigation of risks and hazards.

Other Relevant Practices

Safe practice 12: Patient care information.

Safe practice 15: Discharge systems.

Safe practice 17: Medication reconciliation.

Safe practice 18: Pharmacist leadership structures and systems.

Source: Adapted from Reference 15.

The Leapfrog Group originally developed these safety practices, or Leaps, through an extensive literature review and with input from national subject matter experts and quality researchers, in partnership with National Committee for Quality Assurance (NCQA), TJC, CMS, Agency for Healthcare Research and Quality, NQF, and large national purchasers. The CPOE evaluation tool provides a hospital with a set of patient scenarios, along with a corresponding set of inpatient medication orders that users enter into their hospital's CPOE and related clinical systems. Those conducting the test record the warnings or other responses, if any, from their hospital's CPOE system on an answer sheet, report those results to the Leapfrog Group Web site, and receive immediate scoring and feedback summarizing the results of the test. The scenarios and test protocols include potential drug-drug or drug-diagnosis interactions, drug allergies, therapeutic duplication, and dosage errors. The scenarios included in the test are relevant only to acute care, short-term hospital inpatient settings. Separate test scenarios are available for adult and pediatric populations.[17]

The Leapfrog CPOE testing programs should be considered a work in progress. How to use these empiric approaches to develop a unique method and the degree to which these criteria will actually impact safer, more reliable care is unclear. It is essential that certification approaches be tested and evaluated with respect to their impact on EHR systems, patient care, and patient outcomes. The results of these evaluations should be used to further refine and improve these novel approaches to evaluation and certification of CPOE and EHR systems. The testing program provides the hospital with specific areas of compliance, which should allow the hospital to further develop clinical decision support in areas of low performance (Table 3–4).[18]

TABLE 3–4

Leapfrog CPOE Evaluation Test CDS Categories

Category	Description
Therapeutic duplication	Therapeutic overlap with another active medication; may be the same drug, drug class, or components of a combination product.
Single and cumulative dose limits	Dose that exceeds recommended ranges; dose will lead to cumulative dose that exceeds recommended ranges; includes doses of individual components of combination products.
Allergies and cross-allergies	Documented allergy to medication being ordered or to another drug in the same class.
Contraindicated route of administration	Ordering a medication to be administered by the wrong route.
Drug-drug and drug-food interaction	Medication order results in a known, dangerous interaction with another medication or food group.
Contraindicated/dose limits based on patient diagnosis	Medication is contraindicated on the basis of patient's diagnosis, or diagnosis impacts dosing.
Contraindicated/dose limits based on patient age/weight	Medication is contraindicated on the basis of patient's age or weight.
Contraindicated/dose limits based on laboratory studies	Medication is contraindicated on the basis of laboratory studies, or laboratory studies must be considered for dosing.
Contraindicated/dose limits based on radiology studies	Medication is contraindicated on the basis of radiology studies (interaction with contrast media).
Corollary	Order for an intervention that requires a secondary order to meet standard of care.
Cost of care	Order for a test that duplicates a service provided within a time frame in which there is typically no benefit for repeating the test/service.
Nuisance	Order for an intervention that results in an inconsequential interaction that is usually ignored by clinicians.

CPOE = computerized prescriber order entry; CDS = clinical decision support.
Source: Adapted from Reference 18.

Barriers to HIT Adoption

A study published by Jha et al. describes some of the barriers and facilitators related to the adoption of HIT in the United States. Only 1.5% of U.S. hospitals have a comprehensive electronic record system (i.e., present in all clinical units), and an additional 7.6% have a basic system (i.e., present in at least one clinical unit). CPOE for medications has been implemented in only 17% of hospitals.[19] A survey of directors of pharmacy completed by Pedersen and Gumpper reported similar findings.[20] This survey did not look for barriers to implementation. Larger hospitals, those located in urban areas, and teaching hospitals were more likely to have electronic record systems. Respondents cited capital requirements and high maintenance costs as the primary barriers to implementation, although hospitals with electronic record systems were less likely to cite these barriers than hospitals without such systems.

Among hospitals without electronic records systems, the most commonly cited barriers were inadequate capital for purchase (74%), concerns about maintenance costs (44%), resistance on the part of physicians (36%), unclear return on investment (32%), and lack of availability of staff with adequate expertise in information technology (30%). Hospitals that had adopted electronic record systems were less likely to cite four of these five concerns (all except physicians' resistance) as major barriers to adoption than were hospitals that had not adopted such systems.[19] Regarding the availability of adequate staff with appropriate expertise, a number of reports have highlighted the growing concern that the health care system is woefully understaffed with the necessary personnel to successfully transform the industry from paper to electronic.[21,22] Financing of HIT is a primary barrier for all settings of care. Chapter 8 addresses this topic in more detail.

Most hospitals that have adopted electronic records systems identify financial factors as having a major positive effect on the likelihood of adoption: additional reimbursement for EHR use (82%) and financial incentives for adoption (75%). Other facilitators of adoption include the availability of technical support for implementation of information technology (47%) and objective third-party evaluations of EHR products (35%). Hospitals with and those without these systems were equally likely to cite these factors. High levels of decision support in the absence of a comparable prevalence of CPOE were reported.[19] It is possible that respondents who reported implementation of electronic decision support were including in that category decision support capabilities that are available only for electronic pharmacy systems, thereby overstating the preparedness of hospitals to provide physicians with electronic decision support for patient care.

Other barriers to adoption surround the usability of the technology in the course of patient care. Numerous studies describe the unintended consequences of technology. A study by Campbell et al. describes some of the unintended consequences[23]:

- More/new work for clinicians
- Unfavorable workflow issues
- Never-ending system demands
- Problems related to paper persistence
- Untoward changes in communication patterns and practices
- Negative emotions
- Generation of new kinds of errors
- Unexpected changes in the power structure
- Over dependence on the technology

Any of these consequences could result in the failure of an implemented technology or could be considered a barrier to its adoption. Immature clinical decision support functionality has often introduced many of these unintended consequences.

Role of Pharmacy Organizations and Groups in Enabling HIT Adoption

Most of the pharmacy professional organizations have component groups that are focusing on HIT and how it will affect their core members. Some of the organizations have supported the adoption of HIT to ensure patient safety. Other groups propose that HIT will improve efficiencies in medication ordering, preparation/delivery, and administration as well as patient billing processes and turnaround time. Some groups are interested in expanding the role of the pharmacist as a provider of medication therapy management (MTM). The use of HIT can help facilitate the role of the pharmacist in many of these practice settings. Table 3–5 lists specific pharmacy organizations and their HIT initiatives.

A 2009 initiative of the National Community Pharmacists Association (NCPA) will identify opportunities and recommend actions for community

TABLE 3–5

Pharmacy Organizations and Groups Representing Pharmacists' Interest in HIT

Organization	Web Site	Description
Academy of Managed Care Pharmacy	www.amcp.org	National professional society whose mission is to empower its members to serve society by using sound medication management principles and strategies to improve health care for all.
American Association of Colleges of Pharmacy	www.aacp.org	National organization committed to education and scholarship for improving drug therapy. The association will strengthen its mission of promoting professional and graduate education through effective use of policy, information, advocacy, and programming.
American Association of Pharmaceutical Scientists	www.aapspharmaceutica.com	Professional and scientific society that provides a dynamic international forum for the exchange of knowledge among scientists to enhance their contributions to health.
American College of Clinical Pharmacy	www.accp.com	Professional and scientific society that provides leadership, education, advocacy, and resources that enable clinical pharmacists to achieve excellence in practice and research.
American Pharmacists Association (APhA)	www.pharmacist.com	National professional organization whose members are recognized in society as essential in all patient care settings for optimal medication use that improves health, wellness, and quality of life. Through information, education, and advocacy, APhA empowers its members to improve medication use and advance patient care.
American Society of Consultant Pharmacists	www.ascp.com	International professional organization that empowers pharmacists to enhance quality of care for all older persons through the appropriate use of medication and the promotion of healthy aging.
American Society of Health-System Pharmacists	www.ashp.org	National professional organization that represents pharmacists who practice in hospitals, health maintenance organizations, long-term care facilities, home care, and other components of health care systems to improve medication use and enhance patient safety.

(continued)

TABLE 3-5

Pharmacy Organizations and Groups Representing Pharmacists' Interest in HIT (*Continued*)

Organization	Web Site	Description
National Association of Chain Drug Stores, Inc.	www.nacds.org	National association that provides a wide range of services to meet the needs of the chain drug industry in accordance with its goals and objectives.
National Community Pharmacists Association	www.ncpanet.org	National association dedicated to the continuing growth and prosperity of independent community pharmacy in the United States.
National Council for Prescription Drug Programs, Inc.	www.ncpdp.org	Nonprofit, ANSI-accredited standards development organization consisting of more than 1500 members representing virtually every sector of the pharmacy services industry.
Pharmacist Services Technical Advisory Coalition	www.pstac.org	Organization founded to improve the coding infrastructure needed to support billing for pharmacists' professional services. The coalition works to provide the national leadership needed to position and secure pharmacy's place in the EDI health encounter/claims processing and payment environment concerning all health care providers' professional services.
Pharmacy Quality Alliance	www.pqaalliance.org	An alliance of organizations whose mission is to improve the quality of medication use across health care settings through a collaborative process in which key stakeholders agree on a strategy for measuring and reporting performance information related to medications.

ANSI = American National Standards Institute; EDI = electronic data interchange.
Source: Author.

pharmacy, both organizationally and individually, to connect to the emerging, interoperable HIT infrastructure. The publication *Health Information Technology and the American Recovery and Reinvestment Act of 2009: A Roadmap for Community Pharmacy* summarizes the status of current HIT infrastructure, lists opportunities to reach out to regional and state networks, and outlines changes to the methods used to store and share protected health information in an electronic environment. An invitational conference held in June 2009, Connecting Community Pharmacy to the Interoperable Health Information Technology (HIT) Highway, offered sessions on grants for adoption of HIT, educational grants and training of pharmacists in HIT, funding of pharmacy-based research networks, loan programs to purchase certified EHRs, establishment of partnerships with personal health record vendors, and expanded MTM services.[24]

The Pharmacist Services Technical Advisory Coalition (the coalition) was established to improve the coding infrastructure necessary to support billing for pharmacists' professional services. Coalition activities include updating electronic data interchange standards, modifying coding structures, and supporting provider identifiers. The coalition has worked with the American Medical Association Current Procedural Terminology (CPT) Editorial Panel, which represents all specialties of medicine and allied health care professionals including pharmacists, to establish CPT codes for MTM. These steps have been important in helping pharmacists to bill for MTM services.[25] The coalition has developed professional services billing using the X12N 837 platform and built the infrastructure necessary to bill for services, including providing oversight for the second edition of *Professional Claims. Companion Document to the* ASC X12N *Insurance Subcommittee Implementation Guide* 004010X098 *Health Care Claim: Professional.*[26] These activities are highly integrated within the electronic model for pharmacist MTM services and professional billing.[25]

Conclusion

The focus on improving patient care in the inpatient environment relies on hospitals and health systems adopting technologies that promote patient safety and gain efficiencies in care. Accrediting agencies have not mandated that technology be adopted, but that a process is established for the appropriate use of the technology in caring for patients. The use of HIT in the care of ambulatory patients is important to help pharmacists in documenting

MTM and to improve their reimbursement for cognitive services. The use of automation in retail and community pharmacies remains a useful tool that allows pharmacists to expand their roles in this setting. There are considerable barriers to the adoption of HIT. Each institution or pharmacy will need to evaluate when it is appropriate to implement HIT within its environment to best optimize workflow and provide safe care to patients.

Many drivers of HIT adoption could have been addressed in this chapter. Ultimately, a convergence of factors will determine an organized process for adoption of HIT.

LEARNING ACTIVITIES

1. If you work in a hospital or have rotated through a hospital on a rotation, has the institution adopted TJC's recommendations as stated in the Sentinel Event Alert (www.jointcommission.org/SentinelEvents/SentinelEventAlert/sea_42.htm)?
2. Review the National Quality Forum's "Safe Practices for Better Healthcare-2009 Update" and determine how HIT can support quality patient care (www.qualityforum.org/Publications/2009/03/Safe_Practices_for_Better_Healthcare–2009_Update.aspx).
3. List different barriers to adopting HIT within your current or future practice setting.

References

1. The Joint Commission. About us. Available at: http://www.jointcommission.org/AboutUs. Accessed October 25, 2009.
2. The Joint Commission. Benefits of Joint Commission accreditation. July 22, 2009. Available at: http://www.jointcommission.org/HTBAC/benefits_accreditation.htm. Accessed October 25, 2009.
3. The Joint Commission. Issue 42: safely implementing health information and converging technologies. December 11, 2008. Available at: http://www.jointcommission.org/SentinelEvents/SentinelEventAlert/sea_42.htm. Accessed October 25, 2009.
4. Mitka, M. Joint Commission offers warnings, advice on adopting new health care IT systems. JAMA. 2009;301(6):587–9.
5. The Joint Commission. Accreditation program: hospital. In: 2010 *Portable Comprehensive Accreditation Manual for Hospitals* (CAMH): *The Official Handbook*. Oakbrook Terrace, IL: Joint Commission Resources; 2010. Available to authorized users at: http://www.jointcommission.org/NR/rdonlyres/FC01E2E0-A0CB-4A71-AF0B-137AA77D1BD6/0/AllChapters_HAP.pdf. Accessed October 25, 2009.

6. The Joint Commission. Health care at the crossroads: guiding principles for the development of the hospital of the future. November 2008. Available at: http://www.joint commission.org/NR/rdonlyres/1C9A7079-7A29-4658-B80D-A7DF8771309B/0/Hospital_Future.pdf. Accessed October 25, 2009.

7. Der Gurahian J. DNV setting new standard. *Mod Healthcare.* 2008:2–4.

8. Dror Y, Wise R, Horine P, Scott D. Introduction to DNV healthcare and NIAHO: a new choice for hospital accreditation [PowerPoint slides]. 2009. Available at: http://www.dnv.com/binaries/Introduction%20to%20DNV%20Healthcare%20and%20NIAHO-A%20New%20Choice%20for%20Hospital%20Accreditation-Overview_tcm4-331352.ppt. Accessed October 25, 2009.

9. DNV Healthcare Inc. National Integrated Accreditation for Healthcare Organizations (NIAHO) accreditation requirements. Issue 307-8.0. 2008. Available at: http://www.dnv.com/binaries/NIAHO%20Accreditation%20Requirements-Rev%20307-8%200(2)_tcm4-347543.pdf. Accessed October 25, 2009.

10. International Organization for Standardization. FAQs on ISO 9001:2008. Available at: http://www.iso.org/iso/iso_catalogue/management_standards/iso_9000_iso_14000/iso_9001_2008/faqs_on_iso_9001.htm. Accessed October 25, 2009.

11. National Quality Forum. About NQF. Available at: http://www.qualityforum.org/About_NQF/About_NQF.aspx. Accessed October 25, 2009.

12. National Quality Forum. Health information technology (HIT). Available at: http://www.qualityforum.org/Topics/Health_Information_Technology_(HIT).aspx. Accessed October 25, 2009. Measures for Electronic Healthcare Information Systems.

13. National Quality Forum. Recommended common data types and prioritized performance measures for electronic healthcare information systems. 2008. Available at: http://www.qualityforum.org/Publications.aspx. Accessed April 25, 2010.

14. National Quality Forum. Health Information Technology Expert Panel II—health IT enablement of quality measurement. Available at: http://www.qualityforum.org/projects/hitep2.aspx. Accessed October 25, 2009.

15. National Quality Forum. Safe practices for better healthcare–2009 Update. March 2009. Available at:http://www.qualityforum.org/Publications/2009/03/Safe_Practices_for_Better_Healthcare–2009_Update.aspx. Accessed October 25, 2009.

16. The Leapfrog Group. LHRP reports. Available at: http://www.leapfroggroup.org/lhrpreports. Accessed April 8, 2010.

17. The Leapfrog Group. Leapfrog CPOE evaluation tool. 2009. Available at: https://leapfrog.medstat.com/cpoe/. Accessed October 25, 2009.

18. Classen DC, Avery AJ, Bates DW. Evaluation and certification of computerized provider order entry systems. JAMIA. 2007;14(1):48–55.

19. Jha AK, DesRoches CM, Campbell EG, et al. Use of electronic health records in U.S. hospitals. N *Engl J Med.* 2009;360:1628–38.

20. Pedersen CA, Gumpper KF. ASHP national survey on informatics: assessment of the adoption and use of pharmacy informatics in U.S. hospitals—2007. AJHP. 2008;65(23):2244–64.

21. Hersh W. What workforce is needed to implement the health information technology agenda? Analysis from the HIMSS Analytics Database. In: AMIA *Annual Symposium Proceedings*/AMIA *Symposium.* Bethesda, MD: American Medical Informatics Association; 2008:303–7.

22. Hersh W. Health and biomedical informatics: opportunities and challenges for a twenty-first century profession and its education. In: *Yearbook of Medical Informatics.* Stuttgart, Germany:

Schattauer Publishers; 2008:157–64. Available at: http://www.schattauer.de/en/magazine/subject-areas/journals-a-z/imia-yearbook/imia-yearbook-2008/issue/special/manuscript/9833/download.html. Accessed April 8, 2010.

23. Campbell EM, Sittig DF, Ash JS, et al. Types of unintended consequences related to computerized provider order entry. JAMIA. 2006;13:547–56.

24. National Community Pharmacists Association. Health information technology and the American Recovery and Reinvestment Act of 2009: a roadmap for community pharmacy. In: *Connecting Community Pharmacy to the Interoperable Health Information Technology Highway: Conference Proceedings*. Alexandria, VA: National Community Pharmacists Association. September 2009. Available at: http://www.ncpanet.org/pdf/leg/hitproceedings.pdf. Accessed November 2, 2009.

25. Pharmacist Services Technical Advisory Coalition. Available at: http://www.pstac.org/. Accessed November 2, 2009.

26. Pharmacist Services Technical Advisory Coalition. *Professional Claims. Companion Document to the ASC X12N Insurance Subcommittee Implementation Guide 004010X098 Health Care Claim: Professional, 2nd Edition*. Bellevue, WA: Washington Publishing Company.

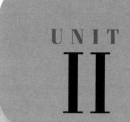
Computing and Telecommunication Fundamentals

UNIT COMPETENCIES

- Discuss the benefits and limitations of systematically processing data, information, and knowledge in health care.
- Describe measures used to ensure the privacy, security, and confidentiality of health information.
- Discuss key issues affecting human-computer interaction.
- Differentiate between spreadsheets, databases, and user interfaces.
- Discuss technologies used to automate the medication delivery process.

UNIT DESCRIPTION

Chapters in this unit address core computing topics that are prerequisite to developing knowledge and skills in pharmacy informatics. Basic computing and networking terminologies, structures, and functions are covered. Telecommunication systems provide an essential function to pharmacy informatics systems; therefore, the reader will be exposed to important telecommunication topics as well.

Personal Computer and Network Systems Fundamentals

Frederick Albright

OBJECTIVES

1. Understand the importance of relevant computer components and their purposes.
2. Build a vocabulary that leads to understanding computer basics, the network-centric nature of systems, and the basis of information technology.
3. Build a conceptual basis to understand and analyze systems graphically. This leads to a better understanding of computer systems and networking, as well as people systems and human-machine systems.
4. Introduce the concepts of interfaces being of importance in building and understanding systems: people, computer, and human-machine.
5. Understand systems and interfaces to provide an intellectual skeleton to analyze current problems and to be proactive in avoiding future problems in systems.
6. Understand the basics of computer data security to protect the data integrity and electronic identity of all users.

7. Build a systematic understanding of how computer systems, networking, and information technology are critical for pharmacy and other health professionals.
8. Understand how these systems are force multipliers for pharmacists, other health care professionals, and the patient in providing higher standards of care and outcomes that are more positive.

Computer and computer networking systems are fundamentally necessary to the delivery of pharmacy and other health care services to patients, clinicians, allied health care workers, insurance providers, government agencies, and caregivers for the purposes of personal/public health, bio-surveillance, and defense. For these principles alone, understanding computer and networking fundamentals is extremely important for the duties of a pharmacist. Developing knowledge and skills with these systems will reinforce the roles of a pharmacist and act as force multipliers for a pharmacist through greater and efficacious meaningful use of electronic data, information, and knowledge in the practice setting.

Pharmacists and other health care providers will find it necessary to have at least a modicum of understanding about computer systems and computer networking. Learning fundamental and necessary higher-ordered concepts about information technology (IT) will multiply the "forces" a pharmacist uses in performance of pharmacy practice. Computers and computer networks are tools in the pharmacist's armamentarium for performing and accomplishing the tasks, duties, and roles of health workers. Patient care and medication safety activities depend on computer, software, and networking systems.

Some computer activities are routine, whereas others require creative and higher-ordered thinking, analysis, and planning by the pharmacist. Computer systems and networks are more than supportive tools; they are integrated into practically every phase of the pharmacy workflow, and are the basis for integration and interoperability between the different domains of electronic health care practice. Knowledge of these systems will be generalizable and indispensible in understanding and effectively using more complex health care computer systems. Accessibility to these systems is extremely important, as is expertise in their utilization for modern pharmacy care.

Miniaturization: Imbedding Computer Systems in Health Care Services

In earlier days when computers were room sized, the computer was a collection of large, heavy circuit boards. A single computer system was massive and perhaps weighed tons. These early digital computers used electrode vacuum tubes to act as electronic switches to store binary data and perform computations. Tubes were prone to electronic failure. Vacuum tubes had larger voltage and current requirements, so larger resistors, capacitors, and other electronic components were required.

Memory was distributed across memory boards, amounting to a few hundred or a few thousand characters for data and/or software. The central processing unit could be on one circuit board, or its functions could be distributed across other dedicated circuit boards. Output and input controls were on boards other than those dedicated to the central processing unit. These boards were connected together via a series of cables or a wired backplane so that intercommunication could occur between the boards.

After invention of the transistor in the 1950s, transistors replaced the vacuum tubes. Transistors required much less electrical power and cooling, and were also orders of magnitude more reliable than vacuum tubes. Discrete transistors along with the other smaller circuit components were mounted on smaller and smaller circuit boards with more and more components on each board (i.e., miniaturization).

The application of microscale photolithography and microminiature circuit masks changed the circuit boards from collections of discrete transistors, capacitors, resistors, connecting wires, and diodes on large boards into collections of computer circuits on a silicon substrate. Computers became more miniaturized, faster, and more powerful, with more memory. As placement of computer components became closer and closer, computing speeds increased. Electrons did not take as long to go from one component to the other. As micro- or even nano-miniaturization continues to evolve, computers will continue to get smaller, faster, and more powerful, and use less energy.

Manufacturing of computer boards and microchips has advanced miniaturization from large-scale integration (thousands of transistors) to very large-scale integration (millions of transistors on a chip) to ultra large-scale integration (ULSI; billions of transistors on a chip). Distances between transistors connecting wires between computer components have dwindled from millimeters (thousandths of a meter) to micrometers (millionths of a meter) to nanometers (billionths of a meter) and soon, perhaps, trillionths of a meter, barring quantum tunneling as described in the next paragraph. Table 4–1 relates the scale of objects to provide a feel for distance on these small scales, compared with familiar objects. The width of the wires connecting transistors and other electronic components on a modern chip approaches the width of a mammalian cell, as will soon the size of transistors in the main computer microprocessor. ULSI puts a computer on a small silicone chip instead of circuit boards in a steel or plastic case.

Miniaturization continues unabated and follows Moore's law (Figure 4–1). Loosely, processing power (transistors) doubles every 2 years.[1] There is a theoretical limit for the proximity of flowing electrons before data are corrupted. For example, if moving electrons flow along wires too closely, they influence each other's quantum energy states (corresponding to the data they represent). Energy states of electrons can be rein-

TABLE 4–1
Relative Scale of Objects

Item	Measured Value	Magnitude Scale (meters)
Mosquito (length)	~1.5 cm	10^{-2}
Red ant (length)	~5 mm	10^{-3}
Paramecium caudatum (length)	~200 µm	10^{-4}
Human hair (diameter)	~100 µm	10^{-4}
Red blood cell (diameter)	~7 µm	10^{-6}
Aerosols (coughing or sneezing)	<5–10 µm	10^{-6}
NIOSH N95 mask (lower bound)	0.3 µm	10^{-7}
H1N1 virus	90 nm	10^{-8}
CPU transistor	≤45 nm	10^{-8}
Cell membrane	6–10 nm	10^{-9}

CPU = central processing unit; NIOSH = National Institute for Occupational Safety and Health.
Rule of thumb: Limit of resolution is approximately 100 µm for most people with normal eyesight.
Source: Adapted from Wikipedia. Order of magnitude. [Click on "length."] Available at: http://en.wikipedia.org/wiki/Orders_of_magnitude; Wikipedia. *Escherichia coli.* Available at: http://en.wikipedia.org/wiki/E_coli; and Clinical Microbiology Reviews. Pandemic threat posed by avian influenza A viruses. Available at: http://www.ncbi.nlm.nih.gov:80/pmc/articles/PMC88966/?tool=pmcentrez. All sites accessed October 24, 2009.

FIGURE 4–1

Moore's law tells us that the number of transistors in a circuit doubles approximately every 2 years. The dashed linear line represents Moore's prediction. The actual doubling of transistors (solid back line with large dots) closely follows the prediction line.

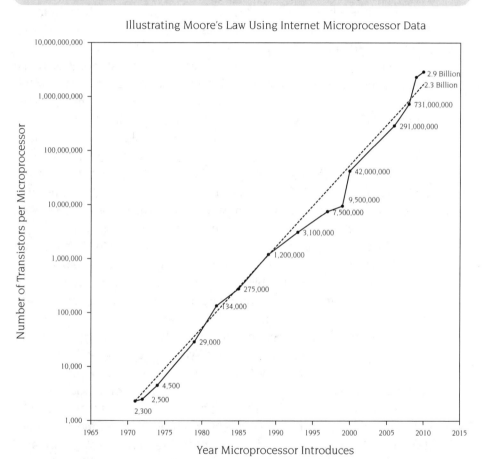

Illustrating Moore's Law Using Internet Microprocessor Data

Source: Adapted from Intel Cooporation. Moore's Law 40th Anniversary Press Kit. 2005. http://www.intel.com/pressroom/kits/events/moores_law_40th. Accessed November 5, 2009.

forced (energy added) or reduced (energy lost). This quantum tunneling can lead to data corruption for electrons traveling along "wires" of the computer or for electrons stored in memory. Presently, the proximity distance limit has not been reached. Historically posited limits have been surpassed. Miniaturization will continue to even smaller scales for the near future until the actual limit is reached.

Bits Make Bytes, and Bytes Make Words to Represent and Store Data

How does a digital computer represent data electronically? The smallest storage unit is a binary digit or bit. A single bit has a value of either 0 or 1, or alternatively, true or false. The **bit** is the smallest parcel of datum stored or used in a computer.

The bit has its analog in a transistorized circuit that stores a charge (electrons). Therefore, by Ohm's law this circuit will have a voltage. If a voltmeter with nanometer-sized probes could be used, it would measure the voltage across the transistorized circuit terminals. Typically, the voltage measured will be a value of 5 volts (a binary digit value of 1) or a value of 0 volts (a binary digit value of 0). Energy saving or "green" digital circuits will use bits with representative voltages less than five (e.g., 3 volts to represent a bit value of 1 and 0 volts to represent a 0 bit value). Smaller transistors store less charge but in a smaller area; therefore, the voltages are smaller, with an implication: less electrical current required and less heat produced.

Bits are organized into 8 consecutive bits to form 1 **byte.** Bytes are collected into words as illustrated in Figure 4–2. Early desktop personal computers were known as 8 bit (1 byte contains 8 bits; each byte can represent one alphabet character) or 16 bit computers (words formed of 2 bytes). Most personal computers today are 32 bit computers (words are 4 bytes for a total of 32 bits). The newest personal computers are now 64 bit computers (64 bit words made of 8 consecutive bytes). Heuristically, as the number of bits in a computer word increases, the computer becomes more powerful and faster because a "large" datum is stored and processed in a larger word instead of across multiple smaller words or bytes that must be linked together, perhaps not consecutively. Data that are more complex (take more bits) can be stored as larger words and read faster compared with stringing bytes and smaller words into larger words, which is a more cumbersome and slow process. The processor using larger words reduces the number of reads/writes needed to transfer data to and from memory.

Conceptual Steps of a Computer System Model

Input is Processed into Output

A simple computer system model consists of input, processing of the input (through the use of program logic or software), and output of the processed input.[2] Figure 4–3 summarizes this with feedback loops. For example, when

FIGURE 4-2

Consecutive bits make bytes. One or more consecutive bytes make words: 16-bit, 32-bit, 64-bit, and so on. The lowest order bit is 0 corresponding to 2^0. The highest order bit is 7 (2^8), 15 (2^{16}), or 31 (2^{32}) depending on the size of the word.

Lowest to highest order bit

0 1 2 3 4 5 6 7 8 9 10 11 12 13 14 15 16 17 18 19 20 21 22 23 24 25 26 27 28 29 30 31

| 1 | 0 | 1 | 0 | 1 | 1 | 0 | 0 | 0 | 0 | 0 | 1 | 1 | 0 | 1 | 0 | 1 | 1 | 1 | 0 | 0 | 0 | 0 | 0 | 0 | 1 | 1 | 1 | 1 | 0 | 1 | 0 | 0 | 1 |

A word composed of 32 consecutive bits is equivalent to a word composed of 4 consecutive bytes.
The number of unique combinations of zeros (0's) and/or ones (1's) is 4,294,967,296 or 2^{32}.
A word this size can represent 4,294,967,296 characters or 4,294,967,295 integers (e.g., 0,1,2, etc.).

Lowest to highest order bit

0 1 2 3 4 5 6 7 8 9 10 11 12 13 14 15

| 1 | 0 | 1 | 0 | 1 | 1 | 0 | 0 | 0 | 0 | 1 | 1 | 0 | 1 | 0 | 1 |

A word composed of 16 consecutive bits is equivalent to a word composed of 2 consecutive bytes.
The number of unique combinations is 65,536 or 2^{16}.
A word this size can represent 65,536 characters or the range of integers between 0 and 65,535.

Lowest to highest order bit

0 1 2 3 4 5 6 7

| 1 | 0 | 1 | 0 | 1 | 1 | 0 | 0 |

A word composed of a single byte is composed of 8 consecutive bits.
The number of combinations is 256 or 2^8.
A word this size can represent 256 characters (ASCII) or a range of integers between 0 and 255.

0

| 1 |

A single bit is either "on" or "off"; it can never be both.
A single order bit can represent a binary number such as 1 or 0, that is, the number of combinations is 2 or 2^1.

ASCII = American Standard Code for Information Interchange.
Source: Author.

FIGURE 4-3

Fundamental representation of a processing system. Input data are processed into output data by a processor. Further, feedback loops are also used to modify the output again, giving additional output. Feedback is often used to control a system.

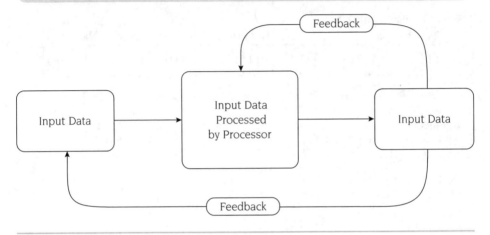

Source: Author.

the command to print (input command) a document from the word processor (using the keyboard or mouse to issue the command) to a selected printer is issued, the command to print the document is interpreted (processing) into a sequence of actions by the computer, with the outcome that the document prints to paper (output). Inside the computer and printer (a computer specialized for printing), a number of feedback loops are present to ensure that the output is printed correctly (e.g., within the margins of the paper and tolerances of other parameters such as ink density, drying time, image resolution, etc.).

These feedback loops are broken down along the basic steps of input, processing, and output. Feedback loops and electronic controls (either hardware and/or software based) are in the computer system to control input and output. The video graphics control card has a video amplifier circuit that incorporates feedback mechanisms to limit the monitor output within the range selected for picture brightness, sharpness, color reproduction, geometry, and other parameters. Feedback and control mechanisms provide the correct phase, voltage, and current to the appropriate computer components. Without feedback, the integrated circuits and/or components would fail because of electrical overcharging and/or undercharging.

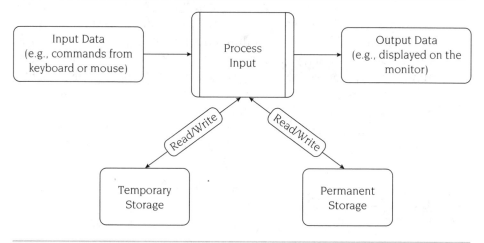

FIGURE 4–4

Fundamental input-processing-output system model (IPO). Starting from the fundamental representation of a processing system model, extend it to include data storage, both permanent and temporary.

Source: Adapted from Wikipedia. IPO model. http://en.wikipedia.org/wiki/IPO_Model. Accessed November 4, 2009.

Computer Memory Stores Data

Computer systems store data as collections of bits in memory. Figure 4–4 represents an extension in the fundamental system conceptual model[2] (as represented in Figure 4–3) by including data storage in a computer system. Computers store data permanently or temporarily in memory, depending on the temporal information utility of the data. The bidirectional arrows between the processor and each type of memory signify that data are transferred (written) to memory after processing by the processor, and/or that the data have been transferred from memory to the processor (read) to be processed. Data can be written to storage (e.g., main memory, disk, or Universal Serial Bus [USB] memory key) or an output device such as the monitor, speakers, or other peripheral output devices.

Important Components in a Computer System

A computer at its most basic level is made up of collections of resistors, capacitors, diodes, inductors, wires (connectors), and other simple electrical components into a meaningfully purposed electronic circuit, often as microchips. These chips and other circuits are mounted on a motherboard, which supports the chips on a flat surface made mostly of plastic and metal, with appropriate wires connecting these components. The wires do more than connect the components. The wires embedded in the motherboard and in the chips not only act as data intercommunication pathways, but other wires carry power to the components from the smallest transistors to the larger multi-component circuits. In addition, it is important that timing signals be transmitted to each component. These timing signals coupled with logic control act as "traffic" signals, synchronizing the operations of different processing components and sharing of computing resources for data intercommunication.

The "blocks" in Figure 4–5 represent some of the most important functional components in a computer. These components are a clock (or clock

FIGURE 4–5

Computer conceptual model.

Data Communication Pathways, Clock, and Power Support Conceptual Matrix

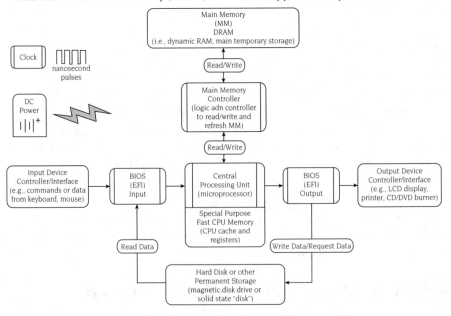

BIOS = basic input/output system; CD = compact disk; CPU = computer processing unit; DC = direct current; DRAM = dynamic random access memory; DVD = digital video disc; EFI = Extensible Firmware Interface; LCD = liquid crystal display; RAM = random access memory.
Source: Author.

generator), direct current power source, generalized input/output device, input/output system controller (basic input/output system [BIOS] or the more modern Extensible Firmware Interface), main processor or central processing unit, main memory, main memory controller, and hard disk (permanent storage). Communication wires are collected into what is known as a communication bus.

Central Processing Unit

The main processing unit of a computer, the **central processing unit** (CPU), is the controlling executor of the computer, as exemplified conceptually in Figure 4–6. The CPU executes program instructions, which are the commands the CPU uses to process the data. All components of importance in

FIGURE 4–6

The central processing unit (CPU) conceptual diagram.

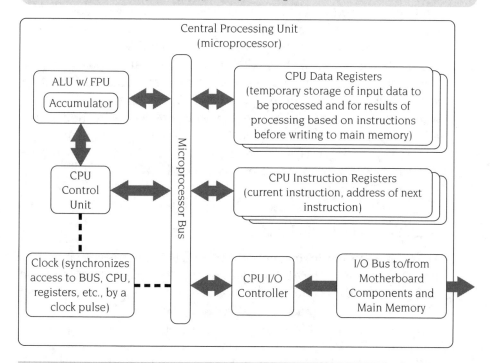

ALU = arithmetic logic unit; CPU = computer processing unit; FPU = floating-point unit; I/O = input/output.
Source: Author.

the CPU are connected together so that data and results can be intercommunicated via the CPU or microprocessor bus. This bus is very fast; data movement from one component of the CPU to another can be measured on the scale of nanoseconds or less. Modern microprocessors have CPU clock speeds in excess of 3 gigahertz (GHz). Data transfers can be measured in billions of transfers per second (giga transfers per second, or GT/sec).[3]

The CPU executes instructions from the operating system and other software, which ultimately originate from the user of the computer. The CPU can perform arithmetic, count, and compare bits, bytes, and computer words using Boolean logic. To perform arithmetic computations, compare numbers, or count, the CPU performs four additional instructions called the "machine cycle"—fetch (data or instructions from memory), decompose (decompose instructions into simpler operations), execute (interpret an instruction to process a datum or data), and writeback (write to memory)—over and over again until the program ends.[4]

After fetching the instruction into the CPU special purpose memory, the instruction is decomposed into elementary instructions (i.e., simpler operations). In addition, if an instruction requires data not already in a CPU register, the CPU fetches the data from system memory. These more elementary operations are then transferred to the other CPU components for execution (e.g., basic and more complex arithmetic and/or logical operations). Once the instruction completes, the results are stored as a finished computation or as an intermediate result. The CPU fetches the "next" instruction from memory to process once the previous instruction's operation(s) have finished. Most instructions and sub-operations complete in one or more "ticks" (cycles) of the CPU clock. The CPU continues to cycle with fetch, decompose, execute, and writeback until it is instructed to stop (e.g., end of program or system shutdown).

Arithmetic and Logic Unit

The **arithmetic and logic unit** (ALU) of the CPU performs arithmetic and logical operations.[5] The ALU operates or processes pairs of integers.[6] The ALU performs only addition and emulates subtraction, multiplication, and division of integers by adding negatives of integers for subtraction, adding multiples of integers for multiplication, and/or subtracting multiples of integers for division. The ALU compares two integers logically for equality (e.g., greater than, less than, and/or equal to), as well as other logical operations such as changing a logical state from true to false.

Floating-Point Unit: Representing and Processing Decimal Numbers

The **floating-point unit** (FPU) processes not integers but decimal numbers (i.e., floating-point numbers). Floating-point numbers have digits to the left and right of the decimal point. Simple examples of floating-point numbers are ½ as 0.5 or 72 ¼ as 72.25, or pi (π) as 3.14159265. A couple of other examples are the molar mass and number of molecules in a mole of a chemical substance such as a drug or other substance to treat patients. The molar mass of glucose is 180.15588. A mole of glucose would have an Avogadro's number of glucose molecules, or 6.022×10^{23} glucose molecules.[7,8] The number of digits before or after the decimal can be assigned to represent a large range of decimal numbers, including negatives. Floating-point arithmetic operations are more complex than integer operations, hence, the development of the FPU of a CPU.[9]

Unlike representations of integers, which are exact on a computer, floating-point numbers are approximations of decimal numbers. Decimal numbers can be represented more exactly with different precisions (i.e., more digits to the right of the decimal point).[10] The FPU adds, subtracts, multiplies, and divides two floating-point numbers or a floating-point number and an integer. Logical operations can also be performed to compare two floating-point numbers. The number of floating-point operations per second (FLOPS) measures approximately the overall speed or power of a floating-point processor.[9] The newer microprocessors have performance ranges from tens of GFLOPS (gigaflops) to hundreds of GFLOPS per second. However, this speed often can be attributed to microprocessors acting in parallel and each having an FPU.

Central Processing Unit Memory

The CPU has onboard special temporary memory that is very quick, meaning CPU memory performs, reads, and writes much faster than main memory. There are two categories of temporary memory in the CPU: register and cache memory. **Registers** are closest to the CPU, adjacent to the CPU computational components. Registers store data to be used immediately (e.g., instructions to direct processing of register data, the current executing instruction, and the next instruction). If the data and instructions are prefetched into the appropriate registers, the CPU is faster. Reads and writes to/from registers are faster than writing to main memory or permanent storage. The quantity of CPU memory is orders of magnitude less than main memory.

Cache is also located on the microprocessor but a bit farther away from the CPU computational components. **Cache** is special purpose memory. Cache is not as fast as register memory, but it is much faster than main or permanent memory.[11] Cache speeds up memory access to data and instructions by storing a large portion of the data and instructions likely to be used next, and it stores results of computations to be written to main memory.[12] Utilizing main memory would slow the computer by one or two orders of magnitude at a minimum.

There are three levels of cache: level 1 (L1), level 2 (L2), and level 3 (L3). As the level of the cache decreases, the cache size becomes smaller and the cache is located geographically closer to the main CPU components. If the CPU does not find the data (or instructions) it needs in one of the CPU registers, it sequentially seeks the data or instructions in L1, L2, and then L3 cache.[12] If the information is not found in the L3 cache, the CPU searches the main memory and, if needed, the hard disk (or other permanent storage component). The CPU can end up in waiting mode as it seeks the data or instructions to fetch from the main memory or a hard disk.

Temporary Storage: Main Memory Unit

The **main memory unit** (MMU) is the computer's primary storage area for temporary memory; storage capacity is typically measured in gigabytes. The MMU uses dynamic random access memory (DRAM), which is mounted on the motherboard. Main memory is categorized as double data rate (DDR) memory (as opposed to earlier random access memory that was single data rate, or SDR). Main memory can be DDR, DDR2, and DDR3 synchronous dynamic random access memory (DDR3 SDRAM). The newest computers at this time use DDR2 SDRAM, and the higher-end personal computers use DDR3 SDRAM for main memory.[13–16] When the computer loses power (power interruption or the computer is turned off), the data degrades from DRAM very quickly, thus the adjective "dynamic" RAM. DRAM data are volatile as is CPU memory.

Memory Controller

Writing data to, and reading data from, memory is an input/output process handled by another subsystem of the computer, called the **memory control**

unit (MCU). The MCU is one of the many specialized computer subsystems in a personal computer that assists the main processing unit in carrying out the millions of tasks that make up the most fundamental processes.

Permanent Storage

Permanent storage includes hard disks, digital video disks (DVD), compact disks (CD), USB flash drive, or other permanent storage devices. Data are stored permanently so that the data can be used at some time in the future. Even without power, the data do not degrade when stored in permanent memory, unlike the volatile state in DRAM. If the computer is turned off gracefully or loses power without warning (even temporarily, as in a power "bump"), permanent storage retains the data. When a word processing program or file is opened, each is loaded from permanent storage into main memory.

Controlling/Managing Input/Output and Bootstrapping

Computers require a means to **bootstrap** (start up and initialize hardware), monitor, and control input/output. For example, the hard disk, graphics card, CD or DVD burner, and other hardware are tested and initialized. *Booting* is short for *bootstrapping*. The bootstrap starts with the BIOS whose firmware is stored in ROM (read only memory; a form of solid state permanent memory). The **BIOS** firmware performs the first phases of the start-up processes. After the BIOS firmware has finished loading and all systems are initialized, BIOS starts the first phase of loading the operating system into main memory from hard disk. Once this phase completes, the control for booting is assumed by the operating system, which completes booting of the system. BIOS continues as an interface for the operating system to monitor and control input/output.

There are different basic input/output control systems for different kinds of personal computers. Over the years, the early input/output control systems have evolved with the computer. Open Firmware, Open BIOS/Open Firmware, and Extensible Firmware Interface (EFI) are now the basic input/output control systems. These "BIOS" standards also provide means to monitor power, make a battery charge last longer (power management), and are built to work with 32 and 64 bit operating and hardware systems.[17]

Main Memory Controller

The **main memory controller** (MMC) manages and controls the read/writes to and from main memory for the CPU using the system clock for timing. The MMC must match the type of main memory on the system in terms of speed and type to control reads/writes.

Operating System

One can imagine the operating system of a computer in a number of ways. Figure 4–7 conceptualizes the operating system as "connecting" the user to the internal hardware of the computer, with the CPU (microprocessor), main memory (temporary storage), hard disk (permanent storage), and user programs running on the computer. An **operating system** is the software system that provides the core interface between a user and the hardware or software on the computer. The operating system acts as the interface between programs, hardware, and systems resources such as the system bus, CPU bus, main memory, and hard disk.

Computer Networks

Meaningful and effective pharmacy or clinical practice is as much a function of computerization as it is a function of computer networking in modern health care practice. **Computer networking,** or for the context of this chapter simply "networking" (not to be confused with social networking), is the supporting connectivity and inter/intra communications between computer systems, networks or other more complex systems. Networks are a core hardware and software technology that provides the medium to interchange and share data (e.g., patient data), applications (e.g., work force scheduling), clinical services (e.g., information retrieval to support evidence-based practice), and/or cyber security (e.g., maintain privacy of personal health information) between computer systems and the people who use them. Networking provides access to computers, data, services, applications, and people in a safe, secure manner, in compliance with the Health Insurance Portability and Accountability Act (HIPAA) and with meaningful use stipulations by the federal government.

A number of networking technologies and standards have been developed. For the purposes of this chapter, networking occurs over two different mediums. The physical medium comprises the Ethernet, which uses special purpose copper cables to connect to a network (at work or home).

FIGURE 4–7

The operating system as an interface. Conceptually the operating system controls the interfaces between system components, software applications, and the user. The major resources shared by the operating system between processes are the motherboard bus, the input/output interfaces/devices, as well as the computer processing unit (CPU) bus, and the central processing unit and its components. The operating system is the master controller for sharing of resources.

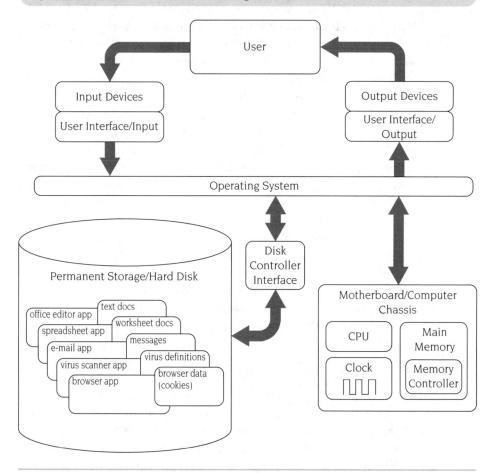

app = application; CPU = computer processing unit; docs = documents; I/O = input/output.
Source: Author.

Ethernet networks are defined by the Institute of Electrical and Electronics Engineers [IEEE] Standard for Networking 802.3. The second medium consists of high-frequency radio waves carrying data to/from a computer through the air. The wireless network standards are currently IEEE 802.11 a, b, g, n. A later alphabetic letter denotes a faster network; 802.11n has the maximum speed (depending on wireless communication conditions) of between 100 and 250 megabytes per second (Mbps).

Both Ethernet and wireless networks require that every system on the network have a unique physical address. The physical address has several synonyms: Ethernet address, hardware address, or media access control (MAC) address. Each computer system uses a network interface control subsystem (NICS) to connect to the network. The NICS manages the network communications for the computer, and it is the computer's interface to the network to allow communication with other networked systems. Each NICS has a unique MAC address. A MAC address consists of a sequence of twelve consecutive hexadecimal numbers grouped into pairs (in a format humans understand; e.g., 00:cb:e3:c2:5f:7f). The computer sees it as a 48-bit-wide pattern of zeros and ones. All devices on the network will have an NICS that connects to either the copper Ethernet cable or the wireless network NICS. Network printers, computers, smartphones, handheld computers, and other devices all have an NICS. Wireless networks use radio waves (microwaves) to communicate. The frequency is approximately 2.5 GHz, the same frequency used by cell phones and microwave ovens. This is why cell phones can disrupt wireless networks or vice versa, or microwave ovens disrupt cellular and wireless communications.

Local Area Network

The smallest collection of networked computers sharing the same range of Internet Protocol (IP) addresses is called a **local area network** (LAN). ISO IP stands for International Standards Organization Internet Protocol. One can think of a LAN as being a collection of computers on a network no farther than a "stone's-throw" away from any other computer on the same network (all are within 300 feet of the central network hub or switch). Computers networked together in a house, a building, or buildings in very close proximity can form a LAN. A typical IP address consists of 4 bytes or 32 bits (i.e., Internet Protocol version 4 [IPv4]). IPv4 is being superseded by IPv6, which uses 128 bits for Internet addressing (4×10^9 vs 3.4×10^{38} addresses).

Components of a Network and Networking

The communication protocol, or standard, governs the sharing of the network physical medium between communicating computers so that no one computer manages to take control of the network unless the protocol allows this action. The **communication protocol** or **standard** can be thought of as a set of rules that each networked device or computer follows so that data can be communicated between systems without error or communication-sharing conflicts. Network connectivity and control hardware provide the physical connectivity and utilize network control logic to enforce sharing of the network medium. The NICS for each computer is designed to the appropriate specification described in the section Computer Networks.

The network control logic uses time intervals determined by the clock to share the physical network medium between other computers on the network in well-defined and equal time chunks. The network interface hardware has a high-speed clock that slices seconds into millions, billions, or hundreds of billions of equal time intervals, depending on the speed capabilities of the network. A clock speed of 100 MHz translates into a maximum network speed of 100 Mbps. A network clock speed of 10 GHz translates into a maximum network speed of 10 Gbps. Each computer has a set amount of time to send and receive data, as defined by the control logic, and can do so only when another computer is not using the network. Network speed can be measured in bits per second ranging from millions of bits (Mbps) or billions (Bbps) of bits per second of data transferred from one computer to another, depending on the logic coupled with the clock's speed.

One other important aspect in terms of the network control logic concerns the ability of the network to detect collisions of data: That is, the receiving computer did not detect the data sent to it or a transmission error occurred. Error correction methodology is part of the communication standard. If collisions occur when a computer attempts to use the network, then the data must be retransmitted. The error detection and correction logic is based on the standard and defines the retransmission of data.

Computer Security and Practices: Basis for Safe and Secure Computing

Computer security compromise can occur through malicious software (malware) executing on a computer or through outright theft of a computer. There are a number of vectors for compromise, such as malware payloads in e-mail attachments, attacks by another compromised system, hackers actively probing a system to discover a "hole" in the system to exploit, and infected software on a USB flash memory key or other digital media, which can release a virus or other malware upon insertion in the computer. Malware includes computer viruses, worms, and Trojan horses.

The weakest link in computer security originates with the user, owing to careless and risky security practices, which range from using weak passwords, not updating or patching the computer system, not running an antivirus program, or not preventing computer theft. Providing training for users in computer security reduces computer security risks substantially and is cost-effective.

Measures and Practices to Protect Computers and Data

A number of necessary and powerful measures can be used to protect a computer and the data it stores. These measures can be physical as well as electronic. The measures will enable the user to readily recover from data loss as well as protect the computer system from being compromised (hacked). Learning how to protect a computer system also provides knowledge of how to protect one's electronic identity. This knowledge will help the user to be more vigilant and prevent computer security compromise at home and at work.

Use of Physical Security
Physical security can be as simple as keeping a computer locked in a room when the user is not present or, when taking a laptop on trips, using an impact-resistant case or pack. Physical security can also be accomplished by locking the computer to the desk via a cable and lock.

Use of Antivirus Software
Modern up-to-date antivirus software protects a computer against malware attacks from the thousands of computer viruses, worms, and Trojan horses. Malware contains specific code fragments known as signatures. Antivirus software scans computer files for these signatures. The virus signatures (generally known as virus definitions) must be updated frequently— sometimes daily—because new and dangerous viruses are released almost daily. Updates can be done automatically by enabling the auto-protection functionality, scanning all file types, and running scans regularly. It is also important that e-mail be scanned. When a virus signature is detected, the

virus checker can do several things: delete, clean, or sequester the file in a quarantined and safe area on the disk, and then notify the user requesting further action.

Additional anti-malware scanners and "cleaners" are available. For example, spyware and adware removal tools can be beneficial. The mechanism for spreading spyware differs from that for malware. Users install spyware without realizing it. Some spyware spreads like a Trojan horse, and other spyware is spread by social engineering in spam e-mail or other means. Spyware can log keystrokes or spy on what Web sites are visited. Spyware is designed to send personal information (e.g., user name and passwords to e-mail or other accounts) to remote sites where such information can be exploited. Adware is more of a nuisance because a system can be bombarded by unsolicited Internet-based advertisements. Adware can hide malware attacks. Caution is warranted when surfing the Internet, especially with regard to which links are followed, and when opening e-mail attachments. Other practices include visit only trusted Web sites; make sure Internet connections are secure when dealing with personal health information, private information, and/or confidential information; and so on. The On Guard Online Web site (www.onguardonline.gov/ topics/ computer-security.aspx), maintained by the federal government, is an excellent site to learn more about measures to prevent the consequences of malware and rogue Web sites.

Some of the signs that a computer system has been infected by malware include frequent and/or unusual system errors, slower system start up, slower shut down, application misbehave or lockup (including the operating system), slow response to keyboard commands, frequent crashes and/or restarts, or inaccessibility of important system resources.

Many types of malware can be removed only if the system hard disk(s) and all data and program files are deleted (by writing 0's or 1's to all permanent memory locations), and then reinstalling the operating system, programs, and user data and files. This is a lengthy process and one runs the risk of losing important data and functionality. The user is advised to know when this is necessary and/or seek advice from a computer professional knowledgeable in such matters. For example, if the anti-virus checker detects a virus, find out how to clean the system for the virus by visiting the Web site of the antivirus software manufacturer or by taking the computer to a professional. Alternatively, one can use a search engine and query the World Wide Web for advice, making sure to visit only legitimate Web sites.

Prompt Installation of System and Software Patches

All software, including the operating system and application software (e.g., word processing or e-mail programs, computerized provider order entry) has imperfect programming code. All software has flaws, weaknesses, errors, or bugs that can be exploited by specialized malware code or hackers targeting systems with software flaws. Companies or organizations that produce operating systems (Microsoft, Apple, and Unix/Linux) regularly release system patches that close the software access routes for malware exploits rooted in the "buggy" code. Operating systems and application software are actively and frequently targeted and exploited. Trojan horses, for example, often spread to other systems because the operating systems have not been updated with the newest system patches or have weak antivirus protection. Security patches should be installed as soon as possible. Enabling the automatic updating feature for the operating system and application software (including the antivirus software) can harden the computer system against new viruses and attack vectors. Using an antivirus checker without promptly installing system and program patches is insufficient. A compromised system is "paralyzed" by malware infection and can greatly hamper pharmacy functions that rely on the computer and other systems, thereby affecting efforts to bring about a better patient outcome.

Enabling of Computer System Firewall

It is important to enable the personal computer system firewall to control unwarranted network traffic to and from a computer even if there is a network firewall for the network. The system firewall prevents unauthorized access into and out of a personal computer. The personal computer firewall is based in software and can be configured via rules chosen by the user to block unwarranted access to the user's electronic identity (in the form of passwords, banking account number, or personal health information) or egress of this information to a crime syndicate's hacking and identity theft system.

Administration Practices for a Secure Computer System

Computer operating systems are no longer as open as they once were by default. Modern systems employ role-based access (administrator, standard user, guest, etc.); user account authentication for log-in (user name with password); firewalls; controlled file access (including execution, read, write privileges), which are based on file ownership or group membership.

Modern operating systems allow creation of more than one user account on a computer. The system can be made more secure by disabling the guest account and creating users with standard accounts instead of administrator accounts. In effect, the standard user account has "training wheels" to prevent the unwary user from making system-wide mistakes (e.g., access to operating system files and accidental deletion). A standard user account also has fewer privileges to create, write, and install programs, which also helps to block would-be attacks from infecting the system if these accounts are used. However, there should be at least one administrator account to manage the system and its users.

Use of Strong Passwords

Authenticating user accounts with weak passwords contributes to users being the weakest link in computer security. Strong passwords should use eight or more characters and consist of upper/lower case letters, one or more digits, and special characters (punctuation, parentheses, brackets, braces, etc.). Other types of weak passwords are those made up of words found in dictionaries of any type (either foreign or domestic), noted or published phrases, published passwords, proper names, or quotes. Such weak password types are prone to successful dictionary attacks. Random character patterns are harder to crack or guess. Passwords are as important as the elements that make up the user's electronic personal identity. If a hacker can guess or methodologically determine a user's password, then that person's electronic and personal identity will very likely be stolen or compromised. This could also apply to health information data for which the user is a steward. Legal consequences could be significant.

Conclusion

Today the plethora of computing resources is more than just pervasive in modern health care. These information technology resources are essential. Without these resources, health care and pharmacy care cannot be provided at the highest standards of practice. Substantial aspects and activities of clinical significance cannot be accomplished or would be compromised without the use of computing resources in the modern health care world. These resources include heart pace makers, magnetic resonance imaging, computed tomography scanning, or simple X-ray imaging, as well as laboratory analyses, kidney dialysis, automated dispensing cabinets, pharmacy information management systems, computerized provider order entry, electronic prescribing, and the electronic health record.

Because these tools so often lie at the core of performing modern standards of practice, as well as automating the pharmacy and other critical and routine services, the efforts of a single person are multiplied in using these systems. Connecting to information resources far from the practice site provides quick and visible access to pharmacy knowledge at a time of need to guide the pharmacist in providing patient care. Computer systems provide quick or remote access to a wealth of meaningfully appropriate pharmacy knowledge such as standards of pharmacy care and practice, the newest information on drug-drug interactions, the newest prices for medications, and new medication warnings. In the past, printed publications provided this information, requiring the pharmacist to use one or more publications and to look up and record the information. Often the information in some publications was out of date, if not dangerous. Computerized resources enable and support the workforce in pharmacy and health care to provide a wider and more in-depth range of services in a safe and secure physical and electronic environment. Using such systems lowers risks to the patient and the pharmacist's employer. Computer systems are interfaces to high standards of care and practice; these systems enable pharmacists to offer a wider and deeper set of services to a greater number of people and organizations in a timelier, meaningful, integrated, and interoperable health care environment. Pharmacists will have a greater measure of assurance that what they do will provide a better outcome for patients. This also reduces clinical or pharmacy care liabilities substantially, giving peace of mind to those who provide patient care and the patient. The abilities and skills of a pharmacist are multiplied with the use of computer and network systems to fill and dispense prescriptions safely and more efficiently, and to manage inventory. The pharmacy work environment will offer more interesting and far-reaching challenges because of computers and networks and how they are evolving to answer the needs of health care.

Acknowledgment

The author wishes to express his appreciation for comments and suggestions from James Frost, MBA, PhD, Assistant Research Professor, Informatics Research Institute, College of Business, Idaho State University, Pocatello, Idaho.

1. What operating system(s) does your home, work, or laptop computer use (Linux, Apple MacOS X, MS WindowsXP/Vista/7)? Have you updated the operating system lately? Can you set up updates to be automatically downloaded to your operating system? US-Cert alerts people to current cyber security threats through a number of means, including e-mail (www.us-cert.gov/ cas/signup.html). Use this link to sign up for these alerts to help lower the risks of compromise on your system(s).

   Other URLs important for securing your operating system include:
   - www.cert.org/homeusers/HomeComputerSecurity.
   - www.microsoft.com/windows/downloads/windowsupdate/ default.mspx.
   - en.wikipedia.org/wiki/Windows_Update.
   - www.cert.org/.

2. On your home network, what type of encryption do you use for your wireless network? There are several: none, WEP, WPA, and WPA2, among others. If you are not using some type of authentication to allow a user on your network at home and no encryption to protect wireless network communications, what dangers are posed to your electronic identity? Which protocol best mitigates the risk of wireless network compromise? Does your equipment allow it?

   Suggested further readings on the Internet about wireless security include:
   - www.wi-fi.org/discover_and_learn.php.
   - www.microsoft.com/windowsxp/using/networking/ security/wireless.mspx.
   - en.wikipedia.org/wiki/Wireless_LAN_security.
   - en.wikipedia.org/wiki/Wireless_security.
   - www.onguardonline.gov/topics/computer-security.aspx.

3. One of the most important connectors for external storage and other peripherals for your computer is the USB. How fast can the data be read from and written to a USB memory device (e.g., personal digital assistant, USB memory key, or external hard disk)? What determines the read and write speeds? You will notice that other peripherals also

connect to the USB. What are these devices? Would you say that USB is a hardware interface standard, a software communication standard, or a networking standard? Explain your answers.

4. Why do you think there is a personal computer market for Linux, WindowsXP/Vista/7, and Apple MacOS X operating systems? How do you determine the version of the operating system on a personal computer? Why is the version important? What would be the consequences if all systems used the same operating system in terms of system security, system integration, system inter-communication and networking, software compatibility, system interoperability, economic impact, health care and administration, training, and business operations and efficiency? What would be the possible consequences and impact on national cyber security, not just health care cyber security, if only one operating system was the standard? Are there advantages in using different operating systems?

References

1. Intel Cooporation. Moore's law 40th anniversary press kit. 2005. Available at: http://www.intel.com/pressroom/kits/events/moores_law_40th. Accessed November 5, 2009.
2. Wikipedia. IPO model. Available at: http://en.wikipedia.org/wiki/IPO_Model. Accessed November 4, 2009.
3. Wasson S. Intel's Core i7 processors. Nehalem arrives with a splash. November 3, 2008. Available at: http://techreport.com/articles.x/15818. Accessed November 4, 2009.
4. Wikipedia. Central processing unit. Available at: http://en.wikipedia.org/wiki/Cpu. Accessed November 4, 2009.
5. Nvidia. Tesla GPU computing solutions for data centers [Tesla preconfigured clusters]. Available at: http://www.nvidia.com/object/preconfigured_clusters.html. Accessed November 5, 2009.
6. Wikipedia. Arithmetic logic unit. Available at: http://en.wikipedia.org/wiki/Arithmetic_logic_unit. Accessed November 4, 2009.
7. Wikipedia. Avogadro constant. Available at: http://en.wikipedia.org/wiki/Avogadro_constant. Accessed November 7, 2009.
8. WikiAnswers. What is the molar mass of glucose? Available at: http://wiki.answers.com/Q/What_is_the_molar_mass_of_glucose. Accessed November 3, 2009.
9. Wikipedia. FLOPS. Available at: http://en.wikipedia.org/wiki/FLOPS. Accessed November 5, 2009.
10. Wikipedia. Floating point. Available at: http://en.wikipedia.org/wiki/Floating_point. Accessed November 2, 2009.
11. Wikipedia. Cache. Available at: http://en.wikipedia.org/wiki/cache. Accessed November 6, 2009.

12. Wikipedia. CPU cache. Available at: http://en.wikipedia.org/wiki/Cpu_cache. Accessed November 8, 2009.
13. Wikipedia. DDR SDRAM. Available at: http://en.wikipedia.org/wiki/DDR_SDRAM. Accessed November 4, 2009.
14. Wikipedia. Dynamic random access memory. Available at: http://en.wikipedia.org/wiki/Dynamic_random_access_memory. Accessed November 7, 2009.
15. Wikipedia. Random-access memory. Available at: http://en.wikipedia.org/wiki/RAM. Accessed November 7, 2009.
16. Wikipedia. DDR3 SDRAM. Available at: http://en.wikipedia.org/wiki/DDR3_SDRAM. Accessed November 4, 2009.
17. Wikipedia. BIOS. Available at: http://en.wikipedia.org/wiki/BIOS. Accessed November 2, 2009.

Essentials of Telecommunication to Support Health Care Delivery

Brent I. Fox

OBJECTIVES

1. Distinguish between telecommunication and data communication.
2. Define common telecommunication terms.
3. Describe the core components and function of a telecommunication system.
4. Describe the characteristics on which telecommunication media are evaluated.
5. Describe the pros and cons of common telecommunication media.
6. Describe common health care applications of telecommunication.

The term *telecommunication* is derived from the Greek word *tele* (which means distant) and *communication*. **Telecommunication,** then, is electronic communication over distance. It is easy to see that our lives—

professional and personal—are permeated with telecommunications. The most obvious example of the role of telecommunication in today's society is arguably the telephone. Today's landline telephone is a descendant of the first electronic device for telecommunication: the telegraph (invented in 1837). The original telephone—patented in 1876—rapidly grew in popularity because it used analog technology. The analog nature of the first telephone allowed anyone to use it without assistance. In comparison, telegraphs are based on digital technology and require specialized skills to operate. Of course, the other driving factor behind telephone adoption was its ability to carry voice, which the telegraph was unable to do.[1]

As the telegraph was usurped by the early telephone, today's cell phone is steadily replacing the traditional landline phone as the preferred method of communication. Although the average consumer did not own a cell phone 20 years ago, it is commonplace today for teenagers (and even younger children) to have their own cell phone. Whereas the original telephone provided the ability to carry voice over distance—making it preferable over the telegraph—today's cell phone provides features that landline phones do not. Portability is one of those key features driving cell phone adoption. Consumers also value the ability to access the Internet from cell phones. An interesting fact is that cell phone-based text messaging has replaced cell phone voice calls in popularity in the United States (Table 5–1).[2]

Telecommunications also supports pharmacists' activities to optimize medication therapy. Many chapters in this book describe medication

TABLE 5-1

Text Messaging Surpasses Voice Calls

Period	Average Monthly Calls	Average Monthly Texts
2006, Q1	198	65
2006, Q3	221	85
2007, Q1	208	129
2007, Q3	226	193
2008, Q1	207	288
2008, Q2	204	357

Q = quarter.
Source: Reference 2.

management tools whose foundations are built on data communication, which is a unique subset of telecommunications. As the phrase indicates, **data communication** is the electronic management and transmission of data. Pharmacists are found throughout the medication use process, with various levels and points of interaction with medications, other providers, patient-specific data (e.g., laboratory results), referential information, and the patient's medical chart. Many of these interactions involve the use of electronic systems that supply, manage, transmit, and store data—the essence of data communication. This chapter addresses the foundations of telecommunications that support these activities, and concludes with a general description of some examples of telecommunications and data communication in pharmacy. Other chapters focus exclusively on the application of telecommunication and data communication to support health care.

Telecommunication Terminology

Two important telecommunication terms were introduced above: *analog* and *digital*. Analog devices, such as the telephone, record sound as oscillating waves with varying amplitude and frequency. Digital devices record sound as a series of discrete pulses, often represented by the numbers 0 (off) and 1 (on). This is a binary messaging system that computers are able to interpret, whereas computers cannot typically interpret analog sound waves. **Modulation** is the process of converting a digital sound wave into analog form. **Demodulation** is the reverse: converting an analog signal into digital.[3] In their personal and professional lives, most individuals are likely familiar with modems (*modulator/demodulator*). These devices convert digital signals to analog form so they can be sent over existing telephone lines, which are analog. On the receiving end of the line, the modem demodulates the signal from analog to digital for interpretation by a computer. In community pharmacies, modems have been extensively used to communicate prescription data to insurance companies for claims processing.

Other commonly encountered telecommunication terms include *synchronous, asynchronous*, and *noise*. **Synchronous** describes two-way communication that occurs in real time (simultaneously). Examples include the telephone, instant messaging, and text messages. **Asynchronous communication** does not occur in real time; the message is sent and received at a later time. E-mail and postal mail are obvious examples of asynchronous communication. **Noise** (also known as interference) is any unwanted signal introduced into a communication system. High signal-to-noise ratios are desired in communication systems because they indicate that the signal is stronger than any noise in the system. Noise can be introduced at virtually any point in a telecommunication system.

Components of Telecommunication Systems

To this point, several characteristics and terms related to communication systems have been addressed. This section fully defines what actually comprises these systems. A **system** can be defined as an independent but interrelated group of parts working toward a common goal. Like other systems, telecommunication systems can be very complex, but at a minimum, all telecommunication systems are composed of a group of core components. These components include the signal, source, encoder, transmitter, receiver, medium, decoder, and destination. The type and purpose of the system often dictate the ultimate configuration of the components. Each of these components is briefly defined below (Figure 5–1).

FIGURE 5–1

A basic data communications system. The signal travels from left to right through a channel on the medium.

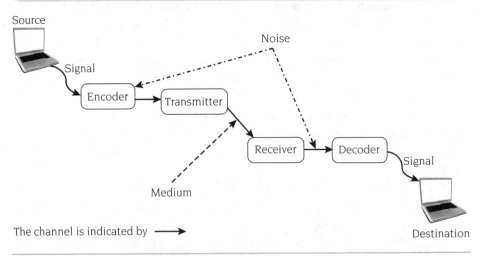

Source

Noise

Signal

Encoder → Transmitter

Receiver → Decoder

Signal

Medium

The channel is indicated by ⟶

Destination

Image source: stock.xchng vi. Stock photo: laptop. Available at: http://www.sxc.hu/photo/802342. Accessed November 10, 2009. (Image is not copyrighted.)

- **Signal:** The message being sent in a telecommunication system is called a signal.
- **Source:** In data communication, the source, or origin, of data signals is most frequently some type of computing system.
- **Encoder:** In data communication, modems function as encoders; they modify the original signal into a form suitable for transmission. In a conversation between two people, the signal originates as an idea in one person's brain and is encoded into audible sounds by that person's mouth.
- **Transmitter:** Transmitters send the encoded signal over the medium.
- **Channel:** The channel is the path of communication between the source and the destination.
- **Medium:** The medium carries the communication signal. In data communication, there are various types of media, which are discussed in the next section. In face-to-face human conversation, air serves as the medium.
- **Receiver:** The receiver accepts the encoded message from the transmitter and passes it along to the decoder.
- **Decoder:** In data communication, modems function as decoders; they convert the received, transmitted signal into the appropriate form for receipt (which is usually the original form). In a conversation between two people, the transmitted signal is decoded by the recipient's ear.
- **Destination:** In spoken communication, the destination is a person. Computing systems are usually the destination in a data communication system.

Within hospital settings, information systems personnel will manage and support telecommunication system components. Pharmacists and pharmacy staff will directly interact with the source and destination computers. In a community pharmacy, pharmacy staff may play a greater role in management of telecommunication system components. In both settings (and in personal life), it is important to understand the actual media through which messages are transmitted.

Telecommunication Media

Anything that can carry an electronic signal from its source to a destination is a **telecommunication medium.** Telecommunication channels comprise the path through which an electronic message travels (on a medium).

Telecommunication media are classified into two categories: cable and broadcast. **Cable media** include twisted-pair, coaxial cable, and fiber-optic cable. **Broadcast media** include infrared, radio, microwave, cellular, and satellite. Cable media rely on physical cables, whereas broadcast media use the air for message transmission. Advantages and disadvantages exist for both types of media. Ultimately, telecommunication media are evaluated (and eventually implemented) on the basis of the needs of the communication system and the characteristics of the media, especially for the subset of data communications. Media evaluation characteristics include cost, bandwidth, resistance to interference (noise), attenuation, security, and ease of installation.

Media Considerations

The cost of a telecommunication medium includes more than the initial purchase price. Purchase price does play an important role in selecting a medium, but the long-term cost of maintenance is an equally—if not more important—consideration. Maintenance costs include activities such as examining the media for damages, repairing damages when they occur, and testing for and counteracting signal degradation (a decrease in quality) in the media. **Longevity** (or operating life) of the medium also impacts maintenance costs. A medium with a lower purchase price and a shorter longevity may ultimately cost more than a medium with a higher purchase price and longer longevity owing to a need for frequent replacement. Decision makers are challenged with balancing initial costs and maintenance costs.

Anyone dealing with telecommunications is likely to encounter the term *bandwidth* on a frequent basis. **Bandwidth** is a measure of the ability to carry increasing data (bits) over time (a second). Internet Service Providers such as your local cable or telephone company usually describe the speed of their residential and commercial Internet connections in terms of megabits per second (Mbps). This number reflects the number of one million bits transmitted per second over the network. This is a measure of the medium's bandwidth, which is its capacity to transmit electrical signals. Bandwidth is also expressed in Kbps (thousand bits per second) and bps (bits per second). A higher bandwidth medium carries more data in the same amount of time than a lower bandwidth medium. Obviously, in pharmacy and any other health care field, greater bandwidth provides the ability to send more information and is a desirable feature.

Noise was discussed previously as a feature of data communication channels. Noise is effectively a property of telecommunication media in that media have varying abilities to resist the introduction of noise into the system. Insulation and twisting of wires are two ways to decrease noise in a system.[3] Although noise introduced into a telephone call is bothersome and distracting, the introduction of noise into a channel that is transmitting health care data can potentially lead to interruption in data transmission or, worse, errors in the data. Therefore, the sensitivity and critical nature of data to be transmitted often play a role in selection of the appropriate transmission medium.

Defined as weakening of an electrical signal over time or distance, **attenuation** is a factor that must be overcome in all telecommunication systems.[3] As a signal attenuates, receivers have trouble separating the original signal from noise that is inherent in the system. Repeaters (also called amplifiers) are frequently used in scenarios in which signal attenuation is a problem. As the word indicates, a **repeater** simply receives the signal and resends it at a stronger power.

Chapter 26 is devoted to the topics of security and privacy. The current chapter will broadly address the importance of maintaining secure telecommunication channels to protect the privacy of the information traveling on them. In the context of telecommunications, **security** is the condition of being free from unwanted or unauthorized access. **Privacy** reflects an individual's ability to control how and what personal information is shared with others.

Most modern societies are comfortable with online banking and the convenience it provides. But, individuals may be less comfortable with their personal health information, including prescription medication history, being electronically available—to authorized providers—from any Internet-connected computer in the world. (Chapter 8 describes current efforts to make this a reality in the United States.) Within the realm of health care data communication, providers are increasingly turning to broadcast media to support mobile providers. The range of security provided by cable and broadcast media varies considerably and is discussed later within the context of each medium. The challenge in health care is to balance security and privacy.

An extremely secure medium with high bandwidth is of little use to the health care system if installation is prohibitively difficult. Media such as twisted-pair copper wire are readily available and very easy to physically manipulate during installation. Fiber-optic cable, on the other hand, is costly, making it more difficult to acquire. Additionally, it is difficult to physically manipulate fiber-optic cable for installation owing to its fragile nature.

The final decision within a health system regarding the choice of telecommunication system media is usually made by a committee, which will determine the telecommunication needs for pharmacists and other clinicians, and then recommend a preferred system based on the factors discussed previously. The owner or an employee in an independent community pharmacy setting could easily be charged with making this decision. In any pharmacy setting, the goal is to select the medium that provides a secure communication channel with sufficient bandwidth for current and future needs while balancing cost and time (for installation and maintenance) with functionality.

Cable Media

Cable and broadcast media are commonly found in devices used in professional and personal settings. Two types of cable media are most likely to be easily recognized: twisted-pair and coaxial. Twisted-pair cable is composed of two insulated wires, usually made of copper, that are twisted together. The wire is twisted to reduce noise in the wires making up the pair, as well as to reduce noise emitted by the pair to neighboring electronic components. Twisted-pair wire can be shielded or unshielded. Shielded twisted-pair wire contains one or more pairs of twisted-pair cable surrounded by an additional layer of insulation, providing further protection against noise. Although unshielded twisted-pair wire lacks this additional layer of insulation, it is frequently used in computer networks and is commonly known as "Cat 5" in this type of implementation.

Despite the use of insulation and twisting, twisted-pair wire is very susceptible to interference. This medium also has considerably lower bandwidth than other types of media, limiting its ability to carry large amounts of data. From a health care perspective, twisted-pair wire is susceptible to unauthorized access ("eavesdropping"), creating a potential insecure environment for the transmission of data. Twisted-pair wire is most commonly found in telephone lines.

Coaxial cable is composed of an inner conductor wire that is surrounded by insulation. The insulation is surrounded by a secondary conductor that acts as a shield and, in turn, is surrounded by conductive insulation, called the "jacket."[5] The physical design gives coaxial cable better resistance to noise, compared with twisted-pair wire, but also makes coaxial cable less flexible and more difficult to work with. Like twisted-pair wire, coaxial cable is susceptible to unauthorized access. Because coaxial cable has significantly greater bandwidth than twisted-pair wire, coaxial cable provides much of the television service found in the United States.

Fiber-optic cable is the final medium in the cable category. It is vastly superior to twisted-pair and coaxial (and many of the broadcast media) in many key characteristics. Fiber-optic cable uses thin strands of glass or high-quality plastic tubing to transmit signals as light waves. These fibers are coated with cladding that functions like a mirror to reflect signals back into the fiber. This results in very little attenuation, even over great distances. An outer jacket surrounds the cladding. Because signals are sent as light waves, fiber-optic cables are immune to noise. Additionally, fiber-optic cable has much higher bandwidth than other cable media, making it ideal for transmitting large amounts of data. From a health care perspective, fiber-optic cable is an ideal medium for transporting private information because it is virtually impossible for an unauthorized person to access the medium without being detected.[1,3]

Fiber-optic cable does have limitations. It is an expensive medium to purchase and maintain. Although the number of cables bundled together can vary according to the specific need, the cables are generally inflexible, making installation difficult. Additionally, because glass (or plastic) fibers are used, it is very difficult to repair the fiber if it is accidentally cut. Figure 5–2 depicts the three types of cable media.

Broadcast Media

Air is actually the medium through which the broadcast media transmit signals. Figure 5–3 shows the relationship between various broadcast media. Like fiber-optic cables, **infrared communication** uses light waves to transfer data. Infrared is the communication medium used in television remotes and to connect computer peripherals such as printers. Infrared has a short range, usually less than a few meters. Among the broadcast media, infrared has a low bandwidth. Because infrared capabilities come standard on many devices, it is inexpensive and easy to install. Infrared is considered an insecure medium.

Radio communication uses radio waves as the medium to transport data. The familiar "WiFi" networks found in coffee shops, airports, offices, homes, and health care facilities use this type of communication. From its use in these settings, the advantages of radio communication are readily

FIGURE 5–2

Twisted-pair (unshielded), coaxial, and fiber-optic cable.

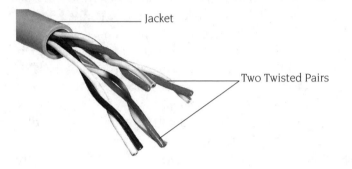

Jacket

Two Twisted Pairs

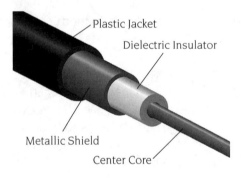

Plastic Jacket

Dielectric Insulator

Metallic Shield

Center Core

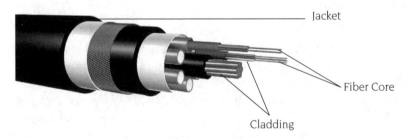

Jacket

Fiber Core

Cladding

Image sources: Wikipedia. Twisted pair. Available at: http://en.wikipedia.org/wiki/Twisted_pair; Wikipedia. Coaxial cable. Available at: http://en.wikipedia.org/wiki/Coaxial_cable; Wikipedia. Optical fiber. Available at: http://en.wikipedia.org/wiki/Fiber_optic. All images accessed November 10, 2009. (Images are not copyrighted.)

FIGURE 5-3

The electromagnetic spectrum depicting the relationship between broadcast media.

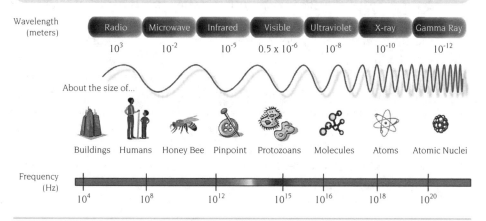

Source: GholamHosseinPour A. The electromagnetic spectrum. Available at: http://mc2.gulf-pixels. com/wp-content/uploads/2009/07/Electromagnetic-Spectrum2.jpg. Accessed August 3, 2009. (Used with the permission of Ali GholamHosseinPour.)

apparent. It provides a relatively high bandwidth signal that easily passes between walls in a building, is easy to set up and configure, and requires minimal running of cables. Radio communication does suffer from interference, and although varying levels of security are available, it is not as secure as fiber-optic cable.[3] Several applications of radio communication in health care are discussed later.

Microwave communication uses antennae that transmit high bandwidth signals between stations usually no more than 30 miles apart. Microwave transmission is "**line of sight,**" meaning that an unobstructed view is required between stations, making this medium susceptible to disruption by weather. The 30-mile limitation is a result of the curvature of the earth. For distances greater than 30 miles, multiple stations are used to receive and then transmit the signal to the next station. Because of its high bandwidth and relative ease of setting up stations, microwave communication is a viable option to transmit large amounts of data over distance when it would be prohibitively expensive to lay cable. However, microwave transmission lacks the security found in fiber-optic cable, requiring the use of encryption when sending protected health information.[3]

This chapter began with a discussion of voice communications over traditional telephone and cellular phones. **Cellular communication** works by organizing geographic regions into defined areas that are covered by a specific cellular tower. As a cellular device travels between the geographic zones serviced by individual cell towers, the transmission is passed between the appropriate towers. This process occurs for both voice and data communications. The most obvious advantage of cellular communication is the broad coverage areas, virtually coast to coast. Yet, the lack of 100% coverage of every square mile in the United States is a tangible limitation of cellular communication. This limitation will continue to exist until cellular coverage extends into rural areas, which often have insufficient coverage.

Cellular communication is a very competitive market, and companies are continually improving bandwidth and available services. The evolution of cellular service is described in terms of "generations" (G), with greater bandwidth and more services as you move from 1G (first-generation) to 4G (fourth-generation). In practical terms, today's cellular service provides both voice and data communication capabilities in a mobile environment, although bandwidth is less than that of radio communication. Encryption is necessary for protection of private health information, and wide variation exists in the fee structures for data transmission among cellular companies.

Satellite communication provides the broadest geographic coverage for telecommunications. In fact, three **geosynchronous** (i.e., orbiting in the same direction and speed as the earth) satellites located 22,300 miles above the earth provide coverage of the entire planet. Like infrared and microwave, satellite communication is line of sight, which means that it is susceptible to disruption by weather. As a means to support voice communication, satellites suffer from a small delay (~¼ second) that can disrupt conversation. Satellites are prohibitively expensive, making them affordable only by governments and large corporations. As a broadcast medium, satellite communication is susceptible to unauthorized access. Therefore, encryption is required to protect the privacy of transmitted information. Table 5–2 compares broadcast and cable media.[3,4]

Telecommunication in Health Care

As described earlier in this chapter, many other chapters in this book describe medication management applications that are built on telecommunication. This chapter will highlight a few common examples of telecommunication in health care. The applications of telecommunication (voice and data) in health care extend over a broad range, from answering a patient's

TABLE 5-2

A Comparison of Cable and Broadcast Media*

Medium	Cost	Security	Installation	Interference	Bandwidth
Cable					
Twisted-pair	$	Poor	Easy	Very susceptible	300 bps–10 Mbps
Coaxial	$$	Poor	Somewhat difficult	Susceptible	56 Kbps–200 Mbps
Fiber-optic	$$$	Excellent	Very difficult	Not susceptible	500 Kbps–25 Tbps
Broadcast					
Infrared	$	Poor[†]	Easy, very short range	Line of sight	115 Kbps
Radio	$$	Several protocols	Easy	Passes through walls	11–100 Mbps
Microwave	$$$	Poor[†]	Easy, short range	Line of sight, weather	256 Kbps–100 Mbps
Cellular	$$	Poor[†]	Infrastructure exists	Coverage area issues	1 G (voice only) 2 G = <20 Kbps 2.5 G = 30–90 Kbps 3 G = 144 Kbps–3 Mbps 4 G = 2–5 Mbps
Satellite	$$$$$	Poor[†]	Very complex	Line of sight, weather	256 Kbps–100 Mbps

Tbps = trillion bits per second.
*Comparisons are relative within media categories.
†Without encryption.
Source: References 3 and 4.

question about his or her most recent refill over the phone to the use of wireless communication to remotely monitor the impact of a medication on a patient's condition. An obvious example of data communication occurs in pharmacies when the pharmacy communicates with its drug wholesaler to place and receive updates on orders for stock medications. This communication occurs between a computer at the pharmacy and a computer at the wholesaler, usually utilizing a cable medium to transport the signal.

Pharmacies also utilize data communication to process third-party payment and clinical screening for prescription medications, with the local pharmacy's computer communicating with potentially multiple computers owned by the patient's insurer. This communication can often occur over hundreds, even thousands, of miles, utilizing multiple communication media, even encrypted signals sent via satellite. An even simpler telecommunication example is the use of **interactive voice response** (IVR) systems that allow patients to use their telephone, keypad, and voice to communicate with the pharmacy's computer system to request refills, determine the status of prescriptions being filled, leave messages for the pharmacy staff, and a host of other activities.

As for hospital clinics and community pharmacy settings, electronic prescriptions are an important example of data communication (see Chapter 10). The United States is making significant strides to replace paper-based prescribing with electronically generated prescriptions that are transmitted over telecommunication media from the prescriber's location to the pharmacy of the patient's choosing. Currently, many of these prescriptions originate in clinics associated with hospitals and health systems. A variety of media may be used, but regardless of the medium, security is a primary concern.

Security is also a primary concern given the increasing trend toward wireless access by providers to patients' health care information. This access is occurring both within the four walls of the health system/pharmacy building and on the go as pharmacists and other health care professionals seek information about their patients wherever they are and whenever they need it. Access could be in the form of a pharmacist using a home computer—connected to a wireless (radio) network—to remotely enter the pharmacy computer system to obtain information to help answer a question for a patient. Or, a prescriber may use a smart phone (3G cellular) to access the latest laboratory results for a patient. In both cases, data communication supports health care delivery, and secure transmission of data is critical.

Within hospital settings, data communication is currently being used to assist in the location of devices, such as pumps that deliver intravenous medications. Pumps are fitted with a transmitter that communicates with a wireless network within the facility, identifying the location of the pump. **Smart pump** is the term used to describe these pumps when they contain drug libraries and dosing parameters for commonly used medications. In an ideal setting, these pumps would communicate wirelessly with the pharmacy computer system, which would contain the most current dosing parameters for the patient's intravenous medications. However, in many implementations, smart pumps are not wirelessly connected to the pharmacy computer system and require manual entry by nursing staff.

It is difficult to discuss telecommunications without discussing "telehealth" (see Chapter 25). **Telehealth** has been defined as "the use of electronic information and telecommunications technologies to support long-distance clinical health care, patient and professional health-related education, public health and health administration."[6] **Telepharmacy** is used to indicate the subset of telehealth activities focused on medication management. As indicated by the definition, telehealth is truly a diverse field focused on education, patient care, and administration. A few examples of telehealth will be mentioned here.

Early telehealth initiatives focused on addressing the need to deliver care and education to rural locations where patients lacked access to providers and where local providers required consultation with distant specialists for their expertise. These initiatives frequently used audio and videoconference capabilities (delivered over various media) to address the specific health care need. Some of the earliest efforts involved the National Aeronautics and Space Administration, the U.S. military, and the Nebraska Medical Center.[7] Today, telehealth activities still focus on providing necessary services to underserved populations and locations.[8]

Current telehealth initiatives are also being implemented to provide pharmacy services in hospitals after regular business hours and on holidays and weekends. Several models exist for this type of telepharmacy activity.[9,10] The common feature is that the hospital partners with a service provider who identifies qualified pharmacists who can remotely enter and/or review prescription orders. They usually work from home or a centralized location. Often, these pharmacists are located in different states than the hospital. The service provider ensures that appropriate privacy and security features are in place to protect patients' information.

One telehealth area poised for significant growth is the wireless monitoring of patients. In the current health care model, patients visit their physicians periodically at best. Various laboratory tests and vital signs are recorded during these visits, providing a snapshot picture of how the patient is doing. Patients on medication therapy see their pharmacists once a month or once every 3 months. Unfortunately during these interactions, very little quantitative data are provided to help the pharmacist assess the patient. A better alternative is to capture—on a daily basis when appropriate—the data during the patient's life between visits with health care providers. This longitudinal data record can then be provided to the appropriate provider at the appropriate time (even in real time) to provide a more complete picture of the patient. The expanding capabilities of cellular communication are anticipated to be the medium through which these data are captured and delivered to providers.

Conclusion

This chapter introduced the technology that supports transmission of voice and data over distance. Many of the technologies discussed in this chapter provide the infrastructure for technologies addressed in other chapters of this book. The U.S. health care system is transitioning from a focus on acute care to an emphasis on the management of chronic conditions. This shift will require the capture and transmission of data generated in the patient's daily life. Secure, efficient, and timely data communication will be critical to the success of this shift. Telecommunications will be the foundation on which these data are communicated across the health care system.

LEARNING ACTIVITIES

1. Go to the CNET Web site (reviews.cnet.com/internet-speed-test), and determine the download speed at your home and pharmacy.
2. Determine the local providers for business and residential Internet service. What transmission media do they use? What speeds do they provide? Do the advertised speeds match the speed you determined in #1?
3. Identify the data communication needs at the pharmacy where you work. What information is transmitted electronically? Who receives the information? What type of security is in place?

References

1. Carr HC, Snyder CA. *The Management of Telecommunications: Business Solutions to Business Problems.* Boston, MA: Irwin McGraw-Hill; 1997:36–42.
2. Nielsenwire. In US, SMS text messaging tops mobile phone calling. Available at: http://blog.nielsen.com/nielsenwire/online_mobile/in-us-text-messaging-tops-mobile-phone-calling. Accessed July 24, 2009.

3. Turban E, Rainer RK, Potter RE. *Introduction to Information Technology*. 2nd ed. Hoboken, NJ: John Wiley & Sons, Inc.; 2003:166–77.
4. CNET. CNET's quick guide. Cellular technology: a brief history. Available at: http://reviews.cnet.com/4520-11288_7-5664933-2.html?tag=rb_content;rb_mtx. Accessed August 8, 2009.
5. Stair RM, Reynolds GW. *Principles of Information Systems: A Managerial Approach*. 5th ed. Boston, MA: Course Technology; 2001:210–20.
6. U.S. Department of Health and Human Services, Health Resources and Services Administration. What is telehealth. Available at: http://www.hrsa.gov/telehealth. Accessed August 7, 2009.
7. Brown N. Telemedicine and telehealth articles. A brief history of telemedicine. Available at: http://tie.telemed.org/articles/article.asp?path=articles&article=tmhistory_ nb_tie95.xml. May 30, 1995. Accessed August 7, 2009.
8. ASHP Foundation. Award for excellence in medication-use safety. 2006: Alaska Native Medical Center. Available at: http://www.ashpfoundation.org/MainMenuCategories/AboutUs/Newsletter/ImpactApril2009/2006.aspx. Accessed August 7, 2009.
9. Keeys CA, Dandurand K, Harris J, et al. Providing nighttime pharmaceutical services through telepharmacy. *Am J Health Syst Pharm*. 2002;59(8):716–21.
10. Stratton TP, Worley MW, Schmidt M, Dudzik M. Implementing after-hours pharmacy coverage for critical access hospitals in northeast Minnesota. *Am J Health Syst Pharm*. 2008;65(18):1727–34.

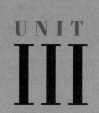
Health Care Data Management and Exchange

CHAPTER 6. Data Management in Pharmacy and Health Care

CHAPTER 7. Health Care Data Communication Standards

CHAPTER 8. The Big Picture: Health Information Exchange, Interoperability, and the U.S. Federal Government

UNIT COMPETENCIES

- Discuss the benefits and limitations of systematically processing data, information, and knowledge in health care.
- Discuss the impact of data quality on health outcomes.
- Discuss legal and ethical issues pertaining to health information.
- Discuss standards for interoperability related to medications, diagnoses, communication, and electronic data interchange.
- Describe the role of information systems in health care management.

UNIT DESCRIPTION

The ability to efficiently and accurately exchange health care data is the core of pharmacy informatics. Moreover, the ability to exchange data in a meaningful manner is even more important. Chapters in this unit address the technical aspects of health care data storage and management. Additional topics include the standards that define health care data exchange and the national movement toward developing a mechanism for meaningful exchange of health care data among all providers.

Data Management in Pharmacy and Health Care

Brent I. Fox

OBJECTIVES

1. Distinguish between core concepts related to data.
2. Describe the importance of management of data and information in pharmacy and health care.
3. Define bits, bytes, fields, records, files, and tables as they relate to databases.
4. Distinguish between the three types of database models.
5. Describe the core components of database management systems.
6. Describe the role of data warehouses, clinical data repositories, and data mining in health care.
7. Describe the potential roles that pharmacists may play in database management.

Data to Wisdom

Is there a difference between data, information, and knowledge? What about understanding and wisdom; are they synonymous? The terms *data* and *information* are commonly used interchangeably in one's personal and professional life, but the terms do represent distinct entities. **Data** (plural of datum) are discrete facts, often taking the form of numbers, descriptions, or measurements. Data are usually recorded in a structured format. When considered alone, data have little to no meaning for the user.

Information is a collection of data that has been interpreted into a relevant form and has meaning. Through the processing of data, information provides more value to the user than the independent data elements do on their own. Information is data that have been processed through relational connections into descriptions to answer questions beginning with words such as *who*, *what*, *when*, *where*, and *how many*. Knowledge is learned, either from instruction or experience, and is "know how," or the ability to transform information into action. Understanding is a higher-level cognitive ability that allows existing knowledge to be used in the creation of new knowledge, often through experience. Wisdom is the highest level of cognition that integrates understanding, morals, values, and compassion into the ability to make meaningful decisions. If one thinks of these terms as existing on a usefulness and complexity continuum, data would be found at the lowest level, followed by information, knowledge, understanding, and wisdom at higher levels.[1,2]

As an analogy, consider a single blood pressure measurement for a patient. This measurement provides a snapshot view of the patient's blood pressure. However, a single blood pressure reading is rarely used to determine if someone is hypertensive. Instead, a health care provider relies on a series of blood pressure readings to determine a chronological trend for the patient. In assessing someone's blood pressure, the provider would also like to know the person's family and social history, and any other environmental factors that could be contributing to the condition. All of these discrete data elements may not provide much value independently. When considered and interpreted collectively, however, these data elements serve as knowledge about the patient's blood pressure.

Continuing the blood pressure example, several pieces, or sets, of information were determined to be useful in ascertaining the person's blood pressure control. This information provides a "picture" of the patient's condition. Pharmacists receive formal education and training in college, possibly in a residency or fellowship program, and additional on-the-job training. Through attendance at professional meetings and completion of live and self-study continuing education programs, pharmacists gain more education about hypertension. For example, they learn about the impact of diet, exercise, and genetics on blood pressure. Understanding allows pharmacists to take patient-specific information, combine it with their education and experiences to identify patterns and determine what is "going on." Wisdom allows a pharmacist to then apply understanding of the patient's information, along with compassion and values, to make the necessary decisions to develop the patient's treatment.

It should be clear that data, information, and knowledge are critical to the ability to maximize medication-related outcomes. Computer systems are extremely efficient at managing data and information, whereas higher-order abilities like understanding and wisdom are characteristics of people. This chapter focuses on the management of data as it relates to pharmacy and health care.

Management of Health Care Data and Information

From a typical day in a community or an institutional pharmacy, it is readily apparent that pharmacy practice is built on the use of data. For example, consider an individual patient who takes Coumadin to prevent clotting. What would the pharmacist who is taking care of the patient like to know? At a minimum, the pharmacist would need to know the Coumadin dose and schedule, historical and recent international normalized ratio (INR) values, any changes in the patient's diet, other prescription medications the patient is taking, and the patient's level of adherence to the Coumadin regimen. Some of these data (Coumadin dose and schedule, INR values, other medications) are likely stored in computers at the patient's physician's office or in pharmacy computer systems. The patient may have to provide, from memory, information about changes and adherence to his or her diet (although some patients do use electronic adherence monitoring devices). Whether the patient is taking any over-the-counter (OTC) medications is also important. However, the pharmacist may not learn about these medications without specifically asking the patient. Patients often do not think of OTC products as medications; therefore, they will not be recorded in the pharmacy's or physician's records.

Now consider that a pharmacy practice realistically involves hundreds, possibly thousands of patients, and that each patient is taking more than a single prescription medication. And, consider that a pharmacist needs to know varying amounts of patient-specific medication, disease, and treatment data to optimize medication-related outcomes. Imagine that all of the needed data are stored and managed in a paper environment; each pharmacy, hospital, physician office, and insurance provider locally stores information about the patient in paper files. If this scenario is true, it quickly becomes a frightening reality. Data exchange in such a paper scenario is a manual process with inherent inefficiencies and opportunities for mistakes.

Although the U.S. health care system does not currently have a nationally implemented structure for electronic health records, the days of relying on paper files for data storage are quickly becoming fodder for history books. Other chapters in this book address this topic in more detail, but the current situation in the United States is a strong movement to fully electronic storage, management, and exchange of health care data and information. Fortunately, pharmacy was the first health care profession to widely adopt computer systems to support its practice. Most departments within hospitals have also adopted computer systems to store data generated and used by the departments. The groups that pay for health care services (public and private insurers) are also realizing the benefits of electronic data management. So, the country as a whole is moving in what is widely agreed upon as the appropriate direction.

Data and information must be maintained in a structured environment that provides a means to store, manipulate, and retrieve its contents to achieve the goal of fully electronic management and transmission of the contents. At the local level, within community pharmacies and hospitals, data are stored in databases. The brief example in the next section illustrates— in a simplified manner—how databases are used in pharmacy.

Databases to Support Pharmacy Practice

A pharmacist receives a new prescription for an existing patient. What data does the pharmacist need to fill the prescription? The data can be divided into three broad categories: patient, medication, and insurer (if applicable). The pharmacist's first step is to locate the patient's record within the pharmacy computer system. To confirm the identity of the patient, the pharmacist may use the patient's name, address, and date of birth. (Medical record number is often a primary method of patient identification in hospitals.) The pharmacist would also like to know the diagnosis (but a community pharmacy is unlikely to have this information), any known medication allergies, and medications the patient is currently taking.

The pharmacist needs to be able to locate the dispensable medication (i.e., the form available to be given to the patient) in the pharmacy computer system. The pharmacist also needs to be able to check the medication against the patient's allergies. Finally, the new medication should also be checked against existing medications for any potential drug-drug interactions. As medication stock runs low, the pharmacist would like to be notified automatically to order more, or simply have an order automatically placed with the wholesaler.

On the business side of the process in a community pharmacy, the pharmacist needs to link the patient to the insurance company. An electronic transaction will occur between the pharmacy and insurer in which the pharmacy submits the patient and medication information. The insurer determines the patient's coverage and checks the medication against other reimbursed medications for potential clinical and administrative problems. The pharmacy receives a message indicating reimbursement status as well as any clinical issues.

Imagine that all of the pieces of data (patient name, drug name, allergies, etc.) for this scenario are stored on paper. Before widespread use of computers, hospital pharmacists handwrote patients' medication information on 5- or 7-day records, creating a medication record for each patient. In community pharmacies, prescriptions were maintained in prescription file boxes, arranged numerically according to the order in which they were filled. Community pharmacies did not maintain actual patient records until they adopted 3 × 5 inch index cards on which the patients' medications were handwritten. In both practice environments, the pharmacist's ability to ensure appropriate medication therapy was limited because there was no structured, efficient means to gather all pertinent patient data together simultaneously for a complete assessment of the patient. A pharmacist concerned about the addition of a new medication to a patient's profile had to search through various paper-based sources to determine if the patient was allergic to the medication, for example. Pharmacists had to rely on their knowledge and information found in reference books to be able to assess appropriateness, the potential for interactions, and virtually any other therapeutic concerns. Additionally, paper-based records were accessible only to individuals located in close proximity to the records.

Databases exponentially expand pharmacists' ability to store, access, and manipulate the data with which they work. Database structure (described in the next section) provides a format for data storage that is consistent and structured. Consider that a community pharmacist receives a notification that a medication has been withdrawn from the market. To identify all patients taking the medication in a paper environment, the pharmacist would have to manually search all patients' records. In a database environment, the pharmacist can simply perform a search to locate all instances of the desired medication. Or, imagine a scenario in which a physician is creating an electronic prescription in a clinic setting. The physician needs to know the formulary status of the medication to ensure a selection that best matches the patient's financial abilities. The physician's prescribing application electronically communicates with the insurer to locate the patient and the patient's prescription plan. It would be virtually impossible to locate the patient, match the medication with the prescription plan, and examine existing medications for duplicate therapy without the use of databases.

As a final example, consider that a patient presents to his or her regular pharmacy with a prescription for Lorcet Plus. The patient is also taking Tylenol #3. Both medications contain acetaminophen, which is hepatotoxic in high doses. In a paper or unstructured electronic environment, a pharmacist or pharmacy technician may not have the necessary information to recognize this potential problem. They may have to rely solely on their memory to determine that the patient is taking Tylenol #3. Storing the patient's records in a database allows the pharmacy computer system to search specific locations for the unique code that represents the ingredient acetaminophen. The use of a code to represent a medication ingredient allows a single point of reference that can be used across any medication that contains the ingredient. It should be apparent that databases form the core of the information systems that support pharmacy practice.

Database Basics

These simple examples illustrate that databases are powerful in their ability to store large amounts of data in a manner that allows organization and retrieval of useful information. A pharmacist combines this information with his or her knowledge, understanding, and wisdom to make patient care decisions. But what actually is a database? In an electronic environment, a **bit** is the smallest amount of data a computer can process; a bit is represented by a numeric zero or one. A **byte** is made up of 8 bits, represents a single character, and can be a number, letter, or symbol. A

field is a grouping of characters into a word, small group of words, or a number. The grouping of characters in a field is done in a manner that is logical to the user. **Records** are made up of data fields that are related. A compilation of related records is called a **file.** Related files are organized in **databases.**[3]

The example in the previous section described a code to represent acetaminophen; this code is stored in a database field. Lortab and Tylenol #3 would each have an entry (in row format) in the database. Each entry would contain fields (columns) that are unique to the two medications. Each drug's entry is a record. A file would contain records for many medications. Other files would contain patient records. Database files such as these are integrated and have logical relationships that make them useful to one or more software applications. For example, the user can combine data from the drug file with data from the patient file to determine the medications that each patient is taking.

Database Models

Database models describe the logical structure (i.e., how the data are related) between the data within separate files. The physical organization describes where data are stored. There are three primary types of logical database models: hierarchical, network, and relational. **Hierarchical databases** are organized in an inverted tree manner, in which data access starts at the top and moves down "limbs" of the tree. This database model uses a parent-child relationship in which a parent record may have multiple child records, but each child record has a single parent. The hierarchical model is limited because real-world data rarely fit the parent-child relationship (known as one-to-many) structure found in hierarchical databases.[3]

The network database model is similar to the hierarchical model except that the owner-member relationship (parent-child in hierarchical model) can be many-to-many. In **network databases,** a member record is linked to an owner field, while simultaneously the member record can function as the owner for multiple other member records. This structure creates a web or net arrangement of records. The network model is a more accurate representation of real work data than the hierarchical model.[3]

Consider a simple example of a pharmacy database of patients and their physicians. In a hierarchical model, a single physician (parent) record can have multiple patient (child) records to which it links. However, in this model, a patient record can link only to a single physician. This does not represent the real world of pharmacy practice. A network model would allow multiple links between physician (owner) and patient (member) records, representing the real world in which a physician has many patients and patients have more than one physician. Although the network model is a better representation of reality, it is also extremely difficult to design and maintain as the volume of data grows. Both the hierarchical and network models require design of the database structure in advance. These models do not allow much flexibility if the original design does not fit the data to be stored.[3]

The relational database model is found widely throughout pharmacy and health care, and will be the focus of the remainder of this chapter. As the name indicates, the **relational model** uses relationships within existing, separate data sets (tables) to store, manage, and retrieve data. Within relational databases, data are stored in tables (files), in which each row is a record and each column is an attribute. The term *entity* is applied to any person, place, or thing for which data are stored. Entities are described by records. A table within a relational database is called a *relation.* For example, in a pharmacy's database, patients are entities and they are described by records. **Attributes** are characteristics of entities. In the pharmacy database example, patient attributes can include drug allergies, date of birth, address, phone number, and so on.

An important feature of databases is that they provide a mechanism for one or more applications to access, organize, and retrieve data. For this mechanism to work, each record requires an identifier field, called the **primary key.** Primary keys are established for each table and are used to uniquely identify each record in the table. Medical record number is a likely primary key in a patient table. Secondary keys can also be used to identify database records. Unlike primary keys, secondary keys are not necessarily unique to an entity. For example, birth date may be a secondary key in a patient table. When used alone to identify a specific record, birth date is not a suitable identifier because more than one record in the file can have the same date of birth. The use of two secondary keys (birth date and address) may sufficiently identify a specific record.

Relational database tables look very much like tables in spreadsheet software applications. This similarity does not indicate that spreadsheets and databases are similar in functionality and capability. In reality, databases are much more powerful and efficient than spreadsheets for storing, managing, retrieving, and updating data. Databases truly outshine spreadsheets when one or more software applications need to search large amounts of data that are (or can be) stored in multiple tables, modify the data, and update the data in batch. The database search function, called a **query,** is especially important because it allows the user to search across multiple tables and extract data that meet predefined, desired parameters. Data within a database can also be sorted and filtered. Formatted reports can also be generated from data within a database.

Database Management Systems

Microsoft Access, FileMaker Pro, Oracle, and Microsoft SQL Server are well-known software applications. These applications are frequently referred to as databases. They actually fall into a category of software known as **database management systems** (DBMS), which can serve two functions: as the interface between a database and application programs, or as the interface between a database and the user. These systems are classified according to the type of data model they support; Access (personal computers) and Oracle (server environment) are both relational DBMS (RDBMS). Regardless of the environment, RDBMS have several core components: the data definition language, the data dictionary, the data manipulation language, and the interface.

The **data definition language** (DDL) defines the data and relationships of the data elements stored in the database files/tables. It is the logical description of the physical model. Data dictionaries are built in the database development process and are critical to the construction of a high-quality health care database. Data dictionaries do not contain application data (data to be accessed by the DBMS). Instead, data dictionaries describe the data tables, including[4]:

- Table and field names
- Definitions of individual data elements (fields)
- Field type (alphanumeric, numeric, etc.)
- Appropriate values for fields (type and number of characters)
- Relationships between fields within and external to the database

Data dictionaries are important because they minimize data redundancy and inconsistency across applications by specifying, for example, a unique name to be used across all applications for a specific formulation of a medication. Data dictionaries streamline database management because programmers do not need to know where data are stored. The data dictionary describes the data attributes that allow the DBMS to access the data and return it to the application (or user) that requested it. The data dictionary is also used to manage changes to data elements across the entire database, serving as a central location for modification.[5] In the health care domain, data dictionaries are critical when combining data from separate databases.

The **data manipulation language** (DML) can be thought of as a functional component that sits on top of the DDL. The DML allows the user to access, query, update, and delete data. Databases and RDBMS do not recognize the structure of human language. Therefore, a unique language is used to perform actions on data within a database. This language is called the **Structured Query Language** (SQL) and is the standard query language in RDBMS. It provides both DDL and DML function using a series of commands such as CREATE, SELECT, UPDATE, and DELETE. As a simple, standard language for RDBMS, SQL is very powerful in that it can be used in any RDBMS, from personal computer software to mainframe usage.[5]

The interface in an RDBMS is the "front end" of the application that serves as the interaction point between the user and the data. The interface is constructed with software applications such as Java and Visual Basic. In Microsoft Access, the interface is constructed with Visual Basic for Applications (VBA). This interface allows the user to build and work with forms as well as reports.[4] An RDBMS interface is the user's view of the database.

Other Database Concepts

Databases are the core of information processing in pharmacy and health care. They support both administration and clinical decision making. Databases range in size and scope, with large databases supporting the work of multiple departments and/or pharmacies. Many other database-related topics could be discussed in this chapter, but three topics will be briefly discussed.

- **Data warehouses:** Data warehouses are large databases that are designed to support organizational decision making. These databases contain data from numerous organizational and external systems in a manner that provides drill-down functionality, allowing the user to search millions of records to identify specific instances of a medical procedure, for example.[4] Data warehouses are specifically designed to provide real-time information to support decision making.

- **Clinical data repository (CDR):** CDRs are conceptually similar to data warehouses but are distinctly different. The CDR houses clinical data from multiple information systems within the hospital, including laboratory, pharmacy, radiology, pathology, progress notes, admission/discharge/transfer dates, and discharge summaries. The goal of the CDR is to provide the health care professional with a complete, real-time view of the specific patient receiving care. The CDR is the core of hospital clinical information systems and is the foundational component of electronic medical records.[6]
- **Data mining:** Data mining is a technique used to examine large databases for underlying trends or patterns in the data. Unlike the query process commonly used to initiate a database search, data mining does not require a defined search query from the user. Data mining is currently more widely used in the business world than in health care.[4] Some health care uses of data mining that have been described include the questionable practice of mining prescription data for prescribers' patterns, examination of diagnoses to identify financial opportunities within a health system, and performance of post-marketing medication safety surveillance.[7-9] As the United States moves toward wide-scale adoption of electronic health records, data mining will increasingly be applied to identify new knowledge related to medication safety and efficacy.

Databases and the Pharmacist

Several examples of how pharmacists use databases in their daily practice environments have been described. Databases support the clinical and administrative functions performed by pharmacists. All pharmacists will likely interact with a database on some level. But, what involvement might a particular pharmacist have with databases? The answer to this question is highly dependent on the practice setting and responsibilities. All pharmacists interact with databases through their daily prescription processing and medication management activities. These databases can include patients, prescription and nonprescription medications, insurers, prescribers, front-end merchandise, large-volume parenteral solutions, and a host of other items that are used in practice. In their interactions with these databases, pharmacists often rely on the database to provide the pertinent data to support their activities, but the pharmacist does not actually interact directly with the data tables. Pharmacists do update databases, for example, by adding new patients or updating a patient's allergy profile in the pharmacy management system, which communicates with the database. This describes the interaction that most pharmacists have with databases; the database supports practice, but the pharmacist is not "hands on" with the database.

Some pharmacists, however, have a direct involvement with databases as a normal course of practice. Often found in health systems, these pharmacists focus on the oversight and maintenance of databases that serve up data to clinical and administrative information systems that support the decisions made by pharmacists, physicians, nurses, and other providers. These pharmacists' activities can include:

- Ensuring consistency of data across clinical applications (e.g., medications in pharmacy applications, prescribing applications, electronic medication administration record, etc.).
- Maintenance of medication databases provided by knowledge base vendors.
- Maintenance of pricing updates in the pharmacy information system.
- Maintenance of the hospital formulary database.
- Maintenance of alerts and other clinical decision support mechanisms.
- Construction of medication order sets and complex medication orders in prescribing applications.
- Construction of queries to retrieve desired information from one or more databases.
- Generation of reports and a host of other responsibilities.

Often the pharmacists who perform these activities have undergone additional training to prepare for these responsibilities, which are not frequently taught in Doctor of Pharmacy programs or PGY1 residencies.

Closing Comments on Databases in the Larger Scheme of Electronic Health Records

Discussion to this point has focused on databases to support the activities of pharmacists at a single location (hospital or community). Databases do play a larger role in pharmacy practice with most large chain pharmacies having a single patient database. These databases are accessible at any of the chain pharmacy's locations and are used to find any patient who had a prescription filled at any pharmacy location. This use of a patient database parallels the role that databases will play in the move toward a national network of electronic health records.

Consider that all of the patient-specific data that pharmacists and other health care professionals need to be able to make informed patient care decisions is stored in databases at thousands of hospitals, pharmacies, clinics, and other locations across the United States. Also consider that the nation's quest for an electronic health record seeks to unite these data to form a complete picture of the patient, regardless of where the patient received care and regardless of where the data are stored. It should quickly become apparent that the accuracy, accessibility, and security of the data contained in these databases are of critical importance. Additionally, the ability to efficiently and securely transfer these data between disparate databases is a key component of an electronic health record that health care professionals and patients can access. For these reasons, health care data must be defined, stored, and communicated in a standardized format.[10] Data standardization is a complex topic that is increasingly being discussed in health care circles because health care professionals recognize that standardization is required for communication among providers, and that any opportunity for misinterpretation of data is an opportunity for error. Data standardization is discussed in detail in Chapter 7.

LEARNING ACTIVITIES

1. Identify three databases that are used in your pharmacy setting. What are the major tables?
2. Take an existing spreadsheet and convert it to a database using your DBMS.
3. Develop a basic database to manage personal information such as exercise activity, your music collection, or your friends.
4. Put yourself in the shoes of a hospital pharmacist whose practice focuses on optimizing drug therapy according to patients' renal function. What data do you need to know to optimize drug therapy? What departments "own" the data? How many databases are you actually accessing to get the information you need to optimize therapy?

References

1. Ackoff R. From data to wisdom. J *Appl Syst Anal.* 1989;16:3–9.
2. Stair RM, Reynolds GW. *Principles of Information Systems: A Managerial Approach.* 5th ed. Boston, MA: Course Technology; 2001:2–7.
3. Turban E, Rainer RK, Potter RE. *Introduction to Information Technology.* 2nd ed. Hoboken, NJ: John Wiley & Sons; 2003:123–62.
4. Wager KA, Lee FW, Glaser JP. *Health Care Information Systems: A Practical Approach for Health Care Management.* 2nd ed. San Francisco, CA: Jossey-Bass; 2009:195–202.
5. Stair RM, Reynolds GW. *Principles of Information Systems: A Managerial Approach.* 5th ed. Boston, MA: Course Technology; 2001:168–209.
6. Sittig DF, Pappas J, Rubalcaba P. Building and using a clinical data repository. February 5, 1999. Available at: http://www.informatics-review.com/thoughts/ cdr.html. Accessed September 21, 2009.
7. Vivian JC. Pharmacists beware: data mining unlawful. June 18, 2009. Available at:http://www.uspharmacist.com/content/d/pharmacy_law/c/13856/. Accessed September 21, 2009.
8. Silver M, Sakata T, Su H-C, et al. Case study: how to apply data mining techniques in a healthcare data warehouse. J *Healthcare Inform Manag.* 2001;15(2):155–64.
9. Trifiro G, Pariente A, Coloma PM, et al. Data mining on electronic health record databases for signal detection in pharmacovigilance: which events to monitor? *Pharmacoepidemiol Drug Saf.* 2009;18(12)1176–84 [Epub ahead of print].
10. AHIMA e-HIM Workgroup on EHR Data Content. Data standard time: data content standardization and the HIM role. J AHIMA. 2006;77(2):26–32.

Health Care Data Communication Standards

Joan E. Kapusnik-Uner

OBJECTIVES

1. Explain how pharmacy computer applications or systems communicate with other health care applications.
2. List two health care-related standards development organizations and a facilitator panel, and describe how their role is promoting optimal communication between computer systems.
3. Describe the differences between messaging standards, terminology standards, and functionality standards.
4. Describe the importance of agreeing upon the "language" that is spoken between systems so that optimal data capture, transfer, and reuse can occur.
5. Describe the RxNorm drug terminology and its intended use within health care applications.
6. Explain the driving forces that are leading to the adoption of RxNorm as an interoperability terminology standard.

Communication Is Everything

It has been suggested by many—and very convincingly—within the decade-old report by the Institute of Medicine (IOM) that enhanced patient safety can be achieved by improving the decentralized and fragmented nature of our health care delivery system, our so-called "nonsystem."[1] Improved patient care and a reduction in medical errors, including adverse drug events, is achievable if there are more effective health care communications, including those that can be facilitated by health care technology solutions. The medication use process provides an example in which implementing better systems and standards will yield better human performance and outcomes. The IOM report has proven to be an effective roadmap for outlining potential influences on quality improvements. The combined goal of the report's recommendations was to motivate and guide external forces to create sufficient pressure to make errors costly to health care organizations and providers so as to compel them to take action to improve safety. This could be attained with legislated or regulated standards of care, as well as by economic and other incentives.

"The problem with communication . . . is the illusion that it has been accomplished" is a quote attributed to George Bernard Shaw that seems especially relevant to our splintered health care system.[2] This is not the case with the banking system, for which new standards of communication have been created to advance the interests of consumers and financial institutions. An example of an important development in banking (possibly now taken for granted) that required new communication standards is automated teller machines (ATMs). The industry decided that ATMs could make transactions between different financial institutions, across states, and even across countries. The business incentives to make the ATMs available *anytime, anywhere* was a great motivation to create new standards that allow these communications and transactions to occur seamlessly and securely. An example is the Banking—Personal Identification Number (PIN) Management and Security standard (ISO/TR 9564-4:2004), which was created for PIN protection.

Messaging Standards

The newer health information systems (HIS) have required new developments in the transmission and messaging standards that focus on ensuring effective communication of data across applications, within and between institutions, and across geographic regions. Patients many times feel that they have been absolutely clear when communicating the drugs they have been taking and that these medications should be made known to all of their health care providers. Physicians writing discharge orders feel that they have been absolutely clear about their discharge plan medication therapies, and yet a significant communication gap exists when patients are seen in long-term care facilities, at outpatient clinic visits, or in community pharmacies.

Because effective communication, including patient care messaging sent between applications, is a cornerstone for enhanced patient safety, the detailed technical requirements for a communication standard must be derived by consensus and agreed upon between business partners (see Table 7–1 for a list of key points related to data communication). Several accredited health care standards development organizations (SDOs) exist to perform this exact task. Organizations like Health Level Seven (HL7) and the National Council on Prescription Drug Programs (NCPDP) are both actively improving standards for the newer and improved health care technology solutions (e.g., the electronic health record [EHR] and electronic prescribing [e-prescribing]).

Government-sponsored initiatives to promote EHR adoption[3] and e-prescribing services[4] also propel the standards organizations even further to reach consensus on practical and achievable standards. Many health

TABLE 7–1
Key Points Related to Data Communication Standards

1. American National Standards Institute-accredited health care standards development organizations: National Council on Prescription Drug Programs and Health Level Seven deliver messaging standards that help deliver more meaningful health care.

2. The Health Information Technology Standards Panel played a leading role in orchestrating and harmonizing various standards options to create constructs that are deemed ready for prioritized use cases.

3. Electronic health record certification is required for verifying data communications and functionality that meet the requirements for "meaningful use" under the American Recovery and Reinvestment Act of 2009, or for more advanced functionality certification by the Certification Commission for Health Information Technology.

4. Non-proprietary drug terminologies, National Drug Codes, and RxNorm are drug terminology standards or "languages" that provide semantic interoperability for medication history information.

Source: Author.

care professionals (i.e., domain experts including pharmacists) participate in these SDOs. They help ensure that pharmacy-practice-use cases (scenarios of real-world application of a particular activity involving health information systems) are accurately represented within the computer messages so that practical requirements are defined within standards. HL7 and NCPDP have technical committees or working groups (usually composed of a large percentage of volunteers) in which member participants discuss creating or modifying the electronic standards for transmission of pharmacy and medical data. This type of volunteer work is usually appreciated and sponsored by employer organizations, and also provides professional satisfaction because of the broad national impact. Pharmacists who are attracted to this type of activity are most often informaticians.

SDOs such as HL7 develop standards for many domains in medicine, including clinical (e.g., pharmacy) and administrative (e.g., insurance claims processing) that can take many forms (e.g., Extensible Markup Language [XML] clinical document structures or decision support rules syntax).[5] A "standard" generally is used to describe the ideal form that something takes, a form that can then be used as a basis of comparison or a reference point against which other things can be evaluated. The details of the standard described in legislation, regulation, or certification documents need to be very specific because the landscape of standards is populated with various *versions* of each given messaging standard (e.g., HL7 version 2.5.1 or the NCPDP SCRIPT 4.3). Different versions implemented in disparate systems that communicate with each other are not necessarily compatible. So, simply by stating that a computer system is "running HL7 messaging" is not sufficient to know whether it is compatible or able to achieve interoperability (see Chapter 8) with other systems.

As progress is made with the IOM roadmap, outcomes studies may reveal messaging standard hazards or gaps. Although it is desirable that a standard should be established, tested, and readily implementable, health care standards are in the early stages of development and they are still maturing. In the case of health care messaging standards, all interfacing systems need to deploy a given messaging standard in a consistent fashion to ensure reliable and bidirectional communications. Incentives even exist to promote system verification and certification that specified standards have been satisfactorily implemented, and that they provide a minimum level of desired functionality. More about certification will be discussed later.

Good Communication Has Special Meaning in Health Care

The Role of ANSI

The ideal landscape is to have all patient health data easily retrievable, viewable, editable, and useable by health care providers, patients, and decision support algorithms. Having ready access to essential patient data (i.e., a patient problem list, allergen list, active medication history, and recent laboratory results) that is codified but has retained its semantic meaning is essential for good communication. To ensure that good communication standards exist, a national accrediting body, the American National Standards Institute (ANSI), acts as a policy forum for the United States consensus standards and is recognized by public and private sectors.[6]

A primary goal of the American National Standards development process is to endorse standards that improve the quality of life in this country, promote U.S. business products and practices globally, and enable a public-private partnership that provides more flexibility than the government rule-making process. The wide acceptance of American National Standards by industry and the government, regardless of the standards development method used, is evidence that the ANSI process is in harmony with the needs of those who use standards. Among other things, ANSI accredits standards developers (e.g., HL7 or NCPDP) and approves standards as American National Standards when the new standards are developed in accordance with the requirements set forth in the ANSI *Procedures for the Development and Coordination of American National Standards*.[6]

ANSI believes that the approval of a document as an "American National Standard" indicates that an SDO (e.g., HL7 or NCPDP) has undertaken steps to ensure that the standard represents a consensus of involved and affected stakeholders and is thus beneficial to the public interest. However, ANSI also recognizes that no single standardization system can address all the needs. Thus, competing SDOs do exist and development, adoption, and use of health care standards can be improved by ensuring that multiple developers and stakeholders (e.g., health care providers, payers, suppliers, integrators, vendors, users, etc.) are aware of existing and ongoing health care standards development and deployment efforts. ANSI does not review or endorse the content of an American National Standard. ANSI's approval of a standard as such provides assurance that the standard was developed in compliance with all of ANSI's due process-based require-ments (i.e., openness, balance, consensus, and due process).[6]

Communication across Systems

Interfacing, *integration*, and *interoperability* are terms often used interchangeably but are better conceptualized as a progression (or refinements) in the level or depth of communication between systems. Semantic interoperability is the current goal for systems, but not long ago simple system interfaces were a challenge. Defining the scope and extent of interoperability between systems has been a major challenge, with rewards and barriers.[7] **Interface** describes two systems or applications that can operate together or perhaps even share information in a bidirectional manner.[8] In 1999, the Vocabulary Technical Committee was formed by HL7 to achieve the goals of semantic interoperability for HL7 standards version 3.0.[9] **Interoperability** in this context goes much further to define structured messages based on a com-mon reference information model. The messages are populated by codes or value sets that are constrained or restricted to those identified by the standard, thus creating a message-specific ***terminology standard*** as well. Although providing semantic interoperability is the Holy Grail, there are critics who cite problems such as insufficient terminology representations and content, on top of the lack of accessible terminology application ser-vices needed to achieve semantic interoperability (see Chapter 8).

NCPDP has had a more measured approach to its messaging standard. NCPDP is the only SDO to focus on the realm of pharmacy; its members rep-resent sectors across the entire pharmacy services industry: chain and independent pharmacies, consulting companies and pharmacists, data-base management organizations, federal and state agencies, health insur-ers, health maintenance organizations, mail service pharmacy companies, pharmaceutical manufacturers, pharmaceutical services administration organizations, prescription service organizations, pharmacy benefit man-agement companies, professional and trade associations, telecommunica-tion and systems vendors, and wholesale drug distributors. NCPDP creates and maintains standards and companion implementation guides. This SDO was named within the Health Insurance Portability and Accountability Act (HIPAA) of 1996.[10] The NCPDP Telecommunication Standard has evolved over several decades from handling off-line batch claims processing to cur-rent, real-time adjudication. Message segments are composed of manda-tory and optional data elements. The Data Element Request Form (DERF) process, which follows due process, is used by members to request standard changes.

The NCPDP SCRIPT standard was developed for e-prescribing applications that transmit prescription information electronically between prescribers, community pharmacies, and payers. The prescription content is transmitted along with some relevant medical history for new or renewal prescriptions, as well as for those that require changes or cancellation. A nonproprietary drug product code generated by manufacturers (i.e., the National Drug Code [NDC]) may be part of the transmission that identifies the dispensed medication, or part of other proprietary drug codes that have been sanctioned as part of the standard. HL7 medication order standards are implemented within HIS at health care facilities such as hospitals and clinics. There has been a concerted effort to harmonize to make these two important standards work together, such as the project that produced an NCPDP-HL7 Electronic Prescribing Coordination mapping guidance document to facilitate inpatient to outpatient information exchange.

Too Many Communication Choices Can Be an Impediment

Health care standards and technology solution requirements are both expanding and evolving at a very fast rate. Therefore, a government-sponsored national oversight panel was created to ensure harmony and consistency in the standards and requirements that are being forwarded as optimal for HIS certification, as well as for regulations and legislation. The Health Information Technology Standards Panel (HITSP) was a cooperative partnership between public and private sectors. HITSP was formed for the purpose of harmonizing and integrating the many available standards that will best suit business and clinical needs for sharing information among organizations and systems. The panel decided how to integrate and constrain selected standards to meet given use cases; it created a road map to incorporate emerging standards that fill gaps and resolves disputes by harmonizing overlapping standards. Interoperability is a special focus that influenced the standards endorsed by HITSP. The panel organized its constructs into various categories, creating a template for *functional standards*:

- Interoperability specifications: For example, IS 01 Electronic Health Record Laboratory Results Reporting, which defines specific interoperability standards to support secure access and transmission or laboratory results and interpretations.

- Capabilities: For example, CAP 117 Communicate Ambulatory and Long Term Care Prescription, which defines transmission of requests for new, changed, or refill medications, as well as dispensed status and eligibility information.
- Service collaborations: For example, SC 111 Knowledge and Vocabulary Service Collaboration, which allows retrieval of vocabulary values sets or other medical knowledge content.
- Transaction packages: For example, TP 43 HITSP Medication Orders Transaction Package used to define transactions between the prescribers and the dispenser, which utilizes two optional methods, including the NCPDP SCRIPT standard for ambulatory and long-term care and also the HL7 version 2.5 Pharmacy/Treatment Orders messages. An XML version of the standard is also supported.
- Transactions: For example, T 42 HITSP Medication Dispensing Status Transaction, which uses the NCPDP SCRIPT standard for new and refill prescriptions.
- Components: For example, the extremely important C 32 HITSP Summary Documents Using HL7 Continuity of Care Document (CCD) Component summarizes patient data that is to be exchanged, such as information related to the demographics and insurance, and health data such as diagnoses or problem list, laboratory results, and allergy/medication history.
- Technical notes: For example, TN 901 Technical Notes for Clinical Documents, which refers to the HL7 Clinical Document Architecture version 2.0 release.
- Requirements design and standard selection: For example, RD SS 144 HITSP Clinical Research Requirements, Design and Standards Selection document, which shows the exchanges of EHR data with a clinical research repository utilizing many diverse standards, including unique stakeholders such as pharmaceutical manufacturers (PhRMA).

HITSP constructs take into account available accredited standards, some of which build on each other. HITSP constructs can be visualized to be the top layer of a wedding cake. The bottom layer may be the broad continuity of care record (CCR) approved by ASTM International; the middle layer is the HL7 CCD that is a refinement of the CCR. The top layer of the wedding cake is the HITSP C32 version of CCD with select constraints such as terminologies, or even select value sets within a single terminology. For example, the CCD specifically calls out Semantic Clinical Drug (SCD) and Brand Names (BN) abstraction value sets for drugs from **RxNorm,** a clinical drug nomenclature standard produced by the National Library of Medicine. RxNorm provides standard names, strengths, and dosage forms for clinical drugs and cross-links these three identifiers, and other modifiers such as flavor, salt, or diluents, to all branded products represented by National Drug Codes. The RxNorm terminology is specifically named in various constructs for medication names and codes.

The contract between HITSP and the Department of Health and Human Services (HSS) concluded on April 30, 2010. The work performed under this contract laid the foundation for the HIT Standards Committee, which is charged with advising the federal government on the technical aspects of achieving nationwide interoperability. This committee is discussed in Chapter 8.

Demonstrating Good Communication with Certification

Because effective communication for patient care messaging sent between applications is fundamental for enhanced patient safety, electronic medical record (EMR) certification has become an essential tool. The Certification Commission for Health Information Technology (CCHIT) was formed to reduce the barriers for entry to deploy HIS. Certification guarantees the system implementation of HITSP-sanctioned messaging and terminology standards, and also tests the availability of functional standards. It is felt to be important to give *some guarantees* to health care providers and administrators who are willing to make significant financial HIS investments and changes in workflow. Certification is akin to having the good housekeeping seal of approval, with which one can anticipate quality enhancement and a perceptible return on the investment.

Certification has been voluntary; it was initially available for ambulatory EMR systems, and later for inpatient EMR systems and other specialty medical systems. Table 7–2 contains a sample of 2011 CCHIT certification criteria for inpatient EMRs.[11] Certification is now quickly moving toward mandatory status as the American Recovery and Reinvestment Act of 2009

TABLE 7-2

Examples of 2011 CCHIT EHR Certification Criteria

Category	Criteria	Year Introduced or Last Modified	2011 Certification*
Problem list	The system shall provide the ability to maintain a coded list of problems using ICD-9 (or later versions of ICD) or SNOMED.	2011	N
Allergy information	The system shall provide the ability to change/add allergies directly from the allergy list and during medication ordering.	2009	N
Allergy information	The system shall provide the ability to modify or inactivate an item on the allergy and adverse reaction list. This could include removal, marking as erroneous, or marking as inactive.	2007	P
Medication list	The system shall provide the ability to record the reason or indication for the medication when recording historical or home medications. Does not require codified data; may be unknown or free-text comments.	2009	N
Medication list	The system shall provide the ability to report on use of high-risk medications (e.g., Beers criteria).	2011	N

CCHIT = Certification Commission for Health Information Technology; EHR = electronic health record; ICD-9 = International Classification of Diseases-ninth revision; SNOMED = Systematized Nomenclature of Medicine.
*P = previous criterion; N = new for year.
Source: Adapted from Reference 11.

(ARRA) is rolled out. It is anticipated that HIS certification will align with the act's "meaningful use" criteria (see Chapter 8). At the time this chapter was written, it was not known if CCHIT or another group would perform the certification necessary to receive ARRA funds. When certified systems are deployed, there will be sufficient proof of quality enhancement capabilities for health care institutions to receive ARRA funds. Certification, however, has not been shown to guarantee that end users have optimal system usability and clinical decision support tools.[12]

Medication Terminology Standards

National Drug Code

The Food and Drug Administration (FDA) approves drug products and labeling. Manufacturers create and register drug product codes, called the National Drug Codes (NDCs), with the FDA. NDCs have been designated by many messaging standards as a valid value set. The FDA has a public NDC directory that is updated as data are available. NDCs are often incomplete and not consistently present in the other FDA sources for NDCs: for example, Drugs@FDA, which is searchable, versus a separate downloadable source. Manufacturers appear to be somewhat lax about notifying the FDA of recent changes or fixing data on incompletely registered drugs. There appears to be little incentive at present for manufacturers to ensure the completeness and correctness of their information in the NDC Directory. Although the NDC is considered a somewhat stable identifier and essential for interoperability, manufactures have been known to "reuse NDCs." Having stable identifiers is critical for usable exchange of medication history information, or for interfacing systems in the medication use process that pass codes, including bar code administration devices. Figure 7–1 is a sample NDC.

Each unique packaged product size is assigned a different 10-digit, three-segment NDC. It is unfortunate that there is embedded meaning in the number series, but this proved in the past to be very useful. The NDC will be one of the following configurations: 4-4-2; 5-3-2; or 5-4-1:

- The labeler code that is assigned by the FDA is in the first segment. A labeler is any firm, including re-packagers or re-labelers, that manufactures or distributes the drug under its firm name.
- The second segment contains the product code, which identifies a specific manufacturer's formulation of ingredients, dose form, and strength. The labeler assigns this segment code.

FIGURE 7–1

Sample entry in the National Drug Code Directory.

NDC 55154-4511-*0
AUGMENTIN TABLETS 500;125MG (CARDINAL HEALTH)

Source: Food and Drug Administration. http://www.accessdata.fda.gov/scripts/cder/ndc/default.cfm.

■ The third segment, the package code, identifies a specific package size and/or type. The labeler assigns this segment code.

An asterisk may appear in either a product code or a package code, as shown in Figure 7–1. The asterisk simply acts as a placeholder and indicates the configuration of the NDC.

Because the NDC is limited to 10 digits, a labeler with a 5-digit code must choose between a 3-digit product code and a 2-digit package code, or a 4-digit product code and a 1-digit package code. Either a 5-4-1 or a 5-3-2 configuration is used for the three segments of the NDC. Because computers do not like asterisks, NCPDP has a formatting standard to create an 11-digit NDC. Most systems pass this standardized format of the NDC, but it is in conflict with the FDA packaging. This can lead to confusion and errors when trying to "reconstitute" the NCPDP-formatted NDC back to its FDA configuration. For example, 12345-0678-09 (11 digits) could be 12345-678-09 or 12345-0678-9 depending on the firm's configuration. By storing the segments as character data and using the asterisk as a place holder, the confusion is eliminated. In the example, FDA stores the segments as 12345-*678-09 for a 5-3-2 configuration or 12345-0678-*9 for a 5-4-1 configuration.

National Library of Medicine

The National Library of Medicine (NLM) produces **RxNorm,** a standardized nomenclature meant to augment the NDCs for interoperability purposes. RxNorm is focused on "clinical drug" formulations and drug delivery devices. It is organized around a set of normalized names (brand and generic) for drugs that are prescribed to patients. In this context, a clinical drug is a pharmaceutical product given to a patient with a therapeutic or diagnostic intent. A drug delivery device is a pack (either generic or brand) that contains multiple clinical drugs and/or devices to be administered in a specified sequence. In RxNorm, each clinical drug, the so-called Semantic Clinical Drug (SCD) level name or abstraction, includes the formulation ingredients, strength amounts, and the dose form information. Although ingredient and strength have straightforward meanings, clarification of what is meant by form is needed. In RxNorm, the form is the physical form by which the drug is administered or is specified to be administered in a prescription or order (e.g., oral suspension *and not* powder for reconstitution). The FDA has in recent years submitted its NDC data set to be included with the RxNorm terminology with relationships to SCD or Semantic Branded

Drug concepts. The Centers for Medicare and Medicaid Services (CMS) has recognized the utility of the RxNorm standard and designated the RxNorm concept unique identifiers (RxCUIs) to be a part of the formulary submission for Medicare Part D sponsors in 2010.

The NLM has an even larger job relative to the RxNorm project because it maintains the entire Unified Medical Language System (UMLS). Included in UMLS is the Metathesaurus that contains several hundred medical terminologies along with derived term synonym relationships. Terms (i.e., a code's description) from the various terminologies are included and given concept unique identifiers (CUIs). When a synonym is detected among the terms, relationships are created by assignment of the same CUI. This allows knowledge base vendors who have disparate source drug vocabularies (e.g., First DataBank's NDDF Plus, RxNorm, and Multum) and who have similar ingredient descriptions, such as "fluconazole," to keep their proprietary code to perform decision support algorithms. But, the code will be linked to a single RxCUI for ingredient message transmission purposes. These semantic relationships and RxCUI assignments by the NLM within RxNorm concept tables are a very useful tool toward achieving medication interoperability within HIS.

The NLM also processes or includes within the UMLS two other important medical terminologies that will be utilized by the HITSP C32 CCD standard. The first is the LOINC (Logical Observation Identifiers Names and Codes) terminology for laboratory test results and procedures. The second is the SNOMED CT (Systematized Nomenclature of Medicine-Clinical Terms) terminology version for the problem list clinical finding (i.e., diagnoses). The latter terminology has mappings to the diagnosis billing code set known as the International Classification of Diseases-ninth revision, Clinical Modification (ICD9-CM), which is used to code and classify morbidity data from inpatient and outpatient records, physician offices, and most National Center for Health Statistics (NCHS) surveys.

Aligning the Desire for Good Communication with Incentives: A Series of Fortunate Events

The following bulleted list contains a series of disparate events or activities that are significant individually for their own unique purpose. However, the additive effects of these events are even more significant in that they are drivers that have moved pharmacy toward standardized communication of health care data. Table 7–3 provides links to many of the organizations and initiatives discussed in this chapter.

TABLE 7–3

Appropriate Online Resources for Data Communication Standards

Resource	Web Site	Description
Health Level Seven	www.hl7.org	An organization that provides a comprehensive architecture framework and related standards for the exchange, integration, sharing, and retrieval of the diverse spectrum of electronic health information that supports clinical and administrative practices.
National Council on Prescription Drug Programs	www.ncpdp.org	A nonprofit organization that creates and promotes the transfer of data related to medications, supplies, and services within the health care system through the development of standards and industry guidance.
Healthcare Information Technology Standards Panel	www.hitsp.org	An organization formed for the purpose of harmonizing and integrating the many available standards that will best suit business and clinical needs for sharing information among organizations and systems.
Certification Commission for Health Information Technology	www.cchit.org	Nonprofit organization founded relatively recently (2004) to reduce perceived barriers to implementation of health information technology by introducing a level of assurance of product quality via certification—somewhat akin to the good housekeeping seal of approval designations by the Good Housekeeping Institute.
Unified Medical Language System	www.nlm.nih.gov/research/umls/about_umls.html	A collection of "knowledge sources" including the Metathesaurus that can be implemented to facilitate the development of computer applications that behave as if they understand medical terminologies and thus can search and query across terms that are synonymous or have other relationships with each other.
National Library of Medicine RxNorm project	www.nlm.nih.gov/research/umls/rxnorm/RxNorm.pdf	RxNorm, a standardized nomenclature for clinical drugs and drug delivery devices produced by the National Library of Medicine. RxNorm's standard names for clinical drugs and drug delivery devices are connected to the varying names of drugs present in many different controlled vocabularies within the UMLS Metathesaurus, including those in

TABLE 7-3		

Appropriate Online Resources for Data Communication Standards (*Continued*)

Resource	Web Site	Description
		commercially available drug information sources. These connections are intended to facilitate interoperability among the computerized systems that record or process data dealing with clinical drugs.
Food and Drug Administration National Drug Code Directory	www.accessdata. fda.gov/scripts/ cder/ndc/ default.cfm	A unique code given to drug products that are distributed by manufacturers and their agents, such as re-labelers, so that the products can be registered and listed with FDA. The three segments of the NDC include the labeler code, the formulation code, and the trade package size information.

FDA = Food and Drug Administration; NDC = National Drug Code; UMLS = Unified Medical Language System.
Source: Author.

■ HIPAA did much to stimulate SDOs and propel government agencies into action toward the goal of enhanced health information exchange. HIPAA specifically mentions NCPDP as a standard setting organization.[10]

■ IOM lays out national goals and a strategy for making quality improvements in health care. It reports on the topic of fragmented systems, rising rates of medical errors including adverse drug events, and highlights systems solutions for which information technology can play a major role.

■ HHS creates the National Committee on Vital and Health Statistics (NCVHS) subcommittees and working groups (e.g., Computer-based Patient Record Working Group) to take testimony and make recommendations on the role of HIS in improving health care. This testimony includes drug terminology standards.[13,14]

■ NCVHS recommends that the messaging standards NCPDP and HL7, as well as UMLS, be the repository and distribution mechanism for government-sponsored terminologies (e.g., SNOMED CT, LOINC, and RxNorm). Enhancement recommendations were also made for improvements in the public availability of the NDC database and mappings to critical private sector drug databases.

- HITSP coordinates standards to be used within voluntary certification criteria for EMR systems through CCHIT. Certification will drive the market toward adoption. HITSP specifies RxNorm use with important CCD 32 construct.
- CMS promotes the adoption of RxNorm by requiring terminology identifiers (i.e., RxCUIs) to be included within formulary submissions of Medicare Part D sponsors.
- ARRA acknowledged the value of HIS certification. The law offers a multi-year series of incentive payment to providers and hospitals for demonstrating "meaningful use" of EMR technology.[15] The total amount in payments projected by the Congressional Budget Office has been reported by some to be as high as 34 to 40 billion dollars.

Conclusion

There is a lot of detail to know and understand about health care communication standards. Standards are at every level of computer programming and interfacing: Messaging, functional, and terminology standards are main categories that together will ensure the type of interoperability and success anticipated with HIS that is comparable to the successes of the ATM banking scenario. Pharmacist involvement as subject matter experts is needed to make the various standards relevant and practical for the profession to deliver best practices in pharmaceutical care.

LEARNING ACTIVITIES

1. Identify in your pharmacy setting the various systems used in the medication use process, and describe the level of interfacing or interoperability achieved between each of them.
2. Go to the FDA's NDC database Web site (www.accessdata.fda.gov/scripts/cder/ndc/default.cfm), and search for common prescription drugs, both parenteral and oral, that are on the shelf in the pharmacy to verify the NDC code and description information. Compare the codes and description information for the same medications as displayed in the pharmacy order entry system.
3. Compare your existing pharmacy system functionality with EHR certification criteria viewable online at CCHIT: www.cchit.org/certify/2011/cchit-certified-2011-inpatient-ehr.

References

1. Kohn LT, Corrigan JM, Donaldson MS, eds. *To Err Is Human: Building a Safer Health System*. Washington, DC: National Academies of Science; 2000.
2. Wisdom Quotes. The problem with communication . . . is the *illusion* that it has been accomplished. Available at: www.wisdomquotes.com/003139.html. Accessed November 12, 2009.
3. Ford EW, Menachemi N, Peterson LT, et al. Resistance is futile: but it is slowing the pace of EHR adoption nonetheless. JAMIA. 2009;16(3):274–81.
4. Halamka J, Aranow M, Ascenzo C, et al. E-Prescribing collaboration in Massachusetts: early experiences from regional prescribing projects. JAMIA. 2006;13(3):239–44.
5. HL7. HL7 standards. Available at: http://www.hl7.org/implement/standards/index.cfm. Accessed November 10, 2009.
6. ANSI. About ANSI. Available at: http://www.ansi.org/about_ansi/overview/overview.aspx?menuid=1. Accessed November 10, 2009.
7. Benge J, Beach T, Gladding C, et al. Use of electronic health record structured text and its payoffs. The approach and barriers to using structured text in EHR to document care encounters. J *Healthc Inf Manag*. 2008;22(1):14–9.
8. Tribble DA. Interfaces 101: unidirectional and bidirectional information exchange. Am J *Health Syst Pharm*. 2009;66(3):214–23.
9. Bakken S, Campbell KE, Cimino JJ, et al. Toward vocabulary domain specifications for health level 7-coded data elements. J Am Med Inform Assoc. 2000;7(4):333–42.
10. Health Insurance Portability and Accountability Act of 1996. The 104th Congress. Public Law 104-191. Available at: http://www.cms.hhs.gov/HIPAAGenInfo/Downloads/ HIPAALaw.pdf. Accessed November 12, 2009.
11. Certification Commission for Health Information Technology. CCHIT certified 2011 inpatient EHR. Available at: http://www.cchit.org/certify/2011/cchit-certified-2011-inpatient-ehr. Accessed November 12, 2009.
12. Wright A, Sittig DF, Ash JS, et al. Clinical decision support capabilities of commercially-available clinical information systems. J Am Med Inform Assoc. 2009;16(5):637–44.
13. Department of Health and Human Services, National Committee on Vital and Health Statistics, Subcommittee on Standards and Security, Work Group on Computer-Based Patient Records. Patient medial record information. October 14, 1999. Available at: http://www.ncvhs.hhs.gov/991014tr.htm. Accessed November 12, 2009.
14. Department of Health and Human Services, National Committee on Vital and Health Statistics. Meeting of Subcommittee on Standards and Security. August 17, 2004. Available at: www.ncvhs.hhs.gov/040817tr.htm. Accessed November 12, 2009.
15. American Recovery and Reinvestment Act of 2009. The 111th Congress. Public Law 111-5. Available at: http://frwebgate.access.gpo.gov/cgi-bin/getdoc.cgi?dbname=111_cong_bills&docid=f:h1enr.pdf. Accessed November 12, 2009.

The Big Picture: Health Information Exchange, Interoperability, and the U.S. Federal Government

Brent I. Fox

OBJECTIVES

1. Describe the current state of electronic sharing of health care information, both clinical and administrative.
2. Define key terms, including *health information exchange, interoperability,* and *semantic interoperability.*
3. Describe key aspects of health information exchange, including drivers, benefits, and challenges.
4. Describe the real-world benefit of semantic interoperability.
5. Describe past, current, and future interoperability efforts in the United States, including the roles of numerous public and private organizations.

6. Describe the significance of Hurricane Katrina and electronic prescribing to interoperability efforts.
7. Describe legislation related to interoperability.
8. Describe anticipated benefits of health information exchange and interoperability.

Much of this book focuses on individual information systems and technologies that are used to support pharmacy practice and patient care. A central theme found across many of the chapters is how to best manage data and information (information, hereafter in this chapter) to support pharmacists, physicians, nurses, and other providers in their quest to deliver safe and effective patient care. A long-standing obstacle to optimal use of information in health care has been an inability to share patient-specific information across episodes and locations of care. In fact, many hospitals today still build and maintain interfaces between disparate systems within the four walls of the facility. Data indicate that roughly one-third of U.S. hospitals have implemented integrated, hospital-wide information systems, meaning that the other two-thirds of hospitals must build interfaces that allow systems from different vendors to share electronic data with each other.[1] Without these interfaces, information stored in the laboratory system would not be accessible in the pharmacy system, for example.

Patient records within hospitals have traditionally been stored in paper format, making it very difficult for providers at other locations to access a complete record that describes all the care a patient has received. In the community pharmacy, computers were adopted many years ago to facilitate the reimbursement process. Pharmacy was actually the first health care profession to widely adopt computers. Today, community chain pharmacies can access centralized patient records, but pharmacies in separate chain organizations cannot exchange patient data with each other. Additionally, community pharmacies do not have access to information about care that has been provided in hospitals, clinics, or the patient's home. And, hospital pharmacies rarely have electronic access to medication information from outside the hospital (although medication reconciliation is attempting to address this limitation). The reality is that a tremendous amount of patient-specific information exists both in the community and in health care institutions that cannot be shared with others.

The inability to share this information is due to several reasons: a reliance on paper records and minimal adoption of electronic medical records (EMRs); a lack of standards to share data when it is available electronically; concerns over information privacy and security; and the lack of a nationwide network on which to share information (e.g., a system similar to the automated teller machine [ATM] network). This chapter will address several of these topics and how they are converging in an effort to create a nationwide health information network. Chapter 7 focuses on the actual standards that are used to allow electronic exchange of health care information to support patient care. Chapter 26 addresses privacy, security, and ethical issues from a global perspective.

The Importance of Health Information Exchange

Health information exchange is defined as "the electronic movement of health-related information among organizations according to nationally recognized standards."[2] The impact of health information exchange has been divided into three broad categories: efficiency, cost, and quality of care. The banking industry is a useful example when discussing efficiency. One can obtain local currency immediately from a bank anywhere in the world, as long as the ATM machine has one of the logos found on the back of the person's debit card (and the account is funded). However, if a person's prescriptions are filled by one pharmacy (chain or independent), a different chain or independent pharmacy across the street will not have access to the person's medication history. Another common scenario concerns a referral to a specialist by a primary care physician; the referred patient must complete registration and insurance paperwork at the specialist's office even though the paperwork was completed at the primary care physician's office. Other scenarios include the refusal of an insurance company to pay for a prescription because it is a legitimate duplication of therapy, and a physician waiting 2 to 3 days to receive the results of laboratory tests that were performed at a hospital just blocks from the physician's office. It is not uncommon for a pharmacy staff member to be almost constantly on the phone trying to resolve insurance coverage issues for patients. These examples of inefficiencies are commonly found in the current health care system. The reality is that this entire chapter could be devoted to a discussion of inefficiencies. The good news is that many of the inefficiencies we see in today's health care environment can be eliminated with electronic exchange of information.

Health care costs are extremely complex, and it would be misleading to suggest that costs can be explained in a few paragraphs. Many factors impact costs, including equipment, personnel, facilities, and medication acquisition fees. Electronic health information exchange is not going to impact some of these costs, such as facilities. However, health care costs are impacted by efficiency of information exchange. For example, consider that time spent looking for existing information leads to increased costs in terms of the personnel who look for the information and to delays in the provision of care. Community practice provides several examples.

Experts have indicated that 30% of prescriptions written annually require calls from community pharmacies to prescribers. With more than 3 billion prescriptions, this represents 900+ million calls annually.[3] An unknown number of calls also occur between pharmacies and insurance companies. These calls usually occur to obtain refill/renewal approvals, discuss clinical issues not known by prescribers, and address a host of eligibility and benefit issues that arise at dispensing. The time spent making and responding to these calls greatly impacts the efficiency of pharmacies and physician offices, leading to delayed care and increased administrative costs for insurance companies, pharmacies, and physician offices. Many of these issues can be addressed at the time of prescribing if prescribers have better access to the patient's clinical, eligibility, and benefit information. Electronic prescribing (Chapter 10) seeks to place critical information in prescribers' hands during prescribing, decreasing overall costs by eliminating sources of inefficiencies.

Reports also indicate problems with information access in physician offices, providing another source of increased costs related to delayed care, inefficiencies, and repeat procedures. In a report of 32 primary care clinics, the following were found[4]:

- Missing clinical information in 13% of visits
- Missing laboratory results in 6% of visits
- Missing letters or dictations in 5% of visits
- Missing history and physical examination in 4% of visits
- Missing radiology results in 4% of visits
- Missing medications in 3% of visits

In more than half (52%) of the cases, the information being sought was reported to exist outside the clinician's clinical system, which was defined as the clinician's practice and affiliated health care institutions. Missing information resulted in delays of care (25% of patients), additional laboratory testing (22%), and additional radiology imaging (11%). Forty-two percent of clinicians reported spending 1 to 4 minutes unsuccessfully searching for the information, whereas 26% reported looking 5 to 10 minutes and 10% reported looking more than 10 minutes. The results of this study of self-reported information access illustrate the need for wide-scale information access to decrease costs related to limited clinician access to patient information.

From an administrative point of view, efficiency and costs are very important because they have far reaching impact on the health care system. The argument can easily be made, however, that quality of care is even more important because it directly impacts the lives of patients. In the cited report, respondents reported that a lack of access to information was at least somewhat likely to adversely impact patients in 44% of visits.[4] Other reports have found that:

- In a single hospital setting, 29% of preventable adverse drug events were due to a lack of drug information for prescribers, and 11% of events were due to a lack of patient information.[5]
- Computerized prescribing systems (Chapter 9) could have prevented adverse drug events.[6]
- Computerized prescribing systems can increase formulary adherence and decrease excessive dosing.[7]
- EMRs (Chapter 18) with decision support (Chapters 11 and 14) can increase adherence to clinical treatment guidelines.[8]

The biomedical literature is consistent on the positive impact of timely, patient-specific information on quality of care. The volume of evidence supporting the need for information exchange is substantial.[9] For example, Medicare beneficiaries see 1.3 to 13.8 different providers each year (average 6.4 providers/year/beneficiary).[10] Yet, these providers do not see each others' records. Drawing on these and other data, the United States is strongly focused on developing a nationwide network to exchange clinical information.

Interoperability: The Concept

Up to this point, this chapter has focused on the general concept of health information exchange—the sharing of information. Digging deeper introduces the term ***interoperability,*** which is the "ability of different information technology systems and software applications to communicate, to exchange data accurately, effectively, and consistently, and to use the information that has been exchanged."[2] Interoperability, then, goes beyond information exchange because it focuses on the ability to *use* the information that is shared (John Poikonen, PharmD; September 23, 2009; written communication). **Semantic interoperability** is the "ability of two (or more) systems to exchange data on the basis of an agreed-upon vocabulary guaranteeing same interpretation (semantics) of notions for the users of the interoperating systems."[11]

Table 8–1 provides additional explanation of interoperability.[10] The table presents stepwise progression of interoperability from the lowest level (1) to the highest level (4). In level 1, information is not electronic in nature and is, accordingly, not shared via information technologies. This level is exemplified by paper- and voice-based communication, which is common in today's health care environment. Level 2 involves the use of electronic information. The information is shared via information technology on both the sending and receiving ends. Examples include e-mail and fax. At level 3, the information being shared is not only sent and received by information technology, but the information is in a structured message identifying the type of information being shared. The highest level of interoperability (level 4) is characterized by information technology systems sharing structured information according to standards that define the structure and content of the message. In the absence of the content standardization found in level 4, a "map" identifies where data ultimately reside in the receiving system. These maps require the construction of unique interfaces between applications, making interoperability very expensive and time consuming (John Poikonen, PharmD; September 23, 2009; written communication).

TABLE 8–1

The Interoperability Taxonomy

Level	Description	Examples
1	Non-electronic data	Voice and paper
2	Machine-transportable data	Fax and e-mail
3	Machine-organizable data	E-mail of structured text with non-standard information
4	Machine-interpretable data	Structured information complying with terminology standards

Source: Adapted from Reference 10.

From the definitions and Table 8–1, it should be clear that the highest level of semantic interoperability offers the greatest opportunity for improvement in the health care system. Level 4 interoperability allows information systems to use the information they receive without the need for interpretation or translation. For example, a physician's EMR application would be able to receive a patient's laboratory results from an external laboratory system and immediately use the results to prevent errors due to oral communication, prevent the ordering of redundant tests, and/or prompt or alert the physician of potential problems. Semantic interoperability (level 4) in community pharmacies could drastically reduce phone calls (saving $2.7 billion annually), support the development of complete medication lists, enable automated refill alerts, inform prescribers of the status of patients' fill histories, and facilitate the completion of insurance forms for certain medications. From a purely financial perspective, health information exchange and interoperability have been estimated to potentially save the U.S. health care system $77.8 billion annually through prevention of redundant procedures and through administrative time saved. The clinical (i.e., quality of care) benefits are believed to be even greater.[10]

Achievement of Interoperability

Given that interoperability is the goal and it can provide real benefits, readers might ask what then is being done to fully realize the benefits? Significant efforts toward health information exchange and interoperability occurred in the 1990s with initiatives called Community Health Information Networks (CHINs). These networks were usually regional in nature and were designed to connect hospitals, clinics, pharmacies, payers, laboratories, and other locations of care to share information electronically. CHINs were often funded through grants, which supported software and hardware purchases, meetings to determine CHIN governance, and other administrative activities.[12]

Ultimately, CHINs were unsuccessful for a number of reasons. Once grant funding was exhausted, CHINs were supposed to support themselves through financial investments by the participating providers, institutions, insurers, and so on. However, CHINs were frequently not able to demonstrate enough value to satisfy the participants (Dennis Tribble, PharmD; October 8, 2009; written communication). Additionally, CHINs were founded on the premise that hospitals and health systems would agree to collaborate. Yet, they were essentially competitors in the business world. Ironically, the key component of CHINs was not technical in nature: It was a history of community collaboration on health-related issues.[13]

Role of the Federal Government

Although CHINs of the 1990s were mostly unsuccessful, efforts in the new millennium—spearheaded by the U.S. government—appear to have all the necessary pieces to realize national health information exchange and interoperability. These efforts formally began January 20, 2004, when in the State of the Union Address, President George W. Bush stated, "By computerizing health records, we can avoid dangerous medical mistakes, reduce costs, and improve care. . . ." Shortly thereafter, on April 27, 2004, President Bush established the Office of the National Coordinator for Health Information Technology (ONCHIT) within the Office of the Secretary of Health and Human Services (HHS) to lead the country's efforts toward interoperable exchange of health information.[14] The two broad goals of ONC were:

1. Widespread adoption (at least half the population) of electronic health records by 2014.
2. The creation of an interoperable health information infrastructure.

Table 8–2 lists specific objectives for ONC. These objectives may seem familiar to readers. They coincide with the challenges and issues identified previously in the discussion of health information exchange.

As the first step toward achieving the objectives in Table 8–2, ONC chartered the American Health Information Community (AHIC) in July 2005 (for a duration of 2 years). Known as "The Community," AHIC was charged with recommending specific actions to ONC that would accelerate the adoption of interoperable electronic health records. AHIC was composed of 18 members (including the HHS Secretary) who represented the broad interests of health care stakeholders, including the public and private sectors as well as patients. AHIC was transitioned to a public-private organization in late 2008, the National eHealth Collaborative (NeHC).

The challenges were clear for the first national coordinator for HIT (David Brailer, MD, PhD): The health care system was fragmented, ineffi-

TABLE 8-2

Goals of the ONC and the National Health Information Network*

1. Ensure that appropriate information to guide medical decisions is available at the time and place of care.

2. Improve health care quality, reduce medical errors, and advance the delivery of appropriate, evidence-based medical care.

3. Reduce health care costs resulting from inefficiency, medical errors, inappropriate care, and incomplete information.

4. Promote a more effective marketplace, greater competition, and increased choice through the wider availability of accurate information on health care costs, quality, and outcomes.

5. Improve the coordination of care and information among hospitals, laboratories, physician offices, and other ambulatory care providers through an effective infrastructure for the secure and authorized exchange of health care information.

6. Ensure that patients' individually identifiable health information is secure and protected.

ONC = Office of the National Coordinator.
Source: Reference 14 [direct quote]*.

cient, and expensive. Under the national coordinator's and AHIC's leadership, efforts to achieve interoperable health records were divided into five key areas: standards, privacy and security, adoption of electronic records (stimulation and measurement of), and infrastructure. Several grants were awarded to numerous coalitions and groups to research and identify methods to successfully address the challenges in these five areas. Four areas are discussed here; the fifth is discussed at the end of this chapter.

Standards

In October 2005, the Health Information Technology Standards Panel (HITSP) was formed under a contract with HHS. Broadly speaking, HITSP's objective was to sort through all of the health care data standards and publish a set of nationally adoptable standards for interoperable health care data storage and communication. HITSP's specific goals were to:

- Identify, define, and resolve standards gaps and overlaps.
- Develop harmonized standards and implementation guides.
- Test implementation guides.
- Develop final versions of implementation guides based on testing results.[15]

Pharmacists jokingly remark that one great aspect of health care standards is that there are so many from which to choose. The reality is that HITSP faced a huge task of identifying competing standards and selecting the best option, determining where standards were absent and then developing suitable standards, and testing and guiding the health care vendor and provider community in implementing the final standards. Readers are encouraged to read Chapter 7 for a thorough discussion of HITSP.

Privacy and Security

The Health Insurance Portability and Accountability Act (HIPAA) of 1996 established baseline privacy and security requirements for patient health information (Chapter 26). At the state level, policies were developed that frequently required stricter requirements than those of HIPAA. Implementation of these privacy and security requirements by health care organizations and providers was further tailored to their specific needs and circumstances. This lack of uniformity creates barriers to nationwide interoperable exchange of health information.

In June 2006, the Health Information Security and Privacy Collaboration (HISPC) was formed under an HHS contract. The group was initially composed of experts in privacy and security law as well as health care management, the National Governor's Association, and about 35 state governments. HISPC was charged with assessing business practices that impacted the interoperable exchange of health information as well as any related privacy and security laws. Their specific objectives were to:

- Assess variations in organization-level business policies and state laws that affect health information exchange.
- Identify and propose practical solutions, while preserving the privacy and security requirements in applicable federal and state laws.
- Develop detailed plans to implement solutions.

Ultimately, HISPC is charged with preserving privacy and security protections in a nationwide, interoperable health information network. Much of HISPC's work was performed through subcontracts at the state and territory level to look at the challenges of sharing information across state and organizational borders.[16]

Adoption of Electronic Records

AHIC and the national coordinator for HIT articulated that a primary challenge to widespread adoption of electronic health records resided within local hospitals and physician offices. The grand vision for national health records was based on hospitals and physicians implementing EMR applications that would share information on a national scale, creating electronic health records (EHR). The reality was that hospitals and physicians have a long history of investing in technology on the basis of the promise that technology will improve efficiency and care, only to be "burned" many times when the technology does not deliver as promised. In recognition of these obstacles, the Certification Commission for Health Information Technology (CCHIT) was formed in July 2004 by the American Health Information Management Association (AHIMA), the Healthcare Information and Management Systems Society (HIMSS), and The National Alliance for Health Information Technology. In September 2005, CCHIT was awarded a 3-year contract from HHS to develop a certification process for HIT.[17]

The certification process involves three broad areas: functionality, interoperability, and security and reliability. Specific criteria were developed for each area via a consensus-based, transparent process with an open comment period. **Functionality criteria** assess an application's ability to perform certain features and functions to support clinical and administrative activities. **Interoperability criteria** assess an application's ability to exchange information using agreed-upon standards. **Security and reliability criteria** assess an application's ability to maintain the privacy of patient data and ensure robustness to prevent data loss. CCHIT certification began with ambulatory records in 2006, progressed to inpatient records in 2007, added specialty applications like emergency departments in 2008, and added health information exchanges in 2009. In October 2009, CCHIT launched preliminary certification against the American Recovery and Reinvestment Act of 2009 (discussed later in the chapter).[17]

Infrastructure

Interoperability occurs at that point where disparate systems exchange and use information. For example, true achievement of the goal occurs when a patient who lives and receives health care in Ocean Springs, Mississippi, can go to Mount Angel, Oregon, and a local provider can access the patient's complete health history. For that to happen, an infrastructure must exist to share this information. The fourth component of the ONC's efforts is the National Health Information Network (NHIN), a program established in 2004 through four contracts awarded by HHS to four consortia to establish a mechanism (technical, policy, governance, specifications, and process) for interoperable sharing of health information. At the time of this writing, prototype architectures have been developed, trial implementations have occurred, and limited production is planned.[18]

ONC Efforts: The Context

Hurricane Katrina

The ONC was established in April 2004 and AHIC was chartered in July 2005. At that time, governmental leaders and especially health care providers recognized the limitations of the current health care system's ability to efficiently and effectively use information. The general public was not fully aware of these limitations. This all changed in the weeks following August 29, 2005, when Hurricane Katrina hit coastal Alabama, Mississippi, and Louisiana. Much of the press on Katrina focused on New Orleans, where devastating floods took the lives of a reported 1800 people and caused billions of dollars in damage. Whereas long-term flooding caused the majority of the damage in New Orleans, coastal Mississippi and Alabama were impacted by the initial tidal surge and winds. In fact, many coastal cities in western Mississippi were completely destroyed.

Approximately 1.5 million people older than 16 years evacuated from these three states because of Katrina, the majority of them from the New Orleans area.[19] Many of the evacuees were displaced hundreds, even thousands, of miles from home and literally left with only the clothes on their backs. An estimated 40% of evacuees were on prescription medications prior to the storm. Anecdotal reports suggest that some evacuees could recall their medications' color and form, but very few could remember their entire medication regimen. An unknown number of evacuees needed new medications after the storm. Pharmacies, physician clinics, hospitals, and public health centers were not spared by the floodwaters. As a result, hundreds of thousands of patients' paper-based records were destroyed, and hundreds of computers housing electronic records were also destroyed. From a pharmacy perspective, the net effect was that hundreds of thousands of people evacuated to cities where no one knew their medication history. This highlighted the need for electronic records and also identified vulnerabilities in health information storage.

KatrinaHealth.org was formed in response. It provided qualified health care professionals with secure access to 90-day medication histories for individuals impacted by the storm. Hundreds of organizations (pharmacy benefit managers; pharmacies, foundations; medical software companies; and local, state, and federal agencies) pulled together to have the service up and running within 10 days after the storm. Not only did Katrina highlight limitations in health care information storage and sharing, but KatrinaHealth.org demonstrated how quickly solutions can be found when significant motivation is present.[20]

Electronic Prescribing

Electronic prescribing (e-prescribing; Chapter 10) is another contextual factor running parallel to the ONC's interoperability efforts. E-prescribing is a key to the adoption of interoperable EHRs because it is believed to be a significant enabler of safer, more efficient care.[21] The Medicare Prescription Drug, Improvement, and Modernization Act of 2003 (MMA) requires the use of certain standards when participating Medicare Part D programs use electronic prescriptions (e-prescribing). Under MMA, prescriber usage of e-prescribing is not required, but if prescriptions are transmitted electronically for Medicare patients, they must comply with standards identified by HHS.[22]

The Medicare Improvements for Patients and Providers Act of 2008 (MIPPA) furthered the push for e-prescribing by authorizing incentives (and penalties) for adoption. Specifically, prescribers who successfully e-prescribe using qualified e-prescribing systems are eligible for the incentives (and penalties) depicted in Table 8–3. The percentages depicted are based on the allowed charges for professional services under Medicare Part B.[21]

TABLE 8–3
Medicare e-Prescribing Incentive Payments

Year	Incentive for Use	Fee Reduction for Not Using
2009–2010	+2.0%	—
2011	+1.0%	—
2012	+1.0%	−1.0%
2013	+0.5%	−1.5%
2014	—	−2.0%

Source: Adapted from Reference 21.

The American Recovery and Reinvestment Act of 2009

Although the stimulus for interoperable health information exchange began under President George W. Bush, sufficient funding was never allocated to ONC to achieve the ambitious goal. In the months leading up to the presidential election of November 2008, the two primary candidates agreed on very few issues, except that health care was in trouble and that health information exchange and interoperability represented key steps to turning health care around. Around the same time, the United States was in the midst of the most significant economic downturn since the Great Depression.

One of the first and most pressing challenges in January 2009 for newly inaugurated President Barack Obama was addressing the economy. On February 17, 2009, he signed The American Recovery and Reinvestment Act of 2009 (ARRA) into law to stimulate the economy by investing billions of dollars in health care, education, energy, and other challenges facing the United States. Specifically, the Health Information Technology for Economic and Clinical Health Act (HITECH) provisions of ARRA included approximately $34 billion for HIT.[23]

Within the HITECH provisions, the ONC was codified (with $2 billion in funding for 4 years) as responsible for achieving the 2014 goal for nationwide, interoperable EHRs. The HITECH Act includes approximately $30 billion in funding for Medicare and Medicaid reimbursement incentives for health systems and physicians who meaningfully use certified EHRs, beginning in 2011. The term *meaningful use* is intended to focus on the use of health information to improve care, not simply the adoption of technology. Under HITECH, the HIT Policy Committee was created to advise ONC on the criteria for meaningful use. An iterative process was used to develop the criteria, including a public comment period. The HIT Standards Committee was also created under HITECH to advise ONC on standards, implementation specifications, and certification criteria for interoperable health information exchange. At this time, the relationships of CCHIT, NeHC, the HIT Standards Committee, and the HIT Policy Committee have not been fully defined. However, for now it appears that some of these groups will—at a minimum—work collaboratively and potentially unite. For example, the HITSP chair was selected to serve as vice chair of the HIT Standards Committee. Several leaders have suggested that NeHC is the ideal organization to serve as the HIT Policy Committee.[24,25] Regardless of what happens with individual organizations, committees, and people, the most important topic within the realm of HIT at this time is meaningful use. The ONC and the HIT standards and policy committees are the critical groups to follow as the movement toward nationwide EHRs progresses.

To What End?

Recall that the first national coordinator for HIT had five focus areas, four of which were described earlier in the chapter. The fifth area is the measurement of EMR/EHR adoption by physicians and health systems. When all of the described efforts are distilled, the bottom line is that all of the resources previously described are being expended to drive adoption and interoperable information exchange. The ONC partnered with George Washington University and Massachusetts General Hospital/Harvard Institute for Health Policy to "characterize and measure the state of EHR adoption and to determine the effectiveness of policies aimed at accelerating adoption of EHRs and interoperability."[26] Table 8–4 contains current adoption data. Clearly, much remains to be done.

What are pharmacists expected to gain from all of these efforts? This is a reasonable question given all of the time, personnel, money, and resources that are focusing on this problem. Many benefits are anticipated, some of which have been demonstrated through research:

- Improved care by basing clinical decisions on evidence-based resources.

TABLE 8–4

EMR Adoption Rates

Setting*	2006	2007	2008
Physician offices (basic)	11%	13%	17%
Physician offices (full)	3%	4%	4%
Hospitals (basic)	N/A	N/A	8%
Hospitals (full)	N/A	N/A	2%

EMR = electronic medical record.
*Basic and full indicate level of functionality, with full providing more advanced features. See reference for more information.
Source: Adapted from Reference 25.

- Improved care by fully informing health care professionals of the patient's condition.
- Improved care by better coordination among providers.
- Improved care through monitoring of patients' receipt of necessary tests, examinations, and so on.
- Decreased costs due to elimination of redundant procedures.
- Decreased costs due to efficiency gains by eliminating manual, paper-based processes.
- Improved clinical research using de-identified patient data housed in EHRs.
- Enhanced clinical surveillance by monitoring symptom outbreaks.
- Improved post-marketing surveillance of medications.
- Improved productivity by streamlining administrative tasks.

The true impact of ARRA, HITECH, and interoperable health information exchange will not be known for many years. Clearly the government has committed substantial resources in an effort to bring connectivity among all locations of care, including pharmacies. The 2014 goal is rapidly approaching, and pharmacists will know in a few years if it was too ambitious. Whether or not the goal is achieved on the desired timeline, pharmacists can expect that efforts to achieve and optimize interoperable health information exchange will continue for much of their career.

ACTIVITIES

1. Visit www.healthit.hhs.gov to determine the latest on the country's quest for interoperability.
2. Assess the current state of e-prescribing in a local community pharmacy. Are prescriptions received directly into the pharmacy computer, or are they received as a fax? Is a fax an e-prescription? What benefits exist for prescriptions received directly into the computer versus via fax?
3. Go to the URL in #1 and locate the "Meaningful Use" section. Locate the criteria and determine how many apply specifically to medications. Which criteria require information that is housed in pharmacy information systems?

References

1. Pedersen CA, Gumpper KF. ASHP national survey on informatics: assessment of the adoption and use of pharmacy informatics in U.S. hospitals—2007. Am J Health Syst Pharm. 2008;65(23):2244–64.

2. Office of the National Coordinator for Health Information Technology. The National Alliance for Health Information Technology report to the Office of the National Coordinator for Health Information Technology on defining key health information technology terms. April 28, 2008. Available at: http://healthit.hhs.gov/portal/ server.pt/gateway/PTARGS_0_10741_848133_0_ 0_18/10_2_hit_terms.pdf. Accessed April 25, 2010.

3. National Committee on Vital and Health Statistics. First set of recommendations on e-prescribing standards. September 2, 2004. Available at: http://www.ncvhs.hhs.gov/ 040902lt2.htm. Accessed October 5, 2009.

4. Smith PC, Araya-Guerra R, Bublitz C, et al. Missing clinical information during primary care visits. JAMA. 2005;293(5):565–71.

5. Leape LL, Bates DW, Cullen DJ, et al. Systems-analysis of adverse drug events. JAMA. 1995;274(1):35–43.

6. Gandhi TK, Weingart SN, Borus J, et al. Adverse drug events in ambulatory care. N Engl J Med. 2003;348(16):1556–64.

7. Teich JM, Merchia PR, Schmiz JL, et al. Effects of computerized physician order entry on prescribing practices. Arch Intern Med. 2000;160(18):2741–7.

8. Khoury AT. Support of quality and business goals by an ambulatory automated medical record system in Kaiser Permanente of Ohio. Eff Clin Pract. 1998;1(2):73–82.

9. eHealth Initiative. *Migrating toward Meaningful Use: The State of Health Information Exchange.* Washington, DC: eHealth Initiative; August 2009.

10. Walker J, Pan E, Johnston D, et al. The value of health care information exchange and interoperability. Health Affairs. January 19, 2005. Available at: http://content.healthaffairs. org/cgi/ content/abstract/hlthaff.w5.10. Accessed March 12, 2010.

11. International Society for Telemedcine and eHealth. Glossary of telemedical terms Q-Z. August 20, 2005. Available at: http://www.isft.net/cms/index.php?q_-_z. Accessed October 6, 2009.

12. Duncan K. Evolving community health information networks. Frontiers Health Serv Manag. 1995;12(1):5–41.

13. Appleby C. The trouble with CHINS (community health information networks). Hosp Health Netw. 1995;69(9):42–4.

14. Bush GW. Executive Order 13335—incentives for the use of health information technology and establishing the position of the National Health Information Technology Coordinator. April 27, 2004. Available at: http://edocket.access.gpo.gov/2004/pdf/04-10024.pdf. Accessed October 7, 2009.

15. Health Information Technology Standards Panel. Available at: http://www.hitsp.org. Accessed October 8, 2009.

16. Health Information Security & Privacy Collaboration. Available at: http://www.rti.org/ page.cfm?objectid=09E8D494-C491-42FC-BA13EAD1217245C0. Accessed March 12, 2010.

17. Certification Commission for Health Information Technology. Available at: http://www. cchit.org. Accessed October 8, 2009.

18. Nationwide Health Information Network. Available at: http://healthit.hhs.gov/portal/ server.pt?open=512&mode=2&cached=true&objID=1142. Accessed October 8, 2009.

19. Groen JA, Polivka AE. Hurricane Katrina evacuees: Who they are, where they are, and how they are faring. *Mon Labor Rev.* 2008;131(3):32–51.

20. KatrinaHealth. Available at: http://www.katrinahealth.org. Accessed October 8, 2009.

21. Health Information Technology. Electronic prescribing (e-prescribing, eRx). Available at: http://healthit.hhs.gov/portal/server.pt?open=512&objID=1220&parentname=CommunityPage &parentid=5&mode=2&in_hi_userid=10741. &cached=true. Accessed October 8, 2009.

22. Medicare Prescription Drug, Improvement, and Modernization Act of 2003. The 108th Congress. Public Law 108-173. Available at: http://frwebgate.access.gpo.gov/cgi-bin/getdoc.cgi?dbname= 108_cong_bills&docid=f:h1enr.txt.pdf. Accessed October 8, 2009.

23. The American Recovery and Reinvestment Act of 2009. The 111th Congress. Public Law 111-5. Available at: http://frwebgate.access.gpo.gov/cgi-bin/getdoc.cgi?dbname=111_cong_bills& docid=f:h1enr.pdf. Accessed October 8, 2009.

24. Health Information Technology. Meaningful use. Available at: http://healthit.hhs. gov/portal/ server.pt?open=512&objID=1325&parentname=CommunityPage&parentid= 36&mode=2&in_ hi_userid=10741&cached=true. Accessed October 8, 2009.

25. American National Standards Institute. HIT Policy and Standards Committees commence work on national health information infrastructure. May 22, 2009. Available at: http://www.ansi.org/ news_publications/news_story.aspx?admin=1&articleid=2204. Accessed October 8, 2009.

26. Health Information Technology. Health IT adoption initiative. Available at: http://healthit. hhs.gov/portal/server.pt?open=512&objID=1152&parentname=CommunityPage&parentid= 12&mode=2&in_hi_userid=10741&cached=true. Accessed October 8, 2009

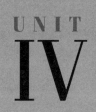

Medication Use Process I: Assessment and Ordering Interventions

UNIT COMPETENCIES

- Discuss standards for interoperability related to medications, diagnoses, communication, and electronic data interchange.
- Describe the structure and key elements of computerized provider order entry and electronic prescribing processes.
- Describe the impact of provider order entry and electronic prescribing on health care outcomes.
- Demonstrate efficient and responsible use of clinical decision support tools to solve patient-related problems.

- Discuss the development of electronic decision support tools and their strengths and limitations.
- Discuss the impact of alerts on workflow and health care outcomes.
- Identify common clinical decision support tools.

UNIT DESCRIPTION

This unit begins the series of units addressing pharmacy informatics within the context of the medication use process. Specifically, this unit includes chapters related to the "prescribing" stage of the medication use process. Topics covered include the prescribing systems used in the acute and ambulatory environments. In both settings, knowledge systems that assist prescribers in making the best prescribing decisions are critical. These knowledge systems are addressed as well.

Computerized Provider Order Entry

Margaret R. Thrower

OBJECTIVES

1. Describe the background of computerized provider order entry (CPOE).
2. Define terminology as it relates to CPOE.
3. Describe data on the impact that CPOE can have on patient safety outcomes.
4. Discuss benefits and limitations/risks associated with CPOE.
5. Provide literature to overcome barriers to adoption and implementation of CPOE.

Computerized **provider order entry** (CPOE) is an important component in health care information systems because it eliminates illegible handwriting, reduces medical errors, and can improve patient care. CPOE is a process of electronic entry of medical provider instructions for the treatment of patients (primarily hospitalized patients) under the provider's care. These orders are communicated over a computer network to the medical staff or to the departments (e.g., pharmacy, laboratory, radiology, etc.) responsible for fulfilling the order. CPOE decreases the delay in order completion, reduces errors related to handwriting or transcription, allows order entry at both the point of care and off-site, provides error checking for duplicate or incorrect doses or tests, and simplifies inventory and charging. CPOE is sometimes referred to as *computerized physician order entry* or *computerized prescriber order entry*, and these terms are often used interchangeably. However, a more accurate term is *computerized provider order entry*. For the purposes of this chapter, the abbreviation CPOE will refer to *computerized provider order entry*.

Importance and Role of CPOE

The deaths per year and many more injuries resulting from medical errors have made patient safety a top priority in U.S. health care.[1] Many medication errors—the most common cause of preventable injuries in hospitals—can be prevented by CPOE systems. These systems have been shown to positively impact patient care and to reduce the incidence of serious medication errors.[2,3] This collective evidence has prompted the LeapFrog Group, a national consortium of Fortune 500 companies, to designate CPOE deployment by hospitals as one of three patient safety goals.[4] Despite the apparent efficacy of CPOE systems, only 12% of hospitals reported using CPOE with clinical decision support systems (CDSS) in 2007.[5] This is expected to change rapidly owing to passage of the American Recovery and Reinvestment Act (ARRA), which was put in place in 2009.[6] ARRA includes a long-awaited, much-needed financial boost to the adoption of electronic medical record (EMR) systems that will incentivize organizations to implement health care information technology (HIT). The economic stimulus package has allotted $34 billion to reward Medicare and Medicaid providers who can prove they are using HIT in a meaningful way. "Meaningful use" has not been fully defined at the time of publication; however, the incentives are scheduled to take effect starting in 2011. These technologies include EMRs and CPOE with clinical decision support as well as other capabilities. (See Chapter 8 for more information on ARRA.)

Overview of CPOE Terminology

Basic CPOE terminology is necessary to understand how this technology works. The following definitions provide a basic understanding of the components of CPOE:

- **Placer:** The application or individual originating a request for the order or services.

- **Order:** A request for a service from one application to a second application. The second application may in some cases be the same; therefore, it is possible that an application is allowed to place orders with itself.
- **Placer order group:** A list of associated orders for a single patient coming from a single location.
- **Order detail segment:** One of the several segments that can carry order information. Future ancillary specific segments may be defined in subsequent releases of the system if they become necessary.
- **Filler:** An application responding to or performing a request for orders or services, or producing an observation. The filler can also originate requests for new orders or services, add additional services to existing orders, replace existing orders, put an order on hold, discontinue an order, release a held order, or cancel existing orders.

Features of CPOE Systems

The ideal features of a CPOE system are described here. Some CPOE systems may not contain all of these features.

Ordering

Provider orders are standardized across the organization, yet they may be individualized for each provider or specialty by using order sets. Orders are communicated to all departments and involve caregivers, improve response time, and decrease scheduling problems and conflicts with existing orders.

Patient-Centered Decision Support

The ordering process includes a display of the patient's medical history, current test results, and evidence-based clinical guidelines to support treatment decisions. The application often requires a medical logic module to facilitate fully integrated CDSS. For clinical decision support (CDS) to be effective, expertise must go into defining and representing medical knowledge. In addition, data that are critical for CDS, such as the patient's weight and allergy information, must be captured and made available to the CDSS. These systems must support, rather than impede, clinical workflows through prompt, available, and usable algorithms that provide clear, concise, and actionable warnings and advice. CDSS are addressed in more detail in Chapters 11 and 14.

Patient Safety Features

The CPOE system allows real-time patient identification, and displays current medications, laboratory values, radiology results, and a listing of the patient's medical conditions. Additional available information identifies drug-dosing recommendations, drug therapy duplication, adverse drug reaction reviews, drug-drug interactions, and also checks allergy, test, or treatment contraindications. Health care providers such as nurses, pharmacists, and physicians can review orders immediately for confirmation.

Interactive Human Interface

The order entry workflow corresponds to familiar "paper-based" ordering to allow efficient use by new or infrequent users. The application must be simple to use from signing in to navigating the system easily.

Regulatory Compliance and Security

Access is secure and a permanent record is created with an electronic signature. An electronic signature is any legally recognized electronic means that indicates that a person adopts the contents of an electronic message. An **electronic signature** is defined as "an electronic sound, symbol, or process, attached to or logically associated with a contract or other record and executed or adopted by a person with the intent to sign the record."[7]

Portability

The system accepts and manages orders for all departments at the point of care from any location in the health system (physician's office, hospital, or home) through a variety of devices, including wired and wireless computers, smartphones, and notebook/laptop and tablet computers.

Management

The system delivers reports online so that managers can monitor and analyze patient census as well as make changes in staffing, replace inventory, and audit utilization and productivity throughout the organization. Data collection for quality initiatives is a priority. Data are collected for training, planning, and **root cause analysis** (RCA) for patient safety events. RCA is a type of problem solving that focuses on identifying the root cause of problems or events. This practice is predicated on the belief that problems are best solved by attempting to correct or eliminate root causes, as opposed to just addressing the immediately obvious symptoms. By focusing corrective measures on the root cause, it is generally thought that the likelihood of the problem recurring will be minimized. Data from CPOE are important in the RCA process given that prevention of a recurrence usually takes multiple interventions.

Billing

Documentation is improved by linking diagnoses to orders at the time of order entry to support appropriate charges. International Classification of Diseases-ninth revision, Clinical Modification (ICD-9-CM) is a classification used in the United States to assign codes to diagnoses associated with inpatient, outpatient, and physician office utilization. The ICD-9-CM is based on the ICD-9 but provides additional morbidity detail and is updated annually. ICD-9-CM was created by the U.S. National Center for Health Statistics as an extension of the ICD-9 system so that more morbidity data could be captured and a section of procedure codes could be added.

Patient Safety Benefits of CPOE

In the past, physicians traditionally hand wrote or verbally communicated orders for patient care, which were then transcribed by various individuals (e.g., nurses, clerks, or pharmacists) before being carried out. Handwritten reports or notes, manual order entry, nonstandard abbreviations, and poor legibility lead to errors and injuries to patients, according to a 1999 Institute of Medicine (IOM) report.[1] A follow-up IOM report in 2001 advised use of electronic medication ordering, with computer- and Internet-based information systems to support clinical decisions.[8] Prescribing errors are the largest identified source of preventable hospital medical errors. A 2006 report by the IOM estimated that a hospitalized patient is exposed to a medication error each day of his or her stay.[9] CPOE with CDSS has been shown to reduce the rates of medication errors and adverse drug events. CPOE systems can provide automatic dosing alerts such as letting the user know that the dose is too high or warnings that a drug-drug interaction is likely. It is very important for pharmacists to work with the medical and nursing staffs at hospitals to improve the safety and effectiveness of medication use during implementation of CPOE systems, as well as after implementation for continuous improvement.

Limitations/Risks of CPOE

CPOE presents several possible dangers by introducing new types of errors.[10,11] Prescriber/provider and staff inexperience may cause slower entry of orders at first, may increase staff time for order entry in general, and may be slower than person-to-person communication. The importance of the interaction between HIT and workflow was highlighted in a pediatric hospital that implemented CPOE and experienced an increase in morbidity after the implementation.[12] Many believe that the increase in morbidity was not due to CPOE implementation but rather to simultaneous changes in workflow. In other settings, shortcut or default selections can override nonstandard medication regimens for elderly or underweight patients, resulting in toxic doses. Frequent alerts and warnings can interrupt workflow, causing these messages to be ignored or overridden owing to alert fatigue. CPOE and automated drug dispensing were identified as a cause of error by 84% of more than 500 health care facilities participating in a surveillance system developed by the United States Pharmacopoeia.[13] Introducing CPOE to a complex medical environment requires ongoing changes in design to cope with unique patients and care settings; close supervision of overrides caused by automatic systems; and training, testing, and re-training of all users.

Implementation of CPOE

CPOE systems can take years to install and configure. Despite sufficient evidence of the potential to reduce medication errors, adoption of this technology by doctors and hospitals in the United States has been slowed by resistance to changes in physicians' practice patterns, costs, and training time, as well as concern for system down time and compliance with future national standards. According to a study by RAND Health, the U.S. health care system could save more than $70 billion annually, reduce adverse medical events, and improve the quality of care if CPOE and other HIT were widely adopted.[14] Use of CPOE will increase as more hospitals become aware of the financial benefits of CPOE and more physicians with computer expertise enter practice. A 2004 survey by the Leapfrog Group found that 16% of U.S clinics, hospitals, and medical practices were expected to be utilizing CPOE within 2 years.[15] Several high-profile failures of CPOE implementation have occurred,[16] so a great deal of effort must be focused on change management, restriction of workflows, dealing with physician resistance to change, and creation of a collaborative environment.

An early success with CPOE was achieved by the U.S. Department of Veterans Affairs (VA) with the Veterans Health Information Systems and Technology Architecture, also known as VistA. A component of VistA, a user interface named computerized patient record system, allows health care providers to review and update a patient's record at any computer in the VA system of more than 1000 health care facilities. This interface also incorporates the ability to place orders by CPOE, including medications, special procedures, X-rays, patient care nursing orders, diets, and laboratory tests and results.[17]

One of the largest projects for a national electronic health record (EHR) is being performed by the National Health Service in England. The project reached a major milestone in February 2010, when one million EHRs were transferred via the GP2GP service of the National Programme for IT.[18]

In 2008, the New England Healthcare Institute published research showing that 1 in 10 patients admitted to a Massachusetts community hospital suffered a preventable medication error. The study argued that Massachusetts hospitals could prevent 55,000 adverse drug events per year and save $170 million annually if they fully implemented CPOE.[19]

Overcoming Barriers to Adopting and Implementing CPOE

In 2004, Poon and colleagues published a paper titled "Overcoming Barriers to Adopting and Implementing Computerized Physician Order Entry Systems in U.S. Hospitals."[20] This was an important publication at the time. The report is still relevant today because it not only highlights the barriers to adopting and implementing CPOE but also addresses how to overcome them. Senior management employees from 26 hospitals were interviewed to help identify ways to overcome these barriers. Some common themes were identified and are summarized in the following pages. The common themes centered around (1) strong hospital leadership, (2) high-quality technology, (3) a high priority on patient safety, and (4) public pressure concerning medication safety.[20]

Barrier 1: Physician and Organization Resistance

A common barrier referenced in interviews was physicians' resistance to CPOE adoption. Several common reasons for this resistance are highlighted in the article[20]:

1. Physicians perceived that paper methods were faster and more efficient, and that CPOE would have a negative impact on their workflow.
2. Although training was generally perceived as helpful, the physicians' low level of computer skills made training challenging.
3. Community hospitals did not employ many of their admitting physicians; therefore, the physicians spent little time in the hospital and were not motivated to learn to use CPOE efficiently. As a result, hospital leaders feared that these physicians would admit patients to other local hospitals that did not use CPOE.
4. Hospitals feared physicians would rebel against CPOE and possibly slow down or impede the entire CPOE implementation. The negative publicity associated with physician rebellion was a common concern for CPOE implementation and a reason for lack of commitment to adopting CPOE.
5. Institutions that were previously unsuccessful in implementing CPOE were fearful of repeated unsuccessful attempts, and the repeated attempts were difficult.

From the survey data, the authors identified four focus areas to overcome resistance. The key points of these four areas are summarized as follows[20]:

1. Strong hospital leadership:
   - In almost all the interviews, strong hospital leadership was identified as an important factor for successful implementation of CPOE.
   - Hospital leaders had to not only be committed to CPOE; they also had to actively demonstrate their belief in the bene-

fits of CPOE and to visibly support and participate in its implementation.

- In addition, hospital leaders needed to feel empowered to mandate CPOE use within their hospitals.
- Finally, hospital leaders needed to communicate a common vision to the hospital staff (this was especially important during setbacks or difficulties), including some of the following key points:
  - Highlighting how CPOE would improve patient safety, quality, and efficiency.
  - Discussing how CPOE would help strengthen the mission of the hospital and demonstrating that implementing CPOE is taking a leadership or "cutting-edge" position in the hospital market.

2. Identify and involve physician champions:
   - The key to successful implementations was physician champions. The authors commented that these physicians were generally well-respected clinicians, who could not only help select the vendor and customize the product, but could provide encouragement to users during implementation and remind users of the benefits of CPOE throughout the process.

3. Address workflow concerns:
   - Throughout the CPOE implementation process, workflow concerns needed to be appropriately addressed and users reassured, especially when set backs or difficulties arose.
   - Frustration with learning a new system was minimized by having support staff readily available and "in person" to assist the users.
   - In the survey, several responses indicated that once physicians had overcome the initial training barrier, they "wondered how they ever did it the other way."

4. Leverage "in house" expertise:
   - In the survey, the important role of the house staff in the implementation process was often discussed.
   - Those physicians that were more comfortable with information technology (IT) or that had previous experience with CPOE seemed to be more motivated to learn strategies that made them more efficient users. They also provided valuable feedback on how to improve the CPOE product and served as facilitators of CPOE adoption.

Barrier 2: High CPOE Cost and Lack of Capital

At the time the survey by Poon et al. was published (2004), the cost of CPOE ranged from $3 million to $10 million, depending on the size of the hospital and existing IT infrastructure. The authors highlighted a few key points from the survey results[20]:

- One chief information officer stated that CPOE was "the most expensive project I had ever done in my twenty-nine years of doing hospital software."
- Difficulties obtaining money to fund CPOE projects were common concerns of those institutions that had not committed to implement CPOE.
- Leaders at institutions that had already implemented CPOE expressed concern that their colleagues at other hospitals might not succeed in securing the money to implement CPOE because (1) there was a perceived absence of a strong and objective business case for CPOE and (2) the uncertainties and high costs associated with implementing CPOE made it easier for hospital leaders to focus on other competing priorities.

In addition, management employees from several institutions shared how they overcame the high cost of CPOE by focusing on the following strategies[20]:

1. Realign the hospital's priorities to focus on patient safety:
    - Respondents to the survey agreed that establishing patient safety as a critical mission of the hospital helped to justify CPOE as a mission-critical project.
    - By making patient safety the top priority, some hospitals were able to move CPOE higher on the priority list, identify funds to implement CPOE, and put other capital projects on hold.
    - One respondent in the interview, a chief financial officer, stated that "patient safety drove all of [their] decisions."
    - Reducing medical errors was an important focus for some hospital boards, which often included community leaders. In some cases, it was easier to obtain approval for the project from the board than to obtain support from hospital staff.

2. Leverage external influence:
   - Respondents to the survey noted that leveraging external resources, such as published literature to increase awareness about patient safety, helped gain support for and drive CPOE adoption.
   - In addition, medical errors and the publicity associated with them were often noted to serve as the initial and/or final motivation for CPOE adoption.
3. Measure CPOE's impact on hospital efficiency:
   - Hospitals that had successfully implemented CPOE experienced improved hospital efficiency by reducing delays in patient care through improved communication and standardization of procedures throughout the hospital or institution.
   - Collecting data early in the implementation is critical, albeit challenging, so that cost savings can be measured. To help drive the success of measuring the impact of CPOE, hospital leaders and physician champions need to take the lead in emphasizing the importance of collecting data during implementation and to establish data collection as a priority.

Many of the survey respondents commented on ways to make CPOE more affordable. These responses centered around two areas[20]:

1. Improve interoperability:
   - Systems from different companies are often unable to communicate directly with each other, and CPOE requires many interfaces with other existing systems. Therefore, hospitals generally have to decide when they implement CPOE whether to purchase it from their primary IT vendor or rebuild their IT infrastructure over time.
   - If system interoperability could be improved, the cost of CPOE implementation would decrease, allowing more hospitals to implement it.
   - The survey showed that participants differed in their opinion regarding the role of the government in improving interoperability.
   - Although some respondents believed that the government was the ideal candidate to mandate standards necessary for improvement, others maintained the opposite view.

2. Provide third-party payers with incentives for implementing CPOE:
   - Respondents to the survey pointed to the benefits of CPOE, especially the decrease in medical costs through prevention of adverse drug events. These improvements actually benefit third-party payers but the cost of implementing CPOE fell entirely on the hospitals. Some participants in the survey felt that financial incentives could help correct that problem, and that the source of these incentives could come from the government or private insurance companies in the form of grants or loans to offset the cost.

Barrier 3: Product/Company Selection

Participants in the 2004 survey conducted by Poon et al. reported that many CPOE products available at that time did not fit the needs of their hospitals, and that significant software customization was required to fit the workflow of their hospitals.[20] Significant improvements have occurred in the 6 years since this article was published; however, some key points from the survey are still relevant to selecting CPOE products/companies. Authors concluded that the product/company should be[20]:

1. Committed to the CPOE market.
2. Ready to identify hospital workflow issues and adapt products accordingly.
3. Committed to a long-term trusting relationship with the hospital because implementation can be a lengthy process.

In addition, the company should[20]:

1. Provide tools to help hospitals evaluate product functionality.
2. Provide information and references for other CPOE implementations performed by the company.
3. Provide direct comparison of the medical knowledge information supported by each product (to aid the hospital in making a product decision and to highlight the level of decision support for each product).

Another important article was published in 2007 by Kuperman and colleagues, "Medication-related Clinical Decision Support in Computerized Provider Order Entry Systems: A Review."[21] This article focused on the CDS portion of CPOE, and the authors suggest that medication-related decision support is probably best introduced into health care organizations in two stages, basic and advanced. Basic decision support includes drug-allergy checking, basic dosing guidance, formulary decision support, duplicate therapy checking, and drug-drug interaction checking. Advanced decision support includes dosing support for renal insufficiency and geriatric patients, guidance for medication-related laboratory testing, drug-pregnancy checking, and drug-disease contraindication checking.

Conclusion

CPOE with CDS can improve patient safety and lower medication-related costs. To realize these benefits, hospitals must overcome significant barriers, but CPOE can be successful if appropriately approached. Hospitals will likely adopt these technologies faster in the future because of important incentives in quality and the increased attention on medication errors and safety. In the near future, increased adoption rates of CPOE due to ARRA are likely. This act will provide incentives for hospitals to adopt more health information technology. Although currently it remains unclear how this technology will be defined, it likely will include EMR, CPOE with CDS, and other health care information technologies.

LEARNING ACTIVITIES

1. List the benefits and limitations to using CPOE. Identify what can be done to overcome the barriers to implementing CPOE.
2. Describe the ideal CPOE system to support your needs as a practitioner. How would this differ among the different health disciplines (e.g., nurses and physicians) that you work with?
3. Identify which pieces of health care technology you have in place in your organization or your place of work.

References

1. Kohn LT, Corrigan JM, Donaldson MS, eds. *To Err Is Human: Building a Safer Health System.* Washington, DC: National Academies of Science; 2000.

2. Kaushal R, Shojania KG, Bates DW. Effects of computerized physician order entry and clinical decision support systems on medication safety: a systematic review. *Arch Int Med.* 2003; 163(12):1409–16.

3. Bates DW, Leape LL, Cullen DJ, et al. Effect of computerized physician order entry and a team intervention on prevention of serious medication errors. JAMA. 1998;280(5):1311–6.

4. Leapfrog Group. 2009 select leapfrog hospital survey results: hospital quality and resource use and what hospitals are doing to improve. Available at: http://www.leapfroggroup.org. Accessed September 1, 2009.

5. Pedersen CA, Gumpper KF. ASHP national survey on informatics: assessment of the adoption and use of pharmacy informatics in U.S. hospitals—2007. *Am J Health Syst Pharm.* 2005; 65(23):2244–64.

6. The American Recovery and Reinvestment Act of 2009. The 111th Congress. Public Law 111-5. Available at: http://frwebgate.access.gpo.gov/cgi-bin/getdoc.cgi?dbname=111_cong_bills& docid=f:h1enr.pdf. Accessed April 6, 2010.

7. Electronic Signatures in Global and National Commerce Act. The 106th Congress. Public Law 106–229. Available at: http://frwebgate.access.gpo.gov/cgi-bin/getdoc.cgi?dbname=106_cong_public_laws&docid=f:publ229.106.pdf. Accessed April 6, 2010.

8. Committee on Quality of Health Care in America, Institute of Medicine. *Crossing The Quality Chasm: A New Health System for the 21st Century.* Washington, DC: National Academies of Science; 2001. Available at: http://www.nap.edu/books/0309072808/html. Accessed September 2, 2009.

9. The Institute of Medicine. *Preventing Medication Errors.* Washington, DC: The National Academies Press; 2006. Available at: http://www.nap.edu/catalog/11623.html. Accessed July 23, 2009.

10. Koppel R, Metlay JP, Cohen A, et al. Role of computerized physician order entry systems in facilitating medication errors. JAMA. 2005;293(10):1197–1203. Available at: http://jama.ama-assn.org/cgi/content/abstract/293/10/1197. Accessed August 12, 2009.

11. Lohr S. Doctors' journal says computing is no panacea. *The New York Times.* 2005. Available at: http://www.nytimes.com/2005/03/09/technology/09compute.html?ei=5089&en=402b79 2e748d99a2&ex=12 68110800&adxnnl=1&partner=rssyahoo&adxnnlx=1150474153-xVix1 BcYkvTKJpuLyHStrQ. Accessed June 23, 2009.

12. Han YY, Carcillo JA, Venkataraman ST, et al. Unexpected increased mortality after implementation of a commercially sold computerized physician order entry system. *Pediatrics.* 2005;116(6):1506–12. Available at: http://pediatrics.aappublications.org/cgi/gca?submit.x= 79&submit.y=13&submit=sendit&gca=116%2F6%2F1506. Accessed August 20, 2009.

13. Santell, JP. Computer-related errors: what every pharmacist should know. United States Pharmacopeia. 2004. Available at: http://www.usp.org/pdf/EN/patientSafety/slideShows2004-12-09.pdf. August 29, 2009.

14. RAND Healthcare. With most comprehensive hospital survey to date, consumers urged to use Leapfrog safety and quality data to make hospital choices: wide variation in use of practices to protect patients from harm Health information technology: can HIT lower costs and improve quality? Available at: http://www.rand.org/pubs/research_briefs/RB9136/index1.html. Accessed on September 23, 2009.

15. The Leapfrog Group. [news release]. 2004. Available at: http://www.leapfroggroup.org/media/file/Leapfrog-Survey_Release-11-16-04.pdf. Accessed August 23, 2009.

16. Connolly C. Cedars-Sinai doctors cling to pen and paper. *The Washington Post.* 2005. Available at: http://www.washingtonpost.com/wp-dyn/articles/A52384-2005Mar20.html. Accessed September 19, 2009.

17. U.S. Department of Veteran Affairs. VistA monograph. July 2008. Available at: http://www4.va.gov/vista_monograph. Accessed June 7, 2010.

18. National Health Service. GP2GP hits one million mark. Available at: http://www.connecting forhealth.nhs.uk/newsroom/news-stories/gp2gpmillion. Accessed March 13, 2010.

19. New England Healthcare Institute. Groundbreaking study details how to reduce medication errors at Massachusetts community hospitals [news release]. Available at: http://www.nehi.net/news/press_releases/16/groundbreaking_study_details_how_to_reduce_medication_errors_at_massachusetts_community_hospitals. Accessed April 6, 2010.

20. Poon EG, Blumenthal D, Jaggi T, et al. Overcoming barriers to adopting and implementing computerized physician order entry systems in US hospitals. *Health Aff.* 2004;23(4):184–90.

21. Kuperman GJ, Bobb A, Payne TH, et al. Medication-related clinical decision support in computerized provider order entry systems: a review. *J Am Med Inform Assoc.* 2007;14(1):29–40.

Electronic Prescribing

Kevin Marvin

OBJECTIVES

1. Define electronic prescribing (e-prescribing).
2. Understand common terminology used with e-prescribing.
3. Describe the components of an e-prescribing system.
4. Understand how and why the government has impacted the use of e-prescribing.
5. Describe how e-prescribing impacts the workflow of prescribers, pharmacists, and patients.
6. Identify important standards used in e-prescribing.
7. Describe what needs exist for future enhancements and functionality of e-prescribing.

The delivery of health care in ambulatory settings is increasing. In 2006, Americans made 902 million physician office visits, or 3.066 visits per patient. Prescriptions were ordered at 70.6% of these visits.[1] Medication prescribing is the most common therapeutic intervention in ambulatory practice settings. Studies have found that 75% of the visits to general practitioners or internists resulted in the continuation or initiation of a medication.[2] Prescription volumes are large and are increasing.

More than 3.5 billion prescriptions are written annually in the United States, and the yearly volumes are increasing.[3]

The increasing volume of prescriptions and the increased costs of prescription drugs have increased the attention to controlling these costs. Errors in prescribing and the management of prescription drug therapy are also costly. Studies estimate that indecipherable or unclear prescriptions result in more than 150 million calls yearly from pharmacists to physicians for clarification.[4] Others estimate the number of prescription-related telephone calls annually at 900 million. Practices report almost 30% of prescriptions require pharmacy callbacks.[5,6] Requesting and receiving approval for refills alone, estimated at nearly 500 million per year, add to the telephone and fax burdens.[7] These interventions by pharmacists often direct prescribers to less costly therapies and prevent medication errors. It is believed that electronic prescribing (e-prescribing) systems will significantly impact prescribers to select less costly therapy and prevent errors before a prescription is sent to the pharmacy. One study estimates possible savings from e-prescribing of $27 billion per year in the United States.[8]

e-Prescribing applications and the processes they support are very prescriber centric. e-Prescribing systems are primarily designed to increase the efficiency of the prescriber in entering new prescriptions and renewing existing prescriptions. In the past, software companies struggled to develop systems that were financially viable. Physicians were generally hesitant to use the new functionality, even if provided at no cost to them. It was difficult to secure funding for e-prescribing from other sources such as insurance companies, pharmacy benefit companies, and others because cost savings and enhanced outcomes had not been well studied.

As part of the Medicare Prescription Drug, Improvement, and Modernization Act of 2003, the Centers for Medicare and Medicaid Services (CMS), under the direction of the Department of Health and Human Services, proposed the adoption of standards for e-prescribing. It was recognized that through the standardization and the use of e-prescribing, there would be better control of costs and medication use under this new program. As a result, CMS has defined and implemented standards and incentives to accelerate the implementation of e-prescribing. This expansion and evolution of e-prescribing will have significant impacts on the practice of pharmacy. e-Prescribing provides the tools and defines how prescribers and pharmacists work together in their support of patients and their therapies. This chapter will describe the components of an e-prescribing system, the standards that enable e-prescribing to exist, workflow components impacted by e-prescribing, and future directions for e-prescribing.

Definitions of e-Prescribing Components

e-Prescribing is commonly defined as "ambulatory computerized provider order entry." Many definitions exist for e-prescribing and each is based on the needs of the definer. The U.S. government's definition according to CMS is "the transmission, using electronic media, of prescription or prescription-related information, between a prescriber, dispenser, PBM, or health plan, either directly or through an intermediary, including an e-prescribing network."[9] This definition specifies only the electronic nature and who is involved in the process. It does not clearly specify who enters the prescription, nor does it state how the electronic data are handled once it reaches the pharmacy. A more complete definition of e-prescribing would be a prescription that is entered directly into an electronic format by a prescriber, and that is verified and processed in electronic format by all required parties, ultimately resulting in a labeled medication product, supportive documentation, and an updated sharable patient electronic medication profile.

It is generally assumed that to fully realize the advantages of e-prescribing, the data should be entered by the prescribing practitioner, and the electronic data should not be manually transcribed into the receiving systems. Few e-prescribing installations currently realize this goal for reasons described later in this chapter. According to CMS, a prescription is not an electronic prescription unless it is transmitted electronically in a standard format. Printed paper prescriptions and electronic faxes are not considered to be electronic prescriptions according to the CMS rule.

Dispenser is a term that CMS uses to specify the pharmacy and pharmacist.[9] It is assumed that the appropriate verifications and patient education are provided by the dispenser in addition to the dispensing of prescription medications.

Surescripts is a company that provides connectivity between the prescriber, the insurance providers, and the pharmacies. This connectivity includes patient insurance verification, insurance plan formulary access, insurance medication profile data, dispensing data, prescription refill requests, and electronic prescriptions. Multiple standards exist to support this connectivity.

The **National Council for Prescription Drug Programs** (NCPDP) is an organization that creates and promotes standards for the transfer of data to and from the pharmacy service sector of the health care industry. NCPDP is American National Standards Institute-accredited and has more than 1450 members representing all areas of pharmacy services.[10] NCPDP has developed standards for provider identification and telecommunication standards for pharmacy claims. It has also developed **SCRIPT,** which consists of multiple standards that support prescription communication and processing.

A **prescriber** is the health practitioner who has the legal authority to order ambulatory medications. This legal authority is generally determined by state government. Prescribers can include physicians, dentists, nurse practitioners, physician assistants, and pharmacist practitioners.

Components of an e-Prescribing System

An e-prescribing system consists of multiple components and entities (Figure 10–1). The software and computer hardware components are certainly necessary, as are the organizations that support transmission and sharing of data, standardization of the data, authorization for payment, communications to the pharmacy, and processing of the prescription within the pharmacy.

This discussion will focus on the software and components that support entry of the prescription by the prescriber, which will include the data server, data sets, interfaces, and user devices. e-Prescribing systems can be stand-alone systems that support only the function of e-prescribing or a functional component of a more comprehensive system that supports other functions within a physician practice. The other functions can be patient registration, billing, appointment scheduling, laboratory, and other ordering as well as full electronic medical record functionality.

The e-prescribing software provides functionality to support the accurate, efficient, and safe entry and communication of prescriptions and supportive information. The design and structure of this software are very important to the success of an e-prescribing application; they determine the usability of the system and how well the system supports the physician, patient, nurse, and pharmacy workflow. The U.S. government incentives for e-prescribing and electronic medical records (EMRs) specify certain minimal requirements that the e-prescribing software must

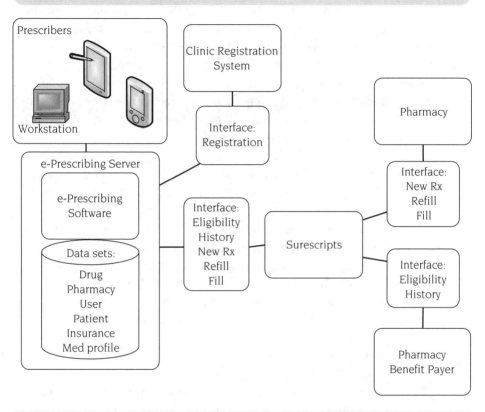

FIGURE 10–1

Components of an e-prescribing system.

e-Prescribing = electronic prescribing; Rx = prescription.
Source: Author.

meet for the health provider to be eligible for the incentives. Such functionality includes[11]:

1. Generating a complete active medication list.
2. Supporting prescription ordering, printing, and electronic transmission.
3. Providing warning alerts for unsafe conditions such as allergies.
4. Providing information on lower cost therapeutically appropriate
   alternatives.
5. Providing information on formulary, patient eligibility, and authorization requirements received from the patient's drug plan.

Additional functionality is required as a component of the U.S. EMR incentives and will evolve over time in accordance with the American Recovery and Reinvestment Act of 2009 (ARRA). The EMR e-prescribing functionality will support additional needs and capabilities within an EMR because additional data are available in an EMR to support order verification and other patient care workflow components. e-Prescribing functionality will be described in more detail later in this chapter in the section e-Prescribing Workflow. The e-prescribing software depends on the management of multiple data sets to support accurate entry and transmission of an electronic prescription. These data sets include:

1. Drug data: A standardized list of medications prescribed by the physician. The drug data include information necessary to support decision support functions, which include therapeutic categories, drug-drug interactions, drug-disease interactions, therapeutic duplications, dose range checking, and allergy warnings.

2. Pharmacy database: A list of pharmacies including pharmacy name, voice and fax numbers, addresses, NCPDP pharmacy identifiers, and other information needed to support selection of the patient's pharmacy and communication of prescriptions to the pharmacy.

3. User database: A list of prescribers, nurses, and other system users. This list includes the authority that each user has to prescribe in the system, each user's Drug Enforcement Agency (DEA) number, and other identifiers needed to support and verify the user's access to the system as well as external communication of this information to pharmacies and others.

4. Patient database: A list of patients, whose data include name, birth date, gender, allergies, addresses, preferred pharmacies, insurance coverage, and other information needed to support the e-prescribing functions.

5. Medication insurance plans/formularies: A list of available insurance plans and the prescription drug coverage supported by the plan. This list includes formulary lists and associated copayment or preauthorization requirements.

6. Medication profile information: This database contains a list of medications prescribed for the patient. This list will contain medication history data as well as a list of currently active prescription orders

for the patient. This information can also be supplemented with dispensing information received from the pharmacy as the patient picks up new prescriptions and refills.

7. Other clinical information: Depending on the functionality of the e-prescribing software and its interfaces, additional patient information may be available, including laboratory results, other test results including radiology, patient problems and diagnoses, information from prior visits, and specialty referral results.

The e-prescribing software can be configured and installed to support the needs of a single prescriber, all prescribers in a medical office, or in a shared mode for multiple sites or facilities that use the same computer equipment and data storage. Shared installations reduce the cost of equipment and maintenance, and will provide better integration of data between prescribers and practice sites. Security configuration and functionality keep the individual practice site's data separate as is required for patient confidentiality. As data and interface standards are better designed and implemented, the differences between the types of shared installations will be less apparent to prescribers. It is common for e-prescribing and EMR vendors to provide their application as an Internet service provider, with the vendor maintaining and supporting the equipment and the e-prescribing system being accessed via the Internet with standard Web browser software.

e-Prescribing systems require a large number of interfaces to support communication to all the involved parties. The interfaces provide for good data integration, resulting in less data entry and more accessible information to the prescriber and others. The interfaces include:

1. Registration: When the e-prescribing system or EMR system is separate from the patient registration or appointment scheduling system, an interface is implemented to create and update the patient demographic and insurance information in the e-prescribing system to keep the data current. Accurate and timely patient demographic information, including name, age, gender, and address, is very important to other interfaces.

2. Patient eligibility: The patient eligibility interface sends a message containing basic patient demographic information to Surescripts, which responds with the patient's prescription benefit plan

information. This eligibility information is then used by the e-prescribing system to verify prescriptions against drug plan formularies and special authorization requirements.

3. Formulary: The formulary interface provides updates to formulary drug lists provided by the prescription benefit companies. The formulary lists in the e-prescribing system are used to notify the prescriber about special authorization requirements, patient prescription copay, and therapeutic formulary alternatives.

4. Medication history: This interface contains a list of prescriptions provided by the prescription benefit companies. This list generally includes only prescriptions that the prescription benefit company is aware of and does not include prescriptions purchased with cash or through other benefit companies for the same patient.

5. **SCRIPT:** The NCPDP SCRIPT interface is a data transmission standard developed to support the communication of prescription information between prescribers and pharmacists. The standard includes support for transmission of electronic prescriptions, refill requests, prescription change requests or clarifications, fill status notifications, and prescription cancellations.

6. Prescriptions: The prescription interface consists of the electronic transactions that occur to send a prescription. In addition, the SCRIPT standard includes transactions and formats to support refill requests, change requests, and clarification requests coming from the pharmacies to the prescriber, as well as the responses returned to the pharmacy from the prescriber.

7. Fill status notification: The purpose of this interface is to support notification to the prescriber that a prescription was filled by the pharmacy and whether the patient picked up the prescription, picked up a partial fill, or never picked up the prescription.

8. Prescription cancellation: This interface allows a prescriber to cancel a previous prescription request.

Electronic prior authorization is another standard to be defined and implemented. The current prior authorization process varies greatly between payer and pharmacy benefit organizations. The type of questions asked and the personnel involved in the prior authorization process also vary and will be difficult to standardize. It is likely that multiple pilot tests involving the prior authorization process will occur before a standard is finalized and implemented. As a result, any standard that might be created likely will not be implemented until at least 2014.[12] **Interface standards** define how the data elements are organized into an electronic transaction that flows between systems. **Codification standards** exist to support accurate interpretation of the individual data elements between systems. Several codification standards are being developed to support interfaces and data integration between e-prescribing applications and pharmacy applications. The primary codification standards for e-prescribing are RxNorm and structured/codified SIG.

RxNorm is a clinical drug nomenclature standard produced by the National Library of Medicine. It provides standard names for clinical drugs, strengths, and dosage forms. It also provides links between the standard semantic clinical description and the branded representation.[13] The RxNorm standard represents the drug entity, strength, and form. For example a drug entity could be represented by acetaminophen or ibuprofen. The form could be represented as a tablet, capsule, or solution. Strength could be 325 mg, 500 mg, 100 mg/mL, or 160 mg/5 mL. The combination of these three identifiers and other modifiers such as flavor, salt, or diluents is then cross-linked by RxNorm to all branded products represented by National Drug Codes (NDCs). The NDC standard is currently used when pharmacies adjudicate or bill patient medications to pharmacy benefit companies. Therefore, RxNorm supports the mapping of prescribed medications to dispensable and billable drug products and vice versa. There are several challenges with regard to national oversight and support of the RxNorm standard and its coordination with the Food and Drug Administration, who oversees NDC assignments. Once these issues are addressed, RxNorm likely will be formalized as an e-prescribing standard.

Structured/codified SIG is also an important standard that has not been finalized as an e-prescribing requirement. Without a structured and codified SIG standard, it is necessary for pharmacists to interpret the SIG that comes from the e-prescribing system and reenter it using the coding system of the pharmacy dispensing system. This translation is inefficient, has potential for error, and makes it difficult to implement good decision support to verify dosing. This complex standard has potential for significant impact on non-medication ordering systems, long-term care systems, and inpatient medication ordering systems. Although a standard has been published and accepted by NCPDP, it is likely to take some time before the standard is universally accepted and implemented in all systems.

e-Prescribing Workflow

An understanding of prescribing workflow is necessary to best comprehend the functions within an e-prescribing system. Workflow includes patient registration and selection, medication history review and reconciliation, prescription entry, decision support, pharmacy selection, prescription transmission to the pharmacy, pharmacy processing and dispensing, and, finally, refill authorization (Figure 10–2).

Patient Registration and Eligibility

Patient registration and eligibility verification are functions that should not be required of a prescriber. These functions generally occur at the front desk of a medical practice, either at the time a patient arrives for an appointment or, ideally, in advance of the patient's arrival. The patient's insurance coverage and address are verified. In addition, the patient visit is opened within the EMR system, which puts the patient on a quick selection list within the e-prescribing or EMR system for caregivers. When registration exists on a separate computer system, the registration data are interfaced with the e-prescribing system.

   With most e-prescribing systems, the prescription eligibility and medication history information is pre-fetched from Surescripts prior to the patient being seen by the prescriber. This pre-fetch occurs in two steps. The first step is a query to Surescripts for patient prescription benefit information. If Surescripts finds that the patient has one or more prescription benefit plans, it will return the information to the e-prescribing application. Once this information is known by the e-prescribing system, the system then requests a medication history profile from the specific benefit plans. When this information is returned, it is stored for prescriber review. As a result, information about current prescription eligibility and medication history is immediately available to the prescriber, with no interface delays, when the prescriber sees the patient.

Medication Entry

The process for prescription entry within a physician practice can vary. In most cases, the clinical practice workflow of prescribers consists of a constant switching between patients as the prescriber supports different aspects of a patient visit. In some cases, the prescriber sees the patient in a single encounter, but in many cases several sub-encounters occur. The

FIGURE 10–2

Workflow for an e-prescribing system.

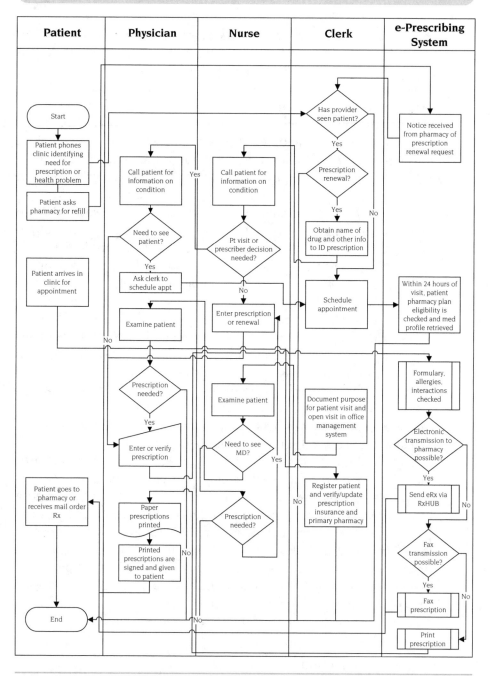

Appt = appointment; e-prescribing = electronic prescribing; eRx = electronic prescription; ID = identify;
MD = physician; Pt = patient; Rx = prescription; RxHUB = proprietary certified e-prescribing system.
Source: Author.

first sub-encounter may consist of data gathering in which patient problems, medication lists, height, weight, blood pressure, and other information are captured. This initial encounter may result in an order for a test or procedure to occur during the visit. A second sub-encounter may be the review of the results of the test or procedure, along with the resulting diagnosis and treatment plan including one or more prescriptions. A physician generally is handling multiple patients in different stages of their office visit along with telephone and other interruptions. The e-prescribing application needs to support the ability of the physician to quickly transition between patients and between data gathering and ordering.

This workflow differs significantly from the workflow shown in a demonstration of an e-prescribing software. The demonstration shows a physician completing e-prescribing functions for a single patient from start to finish with no transitions to other patients. To support this type of workflow, prescribers would need to have portable data entry/display devices or the ability to quickly log into fixed, immobile devices. In addition, they would need the ability to quickly select and switch between patients in the e-prescribing application. Switching between patient records commonly results in errors when prescriptions are entered for the wrong patient in e-prescribing applications. To support transitions from data gathering to e-prescribing, systems need to identify what necessary data gathering has not been completed prior to prescription writing. This data gathering would include allergies, height, weight, laboratory results, medication profile reconciliation, and other diagnosis-specific information.[14]

Initial pilot use of e-prescribing found that many prescribers have clinical support staff (surrogates) enter the prescriptions for the prescriber. Delegating this function to surrogates has potential for error because the surrogates are often reading and translating written prescription orders into the e-prescribing system. With handwritten prescriptions, the pharmacist usually does this translation. Many e-prescribing systems support verification of surrogate-entered prescriptions by the prescriber prior to transmission of the order to the pharmacy. The use of surrogate entry of prescriptions has not yet been directly addressed by U.S. federal regulations but likely will be addressed by state regulations.

Pharmacy Selection

Selection of the dispensing pharmacy by the prescriber is a new workflow component introduced by the U.S. e-prescribing standards. e-Prescribing systems require the prescriber to specify to which pharmacy the pre-scription is to be transmitted. This selection is supported by a searchable database of pharmacies in the e-prescribing system, which is maintained manually and via an interface with Surescripts. e-Prescribing applica-tions do have the ability to specify a default pharmacy for each patient to better support this process. A common e-prescribing error is the transmission of a prescription to the wrong pharmacy. If this error occurs, it is discovered when the patient arrives at the correct pharmacy. Currently, the only way to correct this error is for the pharmacist to telephone the prescriber.

Transmission of Prescription to the Pharmacy

The e-prescribing system transmits the prescription to the pharmacy using standard NCPDP SCRIPT interface transactions. If the electronic interface to the pharmacy is not available, the prescription is sent via fax. After January 1, 2012, prescribers will no longer be allowed to transmit Medicare prescriptions via fax except when temporary or transient net-work transmission failures occur.[15]

Controlled Substance Prescriptions

Current regulations for controlled substances require a signed paper prescription. This requirement creates complicated workflow for pre-scribers and pharmacies because these prescriptions need to be printed on special prescription paper, signed by the prescriber, and given to the patient. The DEA is still in the process of determining specific require-ments to support electronic prescribing of controlled substances. The DEA's preliminary rule has specific requirements for recordkeeping as well as user authentication and registration for e-prescribing of con-trolled substances. Many states also have regulations controlling the e-prescribing of controlled substances. The DEA is being pressured to finalize the controlled substance e-prescribing rule and to create a rule that overrides state requirements.

Prescription Filling Process

The pharmacy workflow components for e-prescribing are less defined. Pharmacy software vendors need to be certified with Surescripts to receive electronic prescriptions. This certification verifies only that the prescription can be viewed in the pharmacy system; it has no specific requirements about how the prescription is processed in the pharmacy system. The standards for drug identification (RxNorm) and structured and codified SIG are not finalized; therefore, the processing of an electronic prescription in a pharmacy system requires transcription of the electronic prescription into the coding supported by the pharmacy system. This involves identifying what stocked medication will be used to fill the prescription, translating the electronic prescription SIG instructions into the coding required by the pharmacy system, and verifying the match of the electronic prescription to the correct patient in the pharmacy system. Some of this transcription is supported by automated matching in pharmacy systems, but the matching still requires pharmacist verification because the automated matching is not always correct. When the electronic prescription is transmitted to the pharmacy, it has a Surescripts-created prescription identification, which is used to match the prescription back to the prescriber in support of fill status messages and prescription renewal requests.

A common problem with pharmacy computer systems is the lack of good integration of e-prescribing workflow into the non-electronic prescription workflow. An example is the identification of incoming electronic prescriptions and the queuing of them into workflow with other prescriptions. Newly arrived electronic prescriptions notices are often not clearly identified in the pharmacy system. It is common that a low-priority electronic prescription is received and is left in the electronic work queue for later processing. This low-priority prescription will then mask the arrival of higher priority electronic prescriptions into the work queue. Once pharmacies and software vendors better understand the workflow requirements of electronic prescriptions, these prescriptions will be better integrated into the pharmacy software systems and fill processes.

Renewal Authorizations

The renewal authorization process in pharmacies and physician practices has great potential for improvement with e-prescribing. Prior to e-prescribing, multiple telephone calls were required to complete a renewal authorization.

Pharmacies can initiate electronic renewal authorization requests that are electronically processed by the prescriber and transmitted back to the pharmacy. This process can significantly reduce the interruption of phone calls between pharmacy and prescriber. Within the prescriber systems, these requests can be pre-screened by nurses and other support staff. The systems can also be configured to allow physicians to cover for each other when refill requests are received and the original prescriber is not available.

Decision Support

The decision support functionalities supported by e-prescribing include allergy checking, drug-drug interactions, therapeutic duplication checking, and dose range checking. All of these functionalities are generally provided by the drug database vendors and are applied at the time of order entry. Because of the high volume of alerts that occur, many prescribers deactivate the decision support functionality or apply parameters that display only the most significant alerts.

In addition to the traditional decision support alerts just described, other e-prescribing functionality also supports drug selection, dosing, and other decisions. Such functionality includes verification of patient benefit formularies and the ability to list alternative formulary drugs in the same therapeutic category. Some e-prescribing systems support problem-based ordering that directs the prescriber to medications commonly prescribed for the diagnoses or problems coded for the patient. e-Prescribing components of EMRs can also cross-reference dosing and prescribing with laboratory results and patient vital signs. Weight-based dosing is also available in many e-prescribing systems to support and document accurate dose calculations.

The prescription verification check provided by the pharmacist is a very important step in the e-prescribing process. These new technologies introduce errors that can be caught only through human intervention and verification. Such errors include errors in transcribing drug names, doses, and frequencies by surrogate prescribers as well as prescriber order entry errors. Errors in patient selection and drug selection by prescribers are common with e-prescribing. Errors in selection of choices from drop-down lists and errors in keyboard entry can result in harm to patients if the errors are not identified and corrected. As pharmacists transition from paper prescriptions to electronic prescriptions, it is important that they continue to be diligent when verifying drug selection against indication, dose, and frequency. Improved decision support functionality within e-prescribing systems will reduce errors but not eliminate them. Pharmacists will prevent the missed errors from occurring.

Future of e-Prescribing

e-Prescribing standards and systems as well as pharmacy systems to best support clinical, operational, and patient workflow are still in the early stages of development. The initial focus has been on supporting prescriber workflow and increasing prescriber adoption of the new technology. As the volume of electronic prescriptions increases, workflow will be refined and better supported by the electronic systems.

As e-prescribing use expands, the experience gathered will further refine the workflow and supporting system tools. Standards and system functionality will also need refinement to support new regulations for controlled substances, pre-authorization, and enhanced integration with EMR systems and patient personal health record (PHR) systems. Implementation of codification standards for drug identification (RxNorm) and structured and codified SIG will close the gap to allow unimpeded flow of prescribing information from the prescriber to the patient's prescription label. New technologies in dispensing and monitoring will support better patient adherence to medication therapies.

As EMR systems continue to be implemented and integrated with e-prescribing, decision support of medication ordering and monitoring will be improved. Laboratory results, problem lists, vital signs, and other clinical data will be available for clinician review and automated verification. Problem-based ordering systems will reduce the errors associated with sound-alike medications. Integration with external medication profiles and shared medication reconciliation will better support verification of current therapies and reduction of duplicative therapies. Integration of EMR data with PHRs will provide the patient with better information and will improve communication with the physician and the pharmacist. System support for documentation of reasons for overriding decision support and the communication of these reasons to the pharmacist will enable better prescriber to pharmacist communication and further reduce phone calls.

Significantly expanded support for patient needs is likely to occur. Patients will be able to request prescription refills and renewal authorizations directly from their PHR, as well as receive recommendations for over-the-counter medications and enter these medications on their PHR medication profile. This profile will then be available to the prescriber and the pharmacist. Better support for pharmacy selection and electronic prescription tracking will be available to patients, prescribers, and pharmacists as this process is refined.

Implementation of RxNorm and structured and codified SIG standards will support the direct integration of e-prescribing into new technologies to support patient compliance. Such support will include prescription containers that remind the patient when medications are due and keep track of when medications are administered. The RxNorm and structured and codified SIG standards will be applied to all patient care areas, including hospitals, to better support medication reconciliation, continuation of medication therapies, and monitoring across care transitions.

This increased integration of patient medication data all the way to the patient will also support a shift toward a more patient-centric health care environment as patients have better access to their health care information.

Conclusion

e-Prescribing is a technology still in its infancy. Much has been accomplished through the development of e-prescribing standards and U.S. government investment in incentives to increase its adoption. To date, most of the e-prescribing efforts have been prescriber centric because they are meant to impact prescribing and manage costs of the new Medicare Part D Prescription Benefit. The additional incentives for adoption of EMRs will positively impact e-prescribing by introducing additional standards support and better integration with other patient information. As e-prescribing workflow and standards are further refined, patients will reap the benefits through better access to information and safer management of their medication therapies. As a result, the focus of e-prescribing will shift from the prescriber to the patient.

LEARNING ACTIVITIES

1. Discuss the impact that adoption of RxNorm and structured and codified SIG will have if they are implemented where you work.
2. Describe the e-prescribing pharmacy selection process to a patient (not a health care worker). Discuss how it can impact the patient who is getting a prescription.
3. In a group discussion, identify possible bottlenecks in the e-prescribing process, what causes the bottlenecks, and how they can be reduced.
4. Talk with a community pharmacist and identify the types of errors they commonly see on written prescriptions and electronic prescriptions. Determine differences that exist between e-prescribing and paper prescription errors.

References

1. Cherry DK, Woodwell DA, Rechtsteiner EA. *National Ambulatory Medical Care Survey: 2005 Summary.* Hyattsville, MD: National Center for Health Statistics; 2007:1–39. Advance Data from Vital and Health Statistics; No. 387.
2. Cypress BW. *Drug Utilization in Office Visits to Primary Care Physicians: National Ambulatory Medical Care Survey, 1980.* Bethesda, MD: Public Health Service; 1982. Department of Health and Human Services Publication No. (PHS) 82-1250.
3. National Association of Chain Drug Stores. *Chain Pharmacy Industry Profile 2008–2009.* Alexandria, VA: National Association of Chain Drug Stores; 2008
4. Institute for Safe Medicine Practices. *A Call to Action: Eliminate Handwritten Prescriptions Within Three Years.* Horsham, PA: Institute for Safe Medicine Practices; 2000.
5. Kohn L, Corrigan J, Donaldson M, eds. *To Err Is Human: Building a Safer Health System.* Washington, DC: National Academy of Sciences; 2000.
6. Torkzadeh G, Chang JC, Hanson G. Identifying issues in customer relationship management at Merck-Medco. *Decis Support Syst.* 2006;42(2):1116–30.
7. Ratliff R. Concurrent Session C4: Prescription Drug: "The Case for E-Prescribing: From Economics to Errors and Emergencies." Presented at the AHQA 2007 Annual Meeting, New Orleans, Louisiana, February 12–15, 2007.
8. Johnston D, et al. E-Health Initiative. *Electronic Prescribing: Toward Maximum Value and Rapid Adoption.* Charlestown, MA: Center for Information Technology Leadership; 2004.
9. Medicare program: e-prescribing and the prescription drug program; final rule. 70(214) *Federal Register* 67571 (November 7, 2005) (codified at 42 CFR § 423).
10. National Council for Prescription Drug Programs. About us. Available at: http://www.ncpdp.org/about/aspx. Accessed October 14, 2009.
11. CMS Centers for Medicare and Medicaid Services. E-prescribing incentive program. Available at: http://www.cms.hhs.gov/ERxIncentive. Accessed October 14, 2009.

12. Agency for Healthcare Research and Quality. E-*Prescribing Standards Expert Meeting Summary*. Rockville, MD: Agency for Healthcare Research and Quality; May 2008. AHRQ Publication No. 08-0062-EF.

13. National Library of Medicine. Unified Medical Language System: an overview to RxNorm. Available at: http://www.nlm.nih.gov/research/umls/rxnorm/overview.html. Accessed 10/12/2009.

14. Dumitru D. e-Prescribing. In: *The Pharmacy Informatics Primer*. Bethesda, MD: American Society of Health-System Pharmacists; 2009.

15. Standards for electronic prescribing. 73(224) *Federal Register* 69938 (November 19, 2008) (codified at 42 CFR § 423.160 subpt. D).

CHAPTER 11

Clinical Decision Support Systems at Prescribing

Shobha Phansalkar

OBJECTIVES

1. Define clinical decision support systems (CDSS).
2. Describe the components of a CDSS.
3. Describe examples of CDSS.
4. Describe clinical settings in which a CDSS has been used.
5. Describe how CDSS and electronic medical records (EMRs) work in conjunction with one another.
6. Describe scenarios in patient care in which the CDSS can be implemented as part of the clinical information system, and provide suggestions to the physician via the EMR.
7. Describe some of the strengths and limitations of CDSS as they are implemented today.

Clinical decision support systems (CDSS) have been used to support decision making in a variety of clinical domains. Several definitions exist for CDSS. One definition proposed by Musen et al. broadly defines a CDSS as "any computer program designed to provide expert support for health professionals making clinical decisions."[1] Johnston et al.'s definition, on the other hand, considers the application of these systems specifically to patient care to provide patient-specific advice.[2] They define CDSS as "computer software employing a knowledge base designed for use by a clinician involved in patient care, as a direct aid to clinical decision making." Yet another definition by Wyatt describes these systems as "active knowledge systems which use two or more items of patient data to generate case-specific advice."[3] In a white paper published by the American Medical Informatics Association in 2006, **clinical decision support** (CDS) was described as "providing clinicians, patients or individuals with knowledge and person specific or population information, intelligently filtered or presented at appropriate times, to foster better health processes, better individual patient care, and better population health."[4] As presented, there are a number of definitions for CDSS, each differing according to the breadth of its application to patient care.

Basic Components of a CDSS

A CDSS consists of three basic components: an inference engine, a knowledge base, and a communication mechanism.[5] The **inference engine,** also called the "reasoning engine," forms the "brain" of the CDSS and works to link patient-specific information with the information in the knowledge base. The **knowledge base** can be composed of assorted clinical knowledge, such as drug interactions, diagnoses, or treatment guidelines. The **communication mechanism** allows the user to enter the patient information into the application and is responsible for communicating the relevant information (e.g., possible drug interaction alerts and preventive care reminders) back to the clinician.

Once a match has been detected between the clinical data and the knowledge base, the inference engine then determines how the system should respond. For example, a physician may enter a prescription for diazepam for a patient who is 70 years old. The inference engine employs logical reasoning and, using the knowledge base, determines whether this is an appropriate prescription. Consider that the knowledge base contains the information that diazepam is contraindicated in patients who are older than 65 years. The inference engine would then instruct the communication mechanism to generate an alert that informs the clinician of the potentially inappropriate prescription. For the system to generate the alert, it is imperative that the inference engine understand the concepts of "age" and the "medication" being prescribed. If even one of these variables was not expressed in a manner clearly understood by the inference engine, or was different from how these concepts were expressed in the knowledge base, then the system would fail to alert the clinician. Therein lies the importance of using a controlled vocabulary and standardized terminology system to express concepts in a CDSS. Without the capability to communicate with each other, the CDSS components would not be able to interact and operate successfully. Specific terminology systems are used in the medical domain for expression of concepts from a given domain. For example, the National Library of Medicine maintains the RxNorm terminology, which provides normalized names for clinical drugs, and the SNOMED CT, which is a comprehensive clinical terminology system for recording diagnoses and problem lists.

There are many types of CDSS depending on the logical reasoning used by the inference engine. One type of expert system is a rule-based system, which uses a series of if-then rules to form a line of reasoning. This process of connecting a set of if-then rules is called ***chaining.*** If the chaining begins from a set of conditions and moves toward arriving at a conclusion, the method is called ***forward chaining.*** However, if the conclusion itself is known but the path to that conclusion is unknown, the system must reason back to the source; this method is called ***backward chaining.*** Figure 11–1 is an example of how a forward chaining inference

---

FIGURE 11–1

Forward chaining process of a clinical decision support system for generating an alert.

   IF   Patient is Female

        AND   High Family History Risk of Breast cancer
        AND   Bilateral Mastectomy NOT on problem list
        AND   Age >40 yrs, <75 yrs
        AND   No mammogram in the past 12 months.

   THEN Generate an alert for overdue mammogram for the specific patient

---

Source: Author.

engine would generate an alert for a patient who is overdue for a mammogram and is at high risk for breast cancer because of her family history.

An early example of a rule-based expert system in medicine was MYCIN. With this system, the user enters patient information and answers a series of yes/no questions, enabling the system to recommend the appropriate dosage of an antibiotic based on patient-specific data such as weight.[6] A rule-based method of designing expert systems has several limitations. Although the process of knowledge acquisition can be slow, tedious, and expensive, the knowledge itself is often incomplete. One approach to overcoming these limitations is to design systems that can "learn" from themselves. This type of expert system utilizes artificial intelligence capabilities, specifically, self-learning algorithms that determine previously established trends and recognize patterns in the clinical data to derive knowledge. One example of such an expert system was developed as early as 1972 by de Dombal et al. to evaluate abdominal pain using Bayesian probability theory.[7] Following the success of systems such as MYCIN, several hybrid systems have been developed that use both deductive rules and probabilistic reasoning. Examples of such hybrid systems include Quick Medical Reference (QMR),[8] DXplain,[9] and Iliad.[10] Further discussion is beyond the scope of this book, but the reader may find more information on ways to develop inference engines from *Clinical Decision Support Systems: Theory and Practice*.[11]

Use of CDSS in Clinical Care

CDSS can also be categorized by the mode in which information is displayed to the user or by the domain of clinical care in which they are applied. CDS can be generated by a variety of modalities that include, but are not limited to, alerts, reminders, guidelines, information displays, computerized provider order entry (CPOE), and electronic templates. CDSS have been employed in various domains of clinical care and have the ability to support a range of complex decisions, from weaning a patient off a mechanical ventilator to a simple reminder about an immunization being due for a patient. CDS takes various forms in clinical information systems; the means of support could be implemented as order sets of clinical guidelines or explicit computerized protocols. Additionally, CDS applications can alert a clinician against prescribing a medication that could result in a drug-drug or drug-allergy interaction. CDSS can support clinical decision making at various stages in the patient care process, from reminders for preventive care medicine to diagnosis and treatment to patient monitoring and follow-up.[5] Examples of the use of CDSS in various stages of the patient care process are provided to highlight the specific and generic nature of these systems.

Preventive Care

CDSS can be used to meet preventive care guidelines by providing reminders for vaccinations and Pap smears, screenings for mammograms, disease management guidelines for smoking cessation, and other services at the point of care. A meta-analysis by Shea et al. identified 16 randomized controlled trials to evaluate computer-based clinical reminder systems for preventive care in the ambulatory setting. The study found six different categories of preventive care services: vaccinations, breast cancer screening, cervical cancer screening, colorectal cancer screening, cardiovascular risk reduction, and other preventive services (e.g., screening for glaucoma, weight, tuberculosis test, etc.). The study found that computerized reminders increased implementation of preventive practices for four of these categories. Overall, for all six categories combined, there was a 77% increase in implementation of preventive practices when computer reminders were used.[12]

Other recent examples of CDS use in preventive care include reminders for foot, eye, renal, blood pressure, and low-density lipoprotein cholesterol screenings for patients with type II diabetes.[13] Although the interruptive nature of these reminders might undermine their utility, a recent study conducted in the Netherlands on screening patients with dyslipidemia showed that computer-generated alerts resulted in a more positive outcome compared with decision support requested on demand. Providing clinicians with reminders for dyslipidemia treatment resulted in 65% of patients receiving treatment for the disease as opposed to 35% in the on-demand group.[14] Thus, preventive care reminders can have a positive impact on appropriate clinical practices when displayed at the point of care. Figure 11–2 illustrates an example of a preventive care reminder in an electronic medical record (EMR).

Diagnosis

Several CDSS have been developed to help clinicians derive conclusions about the diagnosis of a disease on the basis of the signs and symptoms

FIGURE 11-2

Clinical decision support system reminder for Pneumovax generated in an outpatient medical record for a high-risk patient.

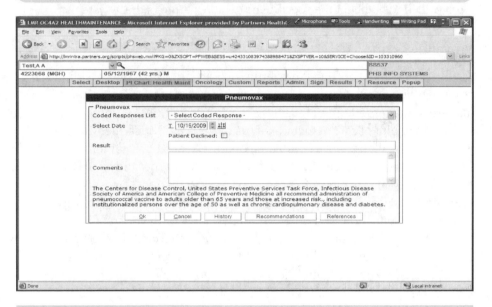

Source: Author.

that the patient may be presenting. These systems provide the potential to reduce diagnostic errors in medicine.[11,15] An early example of a diagnostic CDSS was Iliad, which was developed at the University of Utah. This system employs Bayesian reasoning to calculate probabilities of various diagnoses in internal medicine.[10,16] Iliad contains information on 1200 diseases, 1500 syndromes, and treatment protocols that can be derived from 11,900 findings. Another early system that employed Bayes theorem was developed by DeDombal from Leeds, United Kingdom, to assist in the diagnosis of abdominal pain.[7]

Yet another example of an early diagnostic decision support system was DXplain, which was developed at the Laboratory of Computer Science at the Massachusetts General Hospital.[9,17] DXplain serves the purpose of both an electronic medical textbook and a medical reference system by using a set of clinical findings, such as signs, symptoms, and laboratory data, to produce a list of diagnoses ranked by likelihood. DXplain employs expert rules and probabilistic association for determining the weighted assessments of the disease for a given set of findings. In addition to the probable diagnosis, DXplain allows clinicians to see justifications for each of the potential diagnoses, suggestions to obtain additional clinical information that would be useful and pertinent to the disease, and a list of clinical manifestations that would be atypical for each of the suggested diseases. In addition to being an expert system, DXplain also serves the role of a medical textbook—it can provide a description of more than 2300 different diseases, including the signs and symptoms, the etiology, the pathology, and the prognosis associated with each. DXplain provides up to 10 references for each disease, including clinical reviews when these are available. In addition, DXplain can provide a list of diseases that should be considered for any one of more than 4900 different clinical manifestations (signs, symptoms, and laboratory examinations).[9,18]

QMR is another diagnostic decision support system that uses a rule-based approach and utilizes a knowledge base of diseases, diagnoses, findings, disease associations, and laboratory information.[8,19] QMR was in turn developed from an expert system called INTERNIST-I. Both expert systems rely on the same knowledge base, called the "INTERNIST-1 computerized knowledge base," which describes 570 diseases in internal medicine. However, the two expert systems differ in their intended use: INTERNIST-1 functions solely as a high-powered diagnostic consultant program, whereas the QMR program contains primarily a learning component and allows users to review the diagnostic information available in the knowledge base. QMR provides electronic access to more than 750 diseases representing the vast majority of the disorders seen by internists in daily practice as well a compendium of less common diseases. This program provides information on almost 700 diseases and uses more than 5000 clinical findings, including medical history, symptoms, physical signs, and laboratory test results.[20]

An evaluation by Berner et al. compared the diagnostic capabilities of four internal medicine diagnostic systems: DXplain, Iliad, Meditel, and QMR. The study found that no one system outperformed the others; in fact, on average less than half of the diagnoses suggested by the system concurred with what clinical experts identified as possible diagnoses. However, each program did suggest an average of approximately two additional diagnoses per case that the experts had not initially considered but agreed they were relevant. Rather than using a binary approach, Berner et al. suggested a more comprehensive approach to measure system performance. Metrics used in this evaluation included the ranking of diagnostic hypotheses and other indicators of diagnostic quality such as relevance and comprehensiveness.[21]

Recent advances have led to the development of CDSS that are more specific to the domain of diagnosis, one example being a differential diagnostic tool called ISABEL, which is used in acute pediatric settings.[22] A more recent example of an expert system that is capable of providing point-of-care visual diagnostic decision making is the VisualDx system developed by Logical Images. This system allows clinicians to receive information on patient-centric visual diagnoses based on the patient's signs, symptoms, medical history, and so on. The system contains a library of more than 17,000 images as well as information reviewed by subject matter experts for nearly 1000 visually identifiable diseases.[23]

Early decision support systems have had variable success, primarily because these systems were not integrated with the EMR. Thus, they required that busy clinicians launch another application or go to a separate machine to input the clinical symptoms and receive suggestions on the possible diagnoses. More recently, the importance of linking CDSS with an EMR to achieve their full potential is being realized. This linking allows decision support to occur in the background and the system to make its derivations and present them at appropriate times in the clinical workflow. One example of this is the PRODIGY project in the United Kingdom, which involves integrating decision support systems for medication ordering into many general practice EMRs.

Planning or Implementation of Treatment

Decision support systems are capable of providing guidance to clinicians on the basis of evidence-based medicine. They have been used for this purpose in the inpatient and outpatient setting. The use of CDSS for planning and implementing treatment is more common in the inpatient setting where complex decisions requiring consideration of numerous variables are frequent. This has led to the development of a variety of CDSS for use in acute care settings for complex decisions such as ventilator management in critical care,[24–26] providing postoperative care,[27] or planning parenteral nutrition in the neonatal intensive care unit.[28]

One example of an expert system that is used in the outpatient setting for disease management is the Assessment and Treatment of Hypertension: Evidence-Based Automation (ATHENA) system, which provides guidance to clinicians for the management of hypertension in primary care. The system provides primary care physicians with guidelines on blood pressure control and offers medication recommendations. These recommendations are made in accordance with evidence-based medicine to achieve the desired blood pressure in light of any comorbid diseases or conditions that the patient may have. The system allows clinical experts to customize the knowledge base in accordance with the most up-to-date guidelines and to incorporate new evidence or reflect on local interpretations of guideline ambiguities.[29,30]

Another example of a CDSS used to implement guidelines on a specific diagnosis was developed by Durieux et al., who described a system used for the prevention of thromboembolic disease in postsurgical patients.[31] A systematic review conducted by Shiffman et al. about 10 years ago assessed the effectiveness of CDSS for the implementation of practice guidelines.[32] At that time, the authors found descriptions of 20 systems in the literature that were being used for this purpose. A more recent systematic review by Garg et al. to understand the effectiveness of CDSS on provider performance and patient outcomes revealed that CDSS were used for/in more than 40 disease management studies. Sixty-two percent of these studies showed an improvement in practitioner performance, and of the 27 studies that evaluated patient outcomes, only five (18%) demonstrated improvements.[15,33]

Another aspect of planning treatment in which decision support systems are widely employed is in providing medication decision support. Medication decision support forms a large proportion of the knowledge base of any clinical information system. Kuperman et al. described a framework for the medication decision support interventions that can be employed in a CDSS.[34] The authors categorize these interventions as basic and advanced decision support. Basic decision support includes drug-allergy checking, basic dosing guidance, formulary decision support, duplicate therapy checking, and drug-drug interaction checking. Advanced decision support also includes dosing suggestions for geriatric patients and patients with renal insufficiency, guidance for medication-related laboratory testing, drug-disease contraindication checking, and drug-pregnancy checking.[34] A recent review by Schedlbauer et al. on medication-related decision support and its effect on provider behavior classified 27 types of alerts across 20 studies using Kuperman's framework.[35] This review reported that 23 studies showed an improvement in provider behavior and/or reductions in medication errors when CDS was offered. Figure 11–3 illustrates an example of a drug-drug interaction between warfarin and fluconazole.

Thus, CDS when implemented in a CPOE system can have a positive impact on patient safety and provide useful guidance to clinicians, helping them make informed therapeutic decisions about patient care. In addition, CDSS have the potential to improve the efficiency of tasks such as medication ordering by suggesting appropriate doses, therapeutic alternatives, medications available in the formulary, and so on.

FIGURE 11–3

Clinical decision support system alert for a drug-drug interaction between warfarin and fluconazole. The patient has an existing order for warfarin and the physician is currently prescribing fluconazole. The alert provides the clinician with information on the interaction and asks for a reason if the physician decides to override the alert and continue with the order.

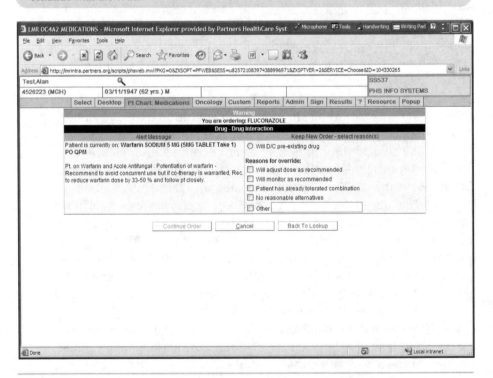

Source: Author.

Follow-up

Once the physician has ordered the medications and tests needed to treat a patient, follow-up is needed to determine if the ordered therapeutic interventions are generating the expected effect. Tests and treatments that are ordered to ameliorate the effects of an intervention or as a consequence of other orders are called ***corollary orders.*** One such example would be ordering an international normalized ratio (INR) test to measure the coagulation time for a patient on anticoagulation therapy such as warfarin. To allow appropriate follow-up with patient care, many clinical information systems incorporate CDS for corollary orders or adverse event monitoring. A study conducted by Overhage et al. to evaluate the impact of corollary orders for adult inpatients in a general medical ward showed a 25% improvement in ordering of corollary medications when physicians were prompted by the CDSS.[36] In this study, physicians used a CPOE system to write orders, with those in the intervention group equipped with an additional CDS component. Physicians in the intervention group were reminded of corollary orders via the CDSS, resulting in one-third fewer pharmacy interventions compared with those experienced by physicians in the control group.[36] The main limitations to the use of corollary orders are that their development and maintenance are resource intensive, and that few organizations can afford to spend the time and money needed for their implementation.

Wright and Sittig proposed a data mining approach to identifying corollary orders by utilizing an automated data mining approach for identifying medication or laboratory orders that were strongly associated with one another. Although these orders are difficult to develop, physicians do recognize their importance and realize the significant role they could play in facilitating appropriate follow-up of patients.[37] One study by Murff et al. studied the attitudes of primary care physicians for receiving CDS to track abnormal test results for their patients in the outpatient setting. Without an electronic tracking system, most of the primary care physicians were dissatisfied with their ability to track abnormal test results.[38]

Thus, CDSS have an important place in a variety of roles in patient care. Previous studies have shown that incorporating decision support at the point of care, where the information provided by the system can be implemented, has the largest impact on patient care. This can be achieved by incorporating decision support systems within an EMR. This linking allows the system to retrieve important pieces of patient information from the EMR and generate suggestions back to the physician in either the EMR or the CPOE system to assist clinicians in clinical decision making.

Strengths and Limitations of CDSS

Previous studies and systematic reviews have described the capabilities of CDSS to have several positive outcomes.[15,39] CDSS have been shown to decrease adverse drug events (ADEs),[40] decrease costs,[40] decrease patient length of stay,[40] and improve clinical practice by providing CDS in accordance with the clinical workflow.[39] A 10-year evaluation of a CDSS used with a CPOE system of a well-known tertiary care center estimated savings of $28.5 million in terms of improving clinical and patient care outcomes.[41] Most importantly, CDSS can improve clinicians' efficiency by providing useful information at the point of care, drawing their attention to possible drug interactions or even reminding them of possible follow-up interventions that can improve patient outcomes. Despite these advantages, CDSS suffer from a number of limitations that have impeded their widespread adoption.

Challenges to CDSS implementation include developing a comprehensive knowledge base and maintaining it to keep it current with clinical guidelines and new evidence in the literature. This is not only time consuming but also a resource-intensive process. If institutions decide they are not able to make this investment for in-house knowledge base development, they can invest in a vendor-maintained knowledge base. However, systems usually fail when these off-the-shelf solutions are implemented for CDS without any tailoring or local customization. Customization of the content driving the CDS is crucial to physicians adopting the decision support provided by these applications. Further, CDSS need to be interoperable with other clinical information systems applications, including but not limited to the EMR, CPOE system, pharmacy system, and so on.

Interoperability between the CDSS and the EMR as well as other systems (e.g., pharmacy and laboratory) poses a significant challenge.[42] Besides technical challenges, CDS also has an impact on the clinical workflow. These systems are designed with the intent to support rather than impede the clinical workflow.[34,42] Several evaluation studies have illustrated the high rate of alert overrides that exists for medication-related decision support in the inpatient and outpatient setting.[34,43,44] Most medication-related decision support alerts are not based on human factors.[34,35] Stratifying these alerts into tiers on the basis of their level of clinical significance has resulted in increased compliance.[43,45] Excessive alerting can desensitize clinicians to the clinical significance of these alerts, potentially leading to disregard and overrides of important messages. This phenomenon is termed "alert fatigue." Several institutions struggle with striking the optimum balance between too many alerts that can lead to alert fatigue and too few alerts, both of which can have an impact on patient safety. Even though recent evidence illustrates that not all overridden alerts lead to ADEs,[44] there is potential for important clinical warnings to be overlooked.[46] This delicate balance of optimal alerting is crucial to provide optimal decision support and can be achieved by tailoring the knowledge base according to clinical significance and local clinical expertise.

Limited evaluation has been conducted to determine the usability of CDS applications. Without rigorous testing of the impact on clinical workflow, customization of the user interfaces, and other human factors that drive effective use, adoption of CDSS will remain limited. Further research is needed to understand optimally functional CDSS that can be effectively assimilated into clinical workflow, to implement user-friendly features that improve clinical efficiency, and to develop standardized alerting messages that can convey the clinical significance to users. Future research in this direction will further understanding of these factors, which are understudied and proven to be barriers to adoption of CDSS.

Conclusion

CDSS have emerged as an important part of any clinical information system. They could serve a variety of functions in helping clinicians to take better care of their patients and in preventing adverse events. The knowledge base incorporated in a CDSS can be tailored to meet the needs of a specific clinical domain or broad enough to encompass various domains. Several examples of CDSS have been discussed; the discussion highlights the specific and generic nature of systems that have been developed and are in use in routine clinical care. The implementation of CDSS in conjunction with an EMR or a CPOE system can help achieve maximum benefit.

CDSS in their current state suffer from several limitations. First and foremost, they are expensive to develop and maintain, thus limiting their wide adoption. Additionally, limited work has been done to understand their impact on clinical workflow, human factors considerations to make them more usable, their impact on provider behavior, and, in general, the socio-technical aspects that govern their adoption. Although it has been the author's intention to present various studies and their results to make the reader aware of evaluations that have been conducted, the description of these is by no means deemed to be complete. Readers are encouraged as they read this chapter to think beyond the clinical and technological aspect of CDSS and to understand the impact of providers' perspectives, issues of behavioral control, governance of systems, and the organizational structure that play an important role in the successful adoption of these systems.

LEARNING ACTIVITIES

1. Define the term *interoperability* in your own words and explain the concept to a colleague. Links to appropriate online resources:
   - The Informatics Review (an online journal; www.informatics-review.com/index.html)
   - Open Clinical (an international organization focused on knowledge management in health care; www.openclinical.org)
   - Chapter by Dr. Eta Berner titled "State of the Art of Clinical Decision Support Systems," available on the Agency for Healthcare Research and Quality Web site (www.healthit.ahrq.gov/images/jun09cdsreview/09_0069_ef.html)
2. Identify one pharmacy system that is used in your clinical setting. Determine what EMR or CPOE system it interfaces with, if any. Then determine what medication knowledge base is used by the EMR or CPOE system for ordering medications.

   Does the pharmacy system use the same medication knowledge base?

   If not, what issues would users face, from a workflow perspective, because the ordering system and the pharmacy system are not truly interoperable?

Acknowledgement

The author would like to acknowledge the contribution of Ms. Monique Bidell, fourth-year pharmacy student at Bouve College of Health Sciences, Northeastern University, Boston, Massachusetts. Ms. Bidell was especially helpful in developing the Strengths and Limitations of CDSS section of this chapter and also proofread the drafts of this chapter.

References

1. Musen MA, Shahar Y, Shortliffe EH. Clinical decision-support systems. In: Shortliffe EH, Perreault LE, Wiederhold G, eds. *Medical Informatics: Computer Applications in Health Care and Biomedicine*. 2nd ed. New York: Springer-Verlag; 2001:573–609.
2. Johnston ME, Langton KB, Haynes RB, et al. Effects of computer-based clinical decision support systems on clinician performance and patient outcome. A critical appraisal of research. *Ann Intern Med*.1994;120(2):135–42.
3. Wyatt J. Computer-based knowledge systems. *Lancet*. 1991;338(8780):1431–6.
4. Osheroff JA, Teich JM, Middleton B, et al. A roadmap for national action on clinical decision support. *J Am Med Inform Assoc*. 2007;14(2):141–5.
5. Berner ES. *Clinical Decision Support Systems: State of the Art*. Rockville, MD: Agency for Healthcare Research and Quality; June 2009. Contract No.: AHRQ Publication No. 09-0069-EF.
6. Shortliffe EH, Davis R, Axline SG, et al. Computer-based consultations in clinical therapeutics: explanation and rule acquisition capabilities of the MYCIN system. *Comput Biomed Res*.1975;8(4):303–20.
7. de Dombal FT, Leaper DJ, Staniland JR, et al. Computer-aided diagnosis of acute abdominal pain. *Br Med J*.1972;2(5804):9–13.
8. Miller R, Masarie FE, Myers JD. Quick medical reference (QMR) for diagnostic assistance. *MD Comput*. 1986;3(5):34–48.
9. Barnett GO, Cimino JJ, Hupp JA, et al. DXplain. An evolving diagnostic decision-support system. *JAMA*.1987;258(1):67–74.
10. Warner HR, Jr. Iliad: moving medical decision-making into new frontiers. *Methods Inf Med*. 1989;28(4):370–2.
11. Berner ES. *Clinical Decision Support Systems: Theory and Practice*. 2nd ed. New York, NY: Springer; 2007.
12. Shea S, DuMouchel W, Bahamonde L. A meta-analysis of 16 randomized controlled trials to evaluate computer-based clinical reminder systems for preventive care in the ambulatory setting. *J Am Med Inform Assoc*. 1996;3(6):399–409.
13. Peterson KA, Radosevich DM, O'Connor PJ, et al. Improving diabetes care in practice: findings from the TRANSLATE trial. *Diabetes Care*. 2008;31(12):2238–43.
14. van Wyk JT, van Wijk MA, Sturkenboom MC, et al. Electronic alerts versus on-demand decision support to improve dyslipidemia treatment: a cluster randomized controlled trial. *Circulation*. 2008;117(3):371–8.
15. Garg AX, Adhikari NK, McDonald H, et al. Effects of computerized clinical decision support systems on practitioner performance and patient outcomes: a systematic review. *JAMA*. 2005;293(10):1223–38.

16. Warner HR, Jr. Iliad: diagnostic tools for general medicine. Interview by Bill W. Childs. *Healthc Inform*.1990;7(4):38.

17. Barnett GO, Hoffer EP, Packer MS, et al. DXPLAIN—demonstration and discussion of a diagnostic clinical decision support system. *Proc Annu Symp Comput Appl Med Care*. 1991:878.

18. Barnett O, Hoffer E, Feldman M, et al. DXplain—20 years later—what have we learned. AMIA *Annu Symp Proc*. 2008:1201–2.

19. Miller RA, McNeil MA, Challinor SM, et al. The INTERNIST-1/QUICK MEDICAL REFERENCE project—status report. *West J Med*. 1986;145(6):816–22.

20. Miller RA, Masarie FE, Jr. Use of the Quick Medical Reference (QMR) program as a tool for medical education. *Methods Inf Med*. 1989;28(4):340–5.

21. Berner ES, Webster GD, Shugerman AA, et al. Performance of four computer-based diagnostic systems. *N Engl J Med*. 1994;330(25):1792–6.

22. Greenough A. Help from ISABEL for paediatric diagnoses. *Lancet*. 2002;360(9341):1259.

23. Tleyjeh IM, Nada H, Baddour LM. VisualDx: decision-support software for the diagnosis and management of dermatologic disorders. *Clin Infect Dis*. 2006;43(9):1177–84.

24. Shahsavar N, Frostell C, Gill H, et al. Knowledge base design for decision support in respirator therapy. *Int J Clin Monit Comput*. 1989;6(4):223–31.

25. Mersmann S, Dojat M, eds. SmartCare—automated clinical guidelines in critical care. In: *Proceedings of the 16th European Conference on Artificial Intelligence* (ECAI'04) 2004. (Valencia, Spain, August 22–27, 2004.) Valencia: IOS Press; 2004.

26. Dojat M, Brochard L, Lemaire F, et al. A knowledge-based system for assisted ventilation of patients in intensive care units. *Int J Clin Monit Comput*. 1992;9(4):239–50.

27. Sawar MJ, Brennan TG, Cole AJ, et al., eds. POEMS (PostOperative Expert Medical System). In: *Proceedings of IJCAI91 One Day Workshop: Representing Knowledge in Medical Decision Support Systems*. (Sydney, Australia, August, 1991.) San Francisco, CA: Morgan Kaufmann Publishers; 1991.

28. Horn W, Popow C, Miksch S, et al. Development and evaluation of VIE-PNN, a knowledge-based system for calculating the parenteral nutrition of newborn infants. *Artif Intell Med*. 2002; 24(3):217–28.

29. Advani A, Tu S, O'Connor M, et al. Integrating a modern knowledge-based system architecture with a legacy VA database: the ATHENA and EON projects at Stanford. *Proc AMIA Symp*. 1999:653–7.

30. Open Clinical. Available at: http://www.openclinical.org/. Accessed October 10, 2009.

31. Durieux P, Nizard R, Ravaud P, et al. A clinical decision support system for prevention of venous thromboembolism: effect on physician behavior. *JAMA*. 2000;283(21):2816–21.

32. Shiffman RN, Liaw Y, Brandt CA, et al. Computer-based guideline implementation systems: a systematic review of functionality and effectiveness. *J Am Med Inform Assoc*. 1999;6(2):104–14.

33. The Informatics Review. Available at: http://www.informatics-review.com/index.html. Accessed October 10, 2009.

34. Kuperman GJ, Bobb A, Payne TH, et al. Medication-related clinical decision support in computerized provider order entry systems: a review. *J Am Med Inform Assoc*. 2007;14(1): 29–40.

35. Schedlbauer A, Prasad V, Mulvaney C, et al. What evidence supports the use of computerized alerts and prompts to improve clinicians' prescribing behavior? *J Am Med Inform Assoc*. 2009;16(4):531–8.

36. Overhage JM, Tierney WM, Zhou XH, et al. A randomized trial of "corollary orders" to prevent errors of omission. *J Am Med Inform Assoc*. 1997;4(5):364–75.

37. Wright A, Sittig DF. Automated development of order sets and corollary orders by data mining in an ambulatory computerized physician order entry system. AMIA *Annu Symp Proc.* 2006:819–23.
38. Murff HJ, Gandhi TK, Karson AK, et al. Primary care attitudes concerning follow-up of abnormal test results and ambulatory decision support systems. *Int J Med Informatics.* 2003;71:137–49.
39. Kawamoto K, Houlihan CA, Balas EA, et al. Improving clinical practice using clinical decision support systems: a systematic review of trials to identify features critical to success. BMJ. 2005;330(7494):765 [Epub].
40. Classen DC, Pestotnik SL, Evans RS, et al. Adverse drug events in hospitalized patients. Excess length of stay, extra costs, and attributable mortality. JAMA.1997;277(4):301–6.
41. Kaushal R, Jha AK, Franz C, et al. Return on investment for a computerized physician order entry system. J *Am Med Inform Assoc.* 2006;13(3):261–6.
42. Berner ES, ed. *Clinical Decision Support Systems.* New York: Springer; 1999.
43. Paterno MD, Maviglia SM, Gorman PN, et al. Tiering drug- drug interaction alerts by severity increases compliance rates. J *Am Med Inform Assoc.* 2009;16(1):40–6.
44. Weingart SN, Toth M, Sands DZ, et al. Physicians' decisions to override computerized drug alerts in primary care. *Arch Intern Med.* 2003;163(21):2625–31.
45. Shah NR, Seger AC, Seger DL, et al. Improving acceptance of computerized prescribing alerts in ambulatory care. J *Am Med Inform Assoc.* 2006;13(1):5–11.
46. Kuperman GJ, Reichley RM, Bailey TC. Using commercial knowledge bases for clinical decision support: opportunities, hurdles, and recommendations. J *Am Med Inform Assoc.* 2006;13(4):369–71.

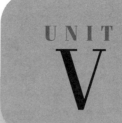

Medication Use Process II: Pharmacist Initiation and Assessment of Medication Interventions

UNIT COMPETENCIES

- Demonstrate efficient and responsible use of clinical decision support tools to solve patient-related problems.
- Apply principles of evidence-based medicine to the medication use process.
- Discuss the development of electronic decision support tools and their strengths and limitations.
- Discuss the impact of alerts on workflow and health care outcomes.
- Identify common clinical decision support tools.
- Describe the role of information systems in health care management.

UNIT DESCRIPTION

This second unit addressing the medication use process focuses on the "transcribing" step. Here, pharmacists use informatics tools to do much more than simply transcribe a medication order. The pharmacy information management system is the core system that supports pharmacists' clinical and administrative activities and is discussed in this unit. Pharmacists (and all clinicians) rely on evidence-based information to make informed decisions that impact patient care. This information is presented to pharmacists through knowledge systems. These topics are addressed in this unit as well.

Pharmacy Information Management Systems: In the Era of Integration

Mark H. Siska

OBJECTIVES

1. Identify the phases of the medication use process primarily supported by current pharmacy information management systems (PIMS).
2. Discuss the limitations of current PIMS in providing closed loop medication ordering and administration.
3. Describe the features required of future PIMS in the era of integration.

npatient and ambulatory pharmacy information management systems (PIMS) have played an integral role in supporting traditional order fulfillment, preparation, distribution, dispensing, and billing functions, which are critical to a pharmacy operation. More recently, these systems have evolved to assist in managing inventory; prioritizing physician and patient orders; screening for and alerting pharmacists of clinically important drug-drug interactions, dosing decisions, allergies, and other potentially harmful medication therapy orders. With the addition of interfaces and supplementary medication management supporting technologies, including automated dispensing devices and order management systems, pharmacies have been able to successfully improve operational efficiencies, as well as medication-related quality initiatives and safety. PIMS have also served as documentation and communication tools for recording pharmacist interventions and other pertinent clinical information, thereby ensuring effective handoffs and continuity of care among pharmacy personnel.

Despite offering a number of significant benefits, past and present-day PIMS that have focused on the traditional pharmacy operations of transcribing, dispensing, and distribution will require dramatic reengineering in the era of integration. These systems will need to serve as the focal point, rather than the end point, for closed loop medication management, thereby adding additional functionality to effectively distribute and exchange medication-related information beyond pharmacy operations and the transcription and dispensing phases of the medication use process.[1] This chapter will summarize the current and future states of PIMS in the era of integration and interoperability.

The Current State of PIMS

Legacy and current PIMS predominantly support traditional pharmacy core functions focused on the transcribing and dispensing phases of the medication use process[2] (Figure 12–1). Integration with supporting and complementary applications or technologies (including automated dispensing cabinets; and hospital information management, accounting, and inventory and work flow management systems) typically involve unidirectional or bidirectional point-to-point interfaces.[3] These loosely integrated best-of-breed applications are effective in streamlining and improving depart-

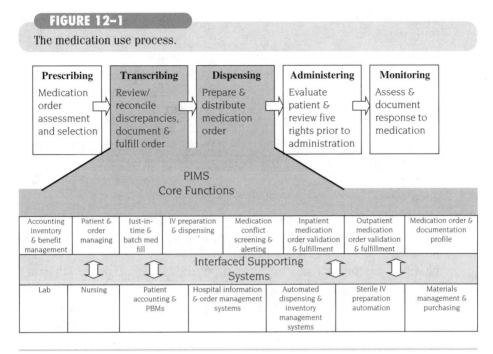

FIGURE 12-1

The medication use process.

PBM = pharmacy benefits manager; PIMS = pharmacy information management systems.
Source: Adapted from Reference 1.

mental operations, and in improving targeted medication-related safety and quality initiatives. However, these applications are limited in their ability to connect or integrate with other systems that support the medication use process, including prescribing and ordering systems, resulting in "siloed" medication management solutions in which continuity and collaboration among pharmacists, nurses, and physicians play an important role in improving medication safety.[3]

The human as well as financial cost of medication errors and recommended solutions for improvement prompted the health care industry, large health care purchasers, and state and federal government to adopt and implement health information technology solutions to minimize medication-related errors.[4] The suggested improvements meant that organizations would need to reengineer existing error-prone medication use processes by introducing additional systems and improving existing applications to support end-to-end management across the continuum of care.[5,6] During the implementation of existing technologies to support the wings of the medication use process—including computerized provider order entry (CPOE) systems, electronic medication administration records (eMARs), and point-of-care bar code medication administration (BCMA) systems—current PIMS were found to be unable to integrate or even interface with these systems, which were predominately designed around paper ordering and medication administration processes.

The emphasis on improving medication continuity and performing medication reconciliation across all episodes of care (outpatient and inpatient) further exposed the limitations of existing PIMS, which were primarily designed to accommodate the inpatient and retail pharmacy environments with stand-alone disparate applications.[2]

Finally, the implementation of electronic medical records (EMRs), personal health records (PHRs), and electronic prescribing (e-prescribing) has forced health care organizations and pharmacies to reengineer existing pharmacy operational models and supporting PIMS to assist in delivering services across the enterprise and other business entities. Current PIMS lack the bandwidth and connectivity to effectively integrate with drug wholesalers', distributors', materials management, and other EMR or PHR systems.[2] The expansion of electronic data resources in health care, including clinical systems in hospitals (CPOE, clinical documentation, eMAR) and pharmacy health information exchanges, has allowed information and knowledge to be delivered at the point of care and utilized to provide concurrent or retrospective clinical decision support. Current PIMS are unable to effectively integrate with these data resources to perform the clinical rules, alerts, and decision support that play significant roles in improving medication-related safety and quality.

The Future of PIMS

To address the multitude of operational transformations driven by supporting medication management systems including CPOE, e-prescribing BCMA, PHRs, and EMRs, the PIMS must be able to facilitate real-time communication, exchange, and understanding of data across all clinical applications supporting the medication use process. PIMS will be required to be part of or tightly coupled with EMR system components to allow the provision of collaborative medication-related data flows.[2] Next-generation PIMS must not have costly, difficult-to-maintain, point-to-point interfaced solutions and must offer **system interoperability,** which is defined in health care as the ability of different information technology systems and software applications to communicate and exchange data accurately, effectively, and consistently, and to use the information that has been exchanged.[6] Beyond their ability to support the acute and ambulatory clinical environments, future PIMS systems will be expected to interoperate with clinical data warehouses and enterprise resource planning systems, including accounts payable, supply chain management, and human resources systems (Figure 12–2).[2] The following sections describe the future PIMS requirements in the context of the medication use process.

Ordering and Prescribing

PIMS must provide interoperable support of order-processing information across the continuum of care including inpatient and ambulatory environments. The electronic handoffs from physician ordering systems (CPOE and e-prescribing) to PIMS must allow for seamless exchange and use of information, without any requirements for transcription. PIMS must tightly integrate medication order management with enterprise-wide process tracking systems, allowing upstream or downstream providers to access information regarding the status of their order. Integration of PIMS and supply chain management systems is also needed to allow real-time inventory administration. The PIMS must provide customizable order views, triaging capabilities, and the ability to communicate delivery or availability time of a particular order to others involved in the medication use process. The PIMS also must provide a variety of mechanisms for notifying performing departments of pending orders, including text and verbal paging.[3]

Transcribing

The PIMS should provide the needed flexibility to support the workflow of pharmacists, technicians, nurses, or other qualified providers or groups of providers. Order verification and confirmation would include the process by which the pharmacist confirms the appropriateness of an ordered medication, including any alerts or patient-specific information such as laboratory tests and results from procedures. With the primary emphasis of medication-related screening and alerting tools shifting to the providers in the ordering systems, future PIMS will play a secondary role in managing this type of clinical decision support. Despite their diminished role in

FIGURE 12–2

Pharmacy information management systems of the future.

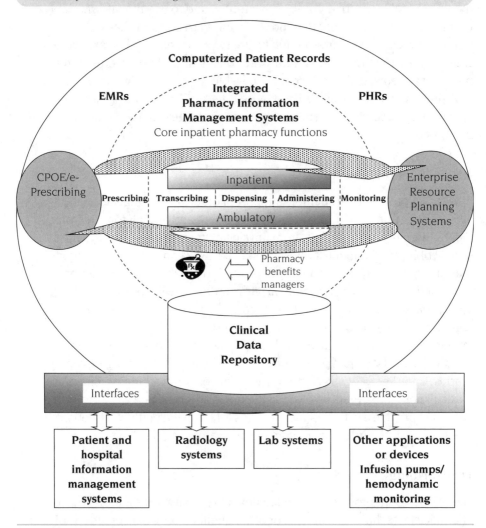

CPOE = computerized prescriber order entry; EMR = electronic medical record;
PHR = personal health record.
Source: Author.

managing these alerts, PIMS must allow for effective communication to downstream providers—including how the alert was reconciled—to minimize needless callbacks. The system must permit the user to defer verification or modification and facilitate communication with the physician or nurse regarding verification status.

The system should allow the pharmacist to fulfill an order with the necessary components to deliver an administrable dose without altering the integrity of the order or requiring additional communication with the ordering provider. The PIMS should allow the pharmacist to edit the provider's medication order during verification and fulfillment, with or without requiring the provider's signature. The fulfillment process should be transparent to the ordering process and should avoid any additional transcription.[3]

Dispensing

Once an order has been verified, confirmed, and fulfilled with the appropriate components for preparation, the PIMS must communicate requirements to the supporting medication preparation, dispensing, patient accounting, and prescription benefit systems that will preserve the medication integrity and security. Such systems might include automated dispensing cabinets, robotic intravenous automation medical devices, and automated dispensing and packaging systems.

These systems must work collectively, prioritize the daily drug preparation and fulfillment processes, and utilize bar code technology at each step to enhance efficiency and dispensing accuracy. PIMS must provide the flexibility to support a number of delivery approaches, focusing on just-in-time, patient-specific distribution and avoiding functionality that promotes unordered drugs on the patient care units.

PIMS must interoperate with supporting medication management automation, such as dispensing cabinets and storage and retrieval systems that manage inventory throughout the receiving, storage, retrieval, and distribution process.[3] Requirements should include:

- The support of electronic procurement and electronic pedigree.
- Real-time, on-hand inventory information at the time of patient-specific medication ordering and/or verification and fulfillment.
- Inventory control across multiple facilities.

■ Automated workflow in the distribution process, with sequenced orders that guide staff through emergency, high-priority, routine, and batch order fulfillment.

Administering

Future PIMS must play a significant role in the drug administration and documentation processes. These systems need to act as an intermediary and facilitator for closing the loop between ordering and medication administration systems by translating what has been ordered and dispensed into a bar code-enabled, administrable dose on an electronic "to do" list. Proper documentation of and/or scanning of these doses should fulfill the eMAR. This record needs to be a continuous document that includes medications administered across all levels and episodes of care within all areas of the organization. The eMAR must also be capable of linking with the organization's billing and financial services systems to improve compliance with billing regulations.

The PIMS must provide a means to reconcile doses from medication administration systems and the order fulfillment and preparation processes with the pharmacy's inventory management systems. PIMS must be able to connect to and exchange information with ordering and drug delivery systems as well monitoring devices, including intravenous infusion pumps, bed scales, and physiological monitoring systems, allowing for real-time communication between systems in multiple directions. Through their ability to interoperate with supporting medication administration technologies, PIMS must be able to recognize when to prepare and send another continuous medication infusion without a nurse or member of the pharmacy intervening. PIMS must provide the capability to send specific medication administration instructions directly to an infusion device to deliver a particular medicine over a specified period of time. These types of requirements reemphasize the need for future PIMS to not only communicate information, but to also use information from other administration-related systems.[3]

Monitoring

PIMS must incorporate functionality to support the documentation and monitoring of pharmacists' clinical interventions as well as adverse drug reaction or event reporting. These systems must interoperate with clinical data repositories and warehouses, and use EMR and other clinical application data to run clinical rules and provide real-time clinical decisions and analytics. PIMS must allow for data mining and extraction, allowing users or managers to develop and run queries spontaneously without dramatically affecting system performance. The ability for pharmacy managers and users to run ad hoc or planned detailed reports helps identify trends in acceptance of interventions, time spent on clinical activities, and avoidance of unnecessary drug costs. The PIMS must provide pharmacy managers with key financial and clinical outcomes data to quantify and improve their clinical programs and staff.[3] Additional features required of future PIMS include:

- Electronic notification or alerting to appropriate caregiver(s) about interventions, adverse drug reactions, and/or medication errors.
- Ability to electronically reconcile or share follow-up information of ongoing monitoring of patients' clinical events.
- Real-time management reporting and trending capabilities that can be exported and graphed.
- The capability to support mobile solutions.
- Integrated in-depth drug information.

Conclusion

Future PIMS must be developed to interoperate with supporting medication management systems and technologies across all disciplines involved in the medication use cycle and throughout the continuum of care.[7] Future PIMS designs must consider the application as the focal point for facilitating medication management interoperability across all supporting systems, eliminating redundant and error-prone practices, reducing the number of opportunities for medication-related mistakes, and effectively closing the loop on the medication use process.[1] These systems must also incorporate designs to interoperate with enterprise resource planning systems, allowing for streamlining of processes such as inventory management and control, billing, and other operations, which will help free pharmacists to conduct patient and physician consultations focused on improved medication therapy management and patient outcomes.

LEARNING ACTIVITIES

1. Identify other business or technology sectors that have successfully created supporting systems that are interoperable.
2. Research and discuss the current technical and semantic standards available for electronic medication management communication and exchange.
3. Identify and discuss current barriers for medication management interoperability. What measures would you put in place to accelerate the development of interoperable systems?

References

1. U.S. Pharmacopeia. The medication use process. 2004. Available at: http://www.usp.org/pdf/EN/patientSafety/medicationUseProcess.pdf. Accessed October 12, 2009.
2. Davis M. *Next-Generation Provider Pharmacy Systems*. Rockville, MD: Gartner Research; June 12, 2002.
3. Siska M. Functional requirements for pharmacy information management systems [serial online]. *Pharm Purch Prod*. November 2006:2–5. Available at: http://www.pppmag.com/documents/V3N8/P2–5.pdf. Accessed October 12, 2009.
4. Bates D. Incidence of adverse drug events and potential adverse drug events. JAMA. 1995;274(1):29–34.
5. Leape L. Systems analysis of adverse drug events. JAMA. 1995;274(1)35–43.
6. Broder C. Healthcare IT groups wrestle with interoperability definition. March 25, 2005. Available at: http://www.healthcareitnews.com/news/healthcare-it-groups-wrestle-interoperability-definition. Accessed October 12, 2009.
7. Evaluating pharmacy information systems: KLAS report provides guidance [serial online]. *Pharm Purch Prod*. 2005;2(4):16, 18–19. Available at: http://www.pppmag.com/documents/V2N4/Klas_May05.pdf. Accessed October 12, 2009.

CHAPTER 13

Evidence-Based Medicine, Clinical Tools, and Evaluation of the Evidence

Valerie Castellani Sheehan

OBJECTIVES

1. Define evidence-based medicine (EBM).
2. Explain the two fundamental principles of EBM.
3. Understand what EBM is and what it is not.
4. Explain the steps involved in applying the principles of EBM to the medication use process.
5. Identify different electronic resources for EBM.
6. Describe why EBM does not replace clinical judgment.

How Can Pharmacists Keep Up?

How many journal articles does a practitioner read each day? MEDLINE indexes more than 17 million articles, with 2000 to 4000 articles added

Editor's Note: MEDLINE is the National Library of Medicine [NLM] bibliographic database that contains references to journal articles in the life sciences with a concentration on biomedicine.

every day.[1,2] A general practitioner would need to read 20 articles every day just to maintain present knowledge.[3] Therefore, it is critical that pharmacists are able to find and use information efficiently and effectively. Evidence-based medicine (EBM) is one method that pharmacists and other clinicians can use to accomplish this goal. **Evidence-based medicine** is the conscientious, explicit, and judicious use of current best evidence in making decisions about the care of individual patients.[4] The first published appearance of the term was in the American College of Physicians' Journal Club in 1991.[5] EBM can be used at the individual patient level to help determine health policy, to manage public health, and to make system-level decisions. For EBM to be useful, it requires not only evaluation of the evidence but clinical expertise and knowledge of the individual patient's situation, beliefs, priorities, and values. Although EBM was first referenced in the medical literature, it has also become an integral part of the pharmacist's decision-making process.

EBM involves two fundamental principles. The first is a hierarchy of evidence to guide clinical decision making. The second principle is that evidence alone is never sufficient to make a clinical decision.[5] The **hierarchy of evidence** is a system of classifying and organizing types of evidence, typically for questions of treatment and prevention. There are different hierarchies of evidence depending on the issue being studied. For example, a study about diagnosis would not randomize patients to different groups; rather, the top of the hierarchy would include studies that enrolled patients about whom clinicians had diagnostic uncertainty, and that undertook a blind comparison between the candidate test and a gold standard.

Another way to think about the hierarchy of evidence is the evidence pyramid (Figure 13–1).[6] With each step up the pyramid, the evidence is of a higher quality and fewer articles of that type are published:

- **Case reports/case series:** Describe reports on the treatment of individual patients. Case reports/series do not use control groups.
- **Case-control studies:** Retrospectively study patients with a specific condition and compare their outcomes with those of a control group who do not have the condition.
- **Cohort studies:** Evaluate a large population and follow patients who have a specific condition or receive a particular treatment over time and compare them with another group that is similar (i.e., have all the same baseline characteristics) but has not been affected by the condition being studied.

FIGURE 13–1

The evidence pyramid.

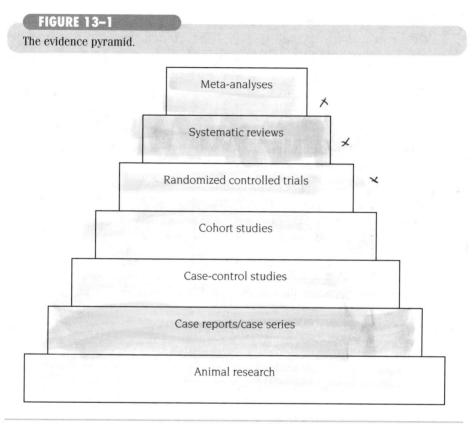

Source: Adapted from Reference 6.

- **Randomized controlled trials (RCTs):** Randomly assign subjects to a treatment, no treatment, or placebo group. Studies are usually blinded (neither the researcher nor the subject knows which intervention the subject received).
- **Systematic reviews:** Evaluate multiple RCTs to answer a specific question. Extensive literature searches are conducted (usually by different researchers) to identify studies with sound methodology. The results are not statistically combined.
- **Meta-analyses:** Use statistical techniques to combine the results of several studies as if they were one large study.

Despite EBM being a relatively new concept in the practice of medicine, it has been fraught with controversy. Some fear that EBM will eliminate the "art" of medicine and the individual clinician's expertise/judgment. Others fear that EBM will be hijacked by purchasers and managers to cut the costs of health care. This would not only be a misuse of EBM but would suggest a fundamental misunderstanding of its financial consequences. Those practicing EBM will identify and apply the most efficacious interventions to maximize the quality and quantity of life for individual patients; this may raise rather than lower the cost of their care. To have a good understanding of EBM, one needs to know what EBM is and what it is not.

EBM *is* integrating individual clinical expertise with the best available external clinical evidence from systematic research. **Individual clinical expertise** means the proficiency and judgment that individual clinicians acquire through clinical experience and practice. Increased expertise is reflected in many ways, but especially in more effective and efficient diagnosis and in the more thoughtful identification and compassionate use of individual patients' predicaments, rights, and preferences in making clinical decisions about their care. **Best available external clinical evidence** means clinically relevant research, often from the basic sciences of medicine, but especially from patient-centered clinical research into the accuracy and precision of diagnostic tests (including the clinical examination), the power of prognostic markers, and the efficacy and safety of therapeutic, rehabilitative, and preventive regimens. Optimal care is delivered through the use of both individual clinical expertise and the best available external evidence—neither alone is sufficient.[4]

EBM *is not* old hat, impossible to practice, or "cookbook" medicine. External clinical evidence can inform, but never replace, individual clinical expertise. It is this expertise that decides whether the external evidence applies to the individual patient at all and, if so, how it should be integrated into a clinical decision. Similarly, any external guideline must be integrated with individual clinical expertise in deciding whether and how it matches the patient's clinical state, predicament, and preferences, and thus whether it should be applied. EBM is not restricted to randomized trials and meta-analyses. It involves tracking down the best external evidence with which to answer clinical questions. The randomized trial, especially the systematic review of several randomized trials, has become the gold standard for judging whether a treatment does more good than harm. However, some questions about therapy do not require randomized trials (successful interventions for otherwise fatal conditions) or cannot wait for the trials to be conducted.[4]

Like most things, EBM is not perfect. Several limitations to EBM are worth noting[6]:

- There is a low yield of clinically useful articles.
- There are frequent conflicts of interest.
- It is often not known who has reviewed an article and how rigorous the review was.
- Different evidence rating systems are used by various organizations.
- Different conclusions may be drawn by experts evaluating the same study.
- It is a time-intensive exercise to evaluate evidence.
- Systematic reviews are limited in topics reviewed and are time intensive to complete.
- Randomized controlled trials are expensive to conduct.
- Studies with negative results are not always published (this is referred to as publication bias).
- Results may not be applicable to every patient population.

Steps Involved in Applying the Principles of EBM to the Medication Use Process

The application of EMB to a specific patient begins after a correct diagnosis is made. The pharmacist then determines that a legitimate, medication-related clinical question exists. Four steps are then followed to apply the EMB process to that pharmacotherapeutic question[7] (Figure 13–2):

1. Recognize information needs and convert them into answerable questions.
2. Conduct efficient searches for the best evidence with which to answer these questions.
3. Critically appraise the evidence for its validity and usefulness.
4. Apply the results to patient situations to best assist clinical decision making.

FIGURE 13-2

An approach to using the medical literature to provide optimal patient care.

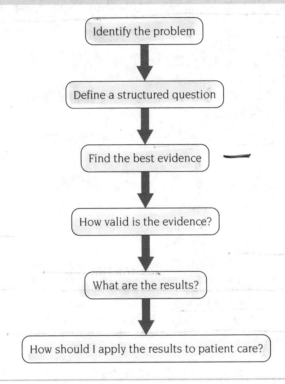

Source: Reference 5.

Step 1: Recognize Information Needs and Convert Them into Answerable Questions

A well-formulated question includes the following elements[8]:

- The **P**atient or problem being addressed: How do you describe the patient group you are interested in? Elderly? Gender? Diabetic?
- The **I**ntervention being considered: What is being introduced? A new drug or test?
- The **C**omparison intervention: Is it another drug or a placebo?
- The **O**utcome of interest: What are you trying to measure? Mortality? Hospitalization?

This method is frequently referred to as the "PICO Method for Framing a Clinical Question."[6] The PICO Method was developed by the NLM. A Web-based PICO tool has been created by the NLM to search MEDLINE.[9]

Once the question is framed, it will likely fall into one of five fundamental categories[5]:

1. **Therapy:** Determining the effect of interventions on patient-important outcomes (symptoms, function, morbidity, mortality, costs).
2. **Harm:** Ascertaining the effects of potentially harmful agents on patient-important outcomes.
3. **Differential diagnosis:** In patients with a particular clinical presentation, establishing the frequency of the underlying disorders.
4. **Diagnosis:** Establishing the power of a test to differentiate between those with and without a target condition or disease.
5. **Prognosis:** Estimating a patient's future course.

Step 2: Conduct Efficient Searches for the Best Evidence with Which to Answer These Questions

Depending on the question, the search may lead to electronic sources, print references, or both. The wide availability and variety of electronic references have made it increasingly difficult for printed references to compete—especially when printed medical references can quickly become out of date (if they are not outdated by the time they are published). Most pharmacy students have access to a diverse collection of electronic references through their affiliation with their school's library. Once in practice, access to references will often depend on the references available at the place of employment.

Ideal medical resources are those that are[6]:

- Evidence-based with references and level of evidence.
- Updated frequently.
- Simple to access with a single sign-on (if electronic).
- Available at the point of care.
- Capable of being embedded into an electronic medical record.
- Likely to produce an answer with only a few clicks (if electronic).
- Useful for primary care practitioners and specialists.
- Written and organized with the end user in mind.

TABLE 13-1

Categories of Clinical Information Resources

Category	Description	How Many Exist	Examples
Systems	Textbook-like resources that summarize and integrate clinical evidence with other types of information directed at clinical practice decisions/directions	Few	UpToDate Merck Manual
Synopses	Summaries of studies and systematic reviews that include guides or advice for application by expert clinicians	Several thousand	ACP Journal Club DARE (Database of Abstracts of Reviews of Effects)
Summaries	Systematic review of articles and clinical practice guidelines; user assesses the information and makes the decision	Fewer than 50,000	National Guideline Clearinghouse Cochrane Database of Systematic Reviews
Studies	Individual studies	Millions	MEDLINE PubMed

Source: Adapted from Reference 5.

Clinical information resources can fall into one of four categories: systems, synopses, summaries, and studies as outlined in Table 13–1. A list of electronic EBM resources can be found in Table 13–2.

Step 3: Critically Appraise the Evidence for Its Validity and Usefulness

A 25-part series called the "Users' Guides to the Medical Literature" was published in JAMA between 1993 and 2000.[10] The purpose of this series was to educate clinicians on how to read clinical journal articles. Even though this series of articles was targeted toward physicians, it can also aid pharmacists in accomplishing the third step in this process.

Step 4: Apply the Results to Patient Situations to Best Assist Clinical Decision Making

Once the evidence is gathered, clinical expertise must be applied and patient characteristics must be evaluated. The pharmacist must look at the whole

TABLE 13–2

Popular EBM Resources for Pharmacy

Resource	Web Site
ACP Journal Club	www.acpjc.org
Agency for Healthcare Research and Quality (AHRQ)	www.ahrq.gov
AHRQ Evidence-Based Practice Program	www.ahrq.gov/clinic/epcix.htm
ASHP Policy Positions and Guidelines (Best Practices)	www.ashp.org/bestpractices
Bandolier	www.medicine.ox.ac.uk/bandolier
Centre for Evidence-Based Medicine (at Oxford)	www.cebm.net
Google Scholar	www.scholar.google.com
Guidelines International Network	www.g-i-n.net
Health Information Research Unit at McMaster University	hiru.mcmaster.ca/hiru
Health Services/Technology Assessment Text	www.ncbi.nlm.nih.gov/books/bv.fcgi?rid=hstat
International Centre for Allied Health Evidence, Division of Health Sciences, University of South Australia	www.unisa.edu.au/cahe/CAHECATS
JAMAevidence	www.jamaevidence.com
Medal.org (medical algorithms)	www.medal.org/visitor/login.aspx
National Guideline Clearinghouse	www.guidelines.gov
Netting the Evidence	www.nettingtheevidence.org.uk
STAT!Ref	www.statref.com
SUMSearch	sumsearch.uthscsa.edu
The Cochrane Library	www3.interscience.wiley.com/cgi-bin/mrwhome/106568753/HOME
Turning Research Into Practice (TRIP) Database	www.tripdatabase.com

ASHP = American Society of Health-System Pharmacists; EBM = evidence-based medicine.
Source: Author.

picture and decide which therapy is best for the individual patient. The decision should be based on the evidence as well as the patient's individual needs, beliefs, and values.

Important Online Resources for Evidence-Based Medicine

Readers are encouraged to visit and explore each Web site in Table 13–2, and to add other sites of interest to the "Favorites" feature of their Internet browser or to their social bookmarking site.

Conclusion

A basic knowledge of EBM—and its integration into one's practice—is essential for any pharmacist who wants to provide quality care to patients. EBM touches every aspect and area of pharmacy—from the retail pharmacist evaluating polypharmacy on a patient's profile, to the hospital pharmacist applying laboratory results to a patient's therapy, to the pharmacist at a pharmacy benefit management (PBM) company who evaluates medications for that PBM's formulary. Establishing an efficient method for keeping up with the literature and applying the principles of EBM are necessary skills for every pharmacist.

LEARNING ACTIVITIES

1. List at least two pros and two cons of EBM.
2. Visit at least three of the Web sites listed in Table 13–2. For each site, identify the benefits of the site and in what circumstances that site would be useful for applying EBM.
3. Apply the EBM process to the following scenario: A physician asks you to help determine which medication would be most appropriate for a patient who is at risk for osteoporosis. The patient is a 63-year-old woman with a history of non-adherence with her current medications. What questions would you ask yourself and the physician to make an evidence-based decision?

References

1. National Library of Medicine. FAQ: finding medical information in MEDLINE. Available at: http://www.nlm.nih.gov/services/usemedline.html. Accessed April 30, 2010.
2. National Library of Medicine. MEDLINE fact sheet. Available at: http://www.nlm.nih.gov/pubs/factsheets/medline.html. Accessed October 11, 2009.
3. Shaneyfelt TM. Building bridges to quality. JAMA. 2001;286(20):2600–1.
4. Sackett DL, Rosenberg WMC, Gray JAM, et al. Evidence based medicine: what it is and what it isn't. BMJ. 1996;312(7023):71. Available at: http://www.bmj.com/cgi/content/full/312/7023/71. Accessed October 15, 2009.
5. Rennie D. *Users' Guides to the Medical Literature*: A Manual for Evidence-Based Clinical Practice. 2nd ed. New York, NY: McGraw-Hill Medical; 2008.
6. Hoyt R, Sutton M, Yoshihashi A. *Medical Informatics: Practical Guide for the Healthcare Professional.* 2008. 2nd ed. Pensacola, FL: University of West Florida, School of Allied Health and Life Sciences, Medical Informatics Program; 2008.
7. Sackett DL. *Evidence-Based Medicine: How to Practice and Teach EBM.* 2nd ed. Edinburgh, Scotland; New York, NY: Churchill Livingstone; 2000.
8. Richardson WS, Wilson MC, Nishikawa J, et al. The well-built clinical question: a key to evidence-based decisions. ACP J Club. 1995 Nov–Dec;123(3):A12–A13.
9. National Library of Medicine. PubMed/MEDLINE via PICO. Available at: http://askmedline.nlm.nih.gov/ask/pico.php. Accessed October 11, 2009.
10. JAMA Web site [search feature]. Available at: http://jama.ama-assn.org/cgi/search?&quicksearch_submit.y=8&quicksearch_submit.x=12&fulltext=Users%27guides+to+the+medical+literature&hits=25. Accessed June 14, 2010.

Clinical Decision Support Systems in Pharmacy Practice

Valerie Castellani Sheehan

OBJECTIVES

1. Define clinical decision support systems (CDSS).
2. List the major elements comprising a CDSS.
3. Distinguish between severity and evidence thresholds with regard to CDSS.
4. Describe several different types of CDSS.
5. Explain the "10 commandments" of effective clinical decision support.
6. Describe important considerations for CDSS use in pharmacy.

With the implementation of computerized provider order entry (CPOE), the topic of clinical decision support systems (CDSS) has become increasingly prevalent in the biomedical literature on health care. CPOE is best able to improve patient safety when combined with CDSS. The focus of much of the CDSS literature is on the impact and interplay of CDSS and CPOE as they pertain to physicians and the creation of prescription and other types of medical orders. (Use of CDSS at prescribing is addressed in Chapter 11; this topic precedes this chapter because the current chapter addresses CDSS as a general tool for pharmacists that is often used after the prescription is created). However, it is important to recognize that pharmacy has utilized CDSS literally for decades. Pharmacy use of CDSS has focused on the evaluation of medication safety in the context of an individual patient's current and new medication orders.

There are many definitions of CDSS. As defined by the MEDLINE Medical Subject Headings (MeSH) scope notes, **clinical decision support systems** refers to "computer-based information systems used to integrate clinical and patient information and provide support for decision-making in patient care."[1] Computer-generated recommendations may be delivered to the clinician, including pharmacists, through the electronic medical record, by pager, or through printouts placed in a patient's paper chart.[2] The most common method of presenting CDSS messages to pharmacists in commentency and institutional settings is through pharmacy information management systems (PIMS).

CDSS Fundamentals

A computer-based CDSS evaluation of medication usage involves the interplay between three complex elements: one or more human intermediaries, an integrated computerized system and its interface, and the knowledge in the decision support system.[3] CDSS have several different functions as outlined in Table 14–1.

According to a 2007 survey conducted by the American Society of Health-System Pharmacists, 12% of U.S. hospitals have implemented CPOE with a robust CDSS.[4] In the same study, up to 90% of hospitals reported that they were planning to look at this technology over the following 3 years. The study did not address CDSS usage within PIMS, but the author's experience is that the overwhelming majority of hospital and community pharmacies (>90%) utilize CDSS in the pharmacist's review of medication orders and patient profiles.

For patients to receive optimal benefit, CDSS must inform medication-related decision making—either directly at prescribing as discussed in Chapter 11, or indirectly during transcribing/order review by the pharmacist, That behavior change should positively affect the outcomes of patients. It

TABLE 14–1

Functions of Computer-Based Clinical Decision Support Systems

Function	Example
Alerting	Notifying user of drug level that is outside the normal range
Reminding	Reminding clinician to administer vaccinations
Critiquing	Rejecting an order for a new drug when a patient has a contraindication to that drug
Interpreting	Analyzing an EEG
Predicting	Calculating pneumonia severity risk using the PSI/PORT score
Diagnosing	Listing a differential diagnosis for a patient with cough
Assisting	Providing dosing recommendations for renal failure patients
Suggesting	Generating suggestions for monitoring INR for a patient receiving warfarin

EEG = electroencephalogram; INR = international normalized ratio; PORT = Pneumonia Patient Outcomes Research Team; PSI = Pneumonia Severity Index.
Source: Reference 3.

is possible that a CDSS could change prescriber behavior but have no influence on patient health outcomes.[3] Research in this area has focused predominantly on the ability of CDSS to change prescriber behavior and not on the systems' impact on pharmacists' decision making. To date, few studies that looked at patient outcomes as a result of those changes have been published; more studies on outcomes are needed. (See Chapter 11 for more details on published literature on outcomes.)

Three major elements comprise a CDSS: (1) a knowledge base, (2) a program for combining knowledge with patient-specific information, and (3) a mechanism to communicate with the user.[5] Many of the issues specific to a CDSS arise in its application, including how it presents the knowledge to the user. These topics are addressed in Chapter 11.

One example of application of CDSS is that it can assist with guideline implementation. Lomas et al. evaluated a series of published guidelines and found that it took an average of approximately 5 years for these guidelines to be adopted into routine practice.[6] Part of this lag time may be due to a lack of knowledge of the guidelines and how to apply them. CDSS can help by identifying appropriate patients and putting the guidelines in front of the provider at the time of decision making.

CDSS must have the ability to be integrated with existing information systems and software. Users must be able to maintain the system, and they must accept the system and ensure that it is kept up to date. Within health systems, building and maintaining interfaces to diverse computer systems is often challenging and sometimes almost impossible. Adding to the complexity is the fact that the inference engine used to compare the rules against the order entered into the database is usually not easily exported to other locations.[3]

Severity and Evidence Thresholds

A primary consideration for pharmacists' use of CDSS is determining the threshold of when messages that indicate the potential need for modification of medication therapy will be presented to pharmacists. There are two types of thresholds: severity and evidence. The **severity threshold** indicates the minimum severity that a drug-related problem must achieve prior to being presented to the pharmacist. For example, the CDSS can be set to present to the pharmacist only drug-related problems with a "high" potential severity. This approach will minimize disruptions in workflow, but it could allow important drug-related problems to "get through" the safety mechanism offered by the CDSS.

The alternative is to lower the severity threshold, thereby presenting potential drug-related problems of minor severity to the pharmacist. This alternative can significantly affect the pharmacists' workflow. Pharmacists who are presented a large number of messages may become desensitized to the messages. This can lead to a situation in which pharmacists are overwhelmed by messages and either miss an important one or simply ignore messages to be able to complete their activities. In either situation, patient safety is compromised.

Chapter 13 addresses the topic of evidence-based medicine (EBM). CDSS applications are frequently the mechanisms by which pharmacists are presented the "evidence" found in EBM. The consideration regarding the **evidence threshold** in CDSS is related to how much evidence should exist to substantiate presenting a drug-related problem message to a pharmacist. For evidence thresholds, the reciprocal holds true compared with the severity threshold. Setting the evidence threshold to "high" will decrease interruptions in workflow but could potentially allow important messages to be suppressed. A lower evidence threshold will allow more messages to be presented to the pharmacist because drug-related problems with less supporting evidence are presented. This leads to more disruptions in pharmacists' activities.

Most CDSS will allow some ability to adjust the severity and evidence thresholds. Adjusting the thresholds presents several challenges. Should a single threshold (severity and evidence) be set for all pharmacists? Can the thresholds be adjusted for each pharmacist on the basis of user log-in to the system? Can the thresholds be modified for specific medications? Can thresholds be adjusted in real time? Who has the ability to control the thresholds? In a hospital setting, the clinical coordinator and pharmacy director may establish policies that dictate the thresholds. Does a management structure exist that can control thresholds in the community environment—if so, does it differ for independent and chain stores? How are thresholds maintained for pharmacists who float among community pharmacies? Obviously, there are many important considerations regarding the use of CDSS within pharmacy. It is important to recognize that the decisions ultimately can impact patient safety.

Cost of CDSS

The cost of CDSS is an important consideration, especially within health systems. Facilities implementing CDSS likely have already begun implementation of CPOE. Optimally, the cost of CDSS should be accounted for during the budgeting for CPOE. Costs associated with CDSS include initial hardware, software, interface, training, maintenance fees, and upgrade costs.[3] Costs associated with non-CPOE CDSS are similar and include vendor maintenance and upgrade fees, time to customize the CDSS (as necessary), and potential impacts on time, which ultimately impact the bottom line in community pharmacies.

Types of CDSS

Several different types of CDSS programs, as defined by their functionality, are available today in institutional and community pharmacy settings. Depending on the product, these systems may or may not be integrated into electronic medical records. The following list reflects the range of CDSS functionality that is found across pharmacy and medicine settings (except #6 and #7, which are specific to physician practice)[7]:

1. Knowledge support: Provides integration of medical resources such as UpToDate.

2. Calculators: Estimate a patient's creatinine clearance, adjust a patient's phenytoin level, or determine a patient's body mass index, and so on.
3. Flow sheets, graphs, patient lists, and registries: Provide the ability to identify and track a trend for laboratory results and vital signs; provide the ability to use a patient list to contact every patient taking a recalled drug.
4. Medication order entry support: Provides rules engines to detect known allergies, drug-drug interactions, and excessive dosages. May also factor in the patient's age, gender, weight, renal and hepatic function, contraindications, and pregnancy and lactation status.
5. Reminders: Provide yearly tracking of preventive health screen measures, such as mammograms.
6. Order sets and protocols: Provide groups of pre-established orders that are related to a symptom or diagnoses. Order sets can reflect best practices.
7. Differential diagnosis: Generates differential diagnosis on the basis of input of patient's symptoms (e.g., chest pain).

The availability of each type of CDSS will largely be influenced by practice setting and available resources. At a minimum, a practice should be supported by a CDSS that checks drug-related problems (interactions, allergies, duplicate therapy, contraindications, etc.) during order review/entry (#4).

Ten Commandments of Effective Clinical Decision Support

Bates et al. have described the lessons they learned over 8 years of implementing and studying the impact of decision support across a variety of domains.[8] They summarized these lessons as the Ten Commandments of Effective Clinical Decision Support and believe that these concepts are key to installing effective CDSS. The list was originally developed on the basis of experience with CDSS to support CPOE. However, many items on the list are clearly applicable to pharmacy practice.

1. Speed is everything: Users value this parameter most. If decision support takes too long to appear on the computer screen, it will be useless.

2. Anticipate needs and deliver in real time: It is not enough for the information that a provider needs to simply be available someplace in the system. Applications must anticipate clinician needs and bring information to the clinicians at the time they need it. Optimal CDSS should also have the capability to anticipate the subtle "latent needs" of the user. **Latent needs** are needs that are present but have not been consciously realized. An example would be notifying a clinician when a patient's medication needs to be dose-adjusted for worsening renal function.

3. Fit into the user's workflow: The clinician's workflow must be considered in the design and implementation of CDSS.

4. Little things can make a big difference: Usability matters—a lot. Usability testing has traditionally not been a routine part of the design of CDSS. A minor change in the way screens are designed can have a major impact on provider actions.

5. Recognize that physicians will strongly resist stopping: Physicians strongly resist suggestions not to carry out an action when they are not offered an alternative. This also applies to pharmacy—a suggestion to stop a medication is not optimally useful if it does not include an alternative agent.

6. Changing direction is easier than stopping: Changing a prescriber's direction/behavior is easier when the issue at hand is part of an order that the prescriber probably does not have strong feelings about, such as the dose, route, or frequency of a medication or the views of a radiographic study.

7. Simple interventions work best: A good rule of thumb is to limit information to one screen. All clinicians are presented with large amounts of information when caring for just one patient. CDSS should minimize the information that is presented and concisely present the most relevant information.

8. Ask for additional information only when you really need it: Examples of this type of information include the weight of a patient and pregnancy status. Experience has shown that the likelihood of success in implementing a computerized guideline is inversely proportional to the number of extra data elements needed. However, key pieces of data, such as patient weight, should be collected as a routine part of care.

9. Monitor impact, get feedback, and respond: There should be a reasonable probability that reminders will be followed when delivered. Providing too many alerts will have a tendency to cause the prescriber to ignore all of them. Achieving the right balance between over and under alerting is difficult. This phenomenon is called "alert fatigue" and is one of the most challenging aspects of CDSS for pharmacists, physicians, and any other clinician who uses CDSS.

10. Manage and maintain your knowledge-based systems: The effort required to monitor and address issues in CDSS is considerable. It is critical to keep up with changing medical practice and ensure that systems are up-to-date. Although this recommendation is offered in the context of institutional practice, it applies to community practice, where pharmacists are the last line of defense before a medication is taken by the patient. An up-to-date knowledge base (CDSS) is critical to ensuring safe and effective medication therapy.

Other Considerations of CDSS

Before they implement CDSS, facilities need to evaluate/consider many elements. Table 14–2 lists important considerations to think about when implementing CDSS. As the core component of the PIMS that supports

---

TABLE 14–2

Important Considerations for Clinical Decision Support Systems

- Budget
- Information system infrastructure
- Use across multiple facilities
- User interface
- User trust in data (user must trust that data are correct)
- Downtime, response time (system must be available when needed)
- Training
- Local language/terminology
- Evidence-based logic
- Updating of logic in a timely manner
- Compatibility with legacy applications
- Methods for testing the system before deployment

Source: Author.

safe medication use, CDSS is a critical piece of an overall approach to patient safety. CDSS selection, maintenance, and management should be a focus of all pharmacy practice settings.

Online Resources for CDSS

Readers are encouraged to visit each of the Web sites in Table 14–3. Explore them and add ones of interest to the "Favorites" or "Bookmarks" feature of the Internet browser.

Conclusion

Pharmacy has a long history of using CDSS to support decision making. Recently, the widespread adoption of CDSS to support physicians' decision making has brought CDSS to the forefront of the biomedical literature. Many of the lessons learned by pharmacists are being applied to CDSS use in other clinical settings. Pharmacists are also learning from these other settings and applying this new knowledge to their use of CDSS.

All pharmacists use CDSS in their practice. It is a core component of a safe practice and its importance cannot be overstated. Pharmacists should understand the current implementation of CDSS in their practice setting. Opportunities to optimize and customize CDSS to the individual pharmacist's use should be explored. Ultimate control over CDSS functionality may not reside with each pharmacist, but all pharmacists have a responsibility to ensure they utilize all tools at their disposal to provide safe and efficacious medication therapy.

TABLE 14–3

Internet Resources for Clinical Decision Support

Resource	Web Site
Agency for Healthcare Research and Quality	www.healthit.ahrq.gov/portal/server.pt?open=514&objID= 5554&mode=2& (click on "Clinical Decision Support" in left navigation pane)
American Medical Informatics Association	www.amia.org/inside/initiatives/cds
Healthcare Information and Management Systems Society	www.himss.org/ASP/topics_clinicalDecision.asp

Source: Author.

LEARNING ACTIVITIES:

1. Write a CDSS rule for a drug allergy and adjustment of a medication on the basis of renal function.
2. If you were going to examine integrating CDSS into your hospital system, name at least five considerations you would need to examine.
3. Within your practice setting, determine the vendor of the CDSS knowledge base. How often is the knowledge base updated? What customization capabilities exist? Can severity and/or evidence thresholds be adjusted?

References

1. National Library of Medicine. Medical subject headings, decision support systems, clinical. Available at: http://www.nlm.nih.gov/cgi/mesh/2009/MB_cgi?mode=&index=18583&field= all&HM=&II=&PA=&form=&input=. Accessed October 11, 2009.
2. Garg AX, Adhikari NK, McDonald H, et al. Effects of computerized clinical decision support systems on practitioner performance and patient outcomes: a systematic review. JAMA. 2005; 293(10):1223–38.
3. Rennie D. *Users' Guides to the Medical Literature: A Manual for Evidence-Based Clinical Practice.* 2nd ed. New York, NY: McGraw-Hill Medical; 2008.
4. ASHP Council on Pharmacy Management. *Board of Directors Report on the Council of Pharmacy Management.* Bethesda, MD: American Society of Health-System Pharmacists; 2009.
5. Berner ES. *Clinical Decision Support Systems: State of the Art.* Rockville, MD: Agency for Healthcare Research and Quality; June 2009. Contract No.: AHRQ Publication No. 09-0069-EF.
6. Lomas J, Sisk JE, Stocking B. From evidence to practice in the United States, the United Kingdom, and Canada. *Milbank Q.* 1993;71(3):405–10.
7. Hoyt R, Sutton M, Yoshihashi A. *Medical Informatics: Practical Guide for the Healthcare Professional 2008.* 2nd ed. Pensacola, FL: University of West Florida, School of Allied Health and Life Sciences, Medical Informatics Program; 2008.
8. Bates DW, Kuperman GJ, Wang S, et al. Ten commandments for effective clinical decision support: making the practice of evidence-based medicine a reality. *J Am Med Inform Assoc.* 2003;10(6):523–30.

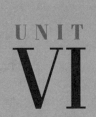

Medication Use Process III: Medication Dispensing and Distribution

UNIT COMPETENCIES

- Discuss standards for interoperability related to medications, diagnoses, communication, and electronic data interchange.
- Discuss technologies used to automate the medication delivery process.
- Discuss the value of bar-coded and radiofrequency identification for medication distribution and administration.
- Describe the role of information systems in health care management.

UNIT DESCRIPTION

After ensuring that safe and efficacious medication therapy has been prescribed, pharmacists manage the systems that dispense and distribute medications to nurses (in hospitals) or to the patients (in the community). Efficiency and safety are two key focus areas of the dispensing and distribution steps. In either setting of care, the acquisition of medications is an important administrative function that pharmacists perform. The chapters in this unit address these topics in the third stage of medication use process.

chapter 15

Pharmaceutical Supply Chain

Margaret R. Thrower

OBJECTIVES

1. Describe key components in the pharmaceutical supply chain.
2. Describe recent data on prescription volume and drug sales in the U.S. pharmaceutical supply chain.
3. Understand the flow of a medication from the manufacturer to the patient.
4. Identify key stakeholders involved in the supply chain.
5. Discuss pedigree and how it relates to the supply chain.

The pharmaceutical supply chain for prescription drugs is important, complex, and not well understood by most health care professionals. The **pharmaceutical supply chain** in its most simplified definition is the means through which prescription medicines are delivered to patients[1] (Figure 15–1). The supply chain begins at pharmaceutical manufacturing sites; the drugs are then transferred to wholesale distributors, which deliver ordered products to all types of pharmacies (e.g., community, mail order, hospital, and other types of pharmacies). Before being dispensed, the products are subject to price negotiations and processed through clinical and utilization management programs by

FIGURE 15-1

The pharmaceutical supply chain.

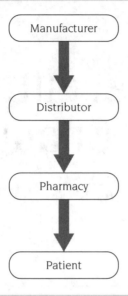

Source: Author.

pharmacy benefit management (PBM) companies (if the prescription is filled in the community pharmacy setting). The products are then dispensed by pharmacies and ultimately delivered to and taken by patients.[1] There are many variations of this basic structure and this structure continues to evolve. The pharmaceutical supply system comprises multiple players whose roles sometimes overlap (e.g., distribution and contracting). The intent of this chapter is to make the U.S. pharmaceutical supply chain transparent and better understood.

Currently, there are few published articles that review the pharmaceutical supply chain in detail. However, a comprehensive article written in 2005, "Follow The Pill: Understanding the U.S. Commercial Pharmaceutical Supply Chain," highlights this topic; key points from that publication can be found throughout this chapter.[1] Other chapters address various information technologies that support much of the information that flows through the pharmaceutical supply chain. These chapters focus on those components of the chain that occur after medications leave the manufacturer.

First, to properly emphasize the importance of the supply chain, one must quantify the total volume of the prescription drug market, given that it is one of the largest expenditures in the United States. In 2009, the total U.S. prescription market was more than $300 billion[2] and grew by 5.1% from 2008 to 2009. IMS Health is a global organization that collects pharmaceutical data from many sources, including wholesalers, drug manufacturers, community pharmacies, hospitals, long-term care facilities (LTCs), and health care professionals. IMS Health projects that in 2010 the global pharmaceutical market will increase by 4% to 6% . The organization also projects that the global pharmaceutical market is expected to continue growing at a rate of 5% to 8% annually through 2014.[3] (Tables 15–1 and 15–2 list the top U.S. prescription drug sales by volume

TABLE 15-1

Top Therapeutic U.S. Classes in 2009

	Ranked by Sales*		Ranked by Dispensed Prescriptions†	
Rank	Therapeutic Class	US$ (billions)	Therapeutic Class	Volume (in millions)
1	Antipsychotics, other	14.6	Lipid regulators	210.5
2	Lipid regulators	14.3	Codeine & combinations	200.2
3	Proton pump inhibitors	13.6	Antidepressants	168.7
4	Antidepressants	9.9	ACE inhibitors	162.8
5	Angiotensin II antagonists	8.4	Beta blockers	128.3
6	Antineoplastic monoclonal antibodies	8.0	Proton pump inhibitors	119.4
7	Antiarthritics, biological response modulators	6.3	Seizure disorders	104.5
8	Erythropoietins	6.3	Thyroid hormone, synthetic	103.3
9	Insulin analogues	6.3	Calcium blockers	91.9
10	Antiplatelets, oral	6.0	Benzodiazepines	87.9

ACE = angiotensin-converting enzyme.
*Total U.S. market is $300.3 billion.
†Total U.S. market is 3,922 million.
Source: IMS Health, Natural Sales Perspectives™ 2009, 660 W. Germantown Pike, Plymouth Meeting, PA 19462-0905. Used with permission. Available at: http://www.imshealth.com. Accessed May 5, 2010.

TABLE 15-2

Top U.S. Pharmaceutical Products in 2009

	Ranked by Sales		Ranked by Dispensed Prescriptions	
Rank	Product	US$ (billions)	Product	Number Dispensed (in millions)
1	Lipitor	7.5	Hydrocodone/acetaminophen	128.2
2	Nexium	6.3	Simvastatin	83.0
3	Plavix	5.6	Lisinopril	81.3
4	Advair Diskus	4.7	Levothyroxine sodium	66.0
5	Seroquel	4.2	Azithromycin	53.8
6	Abilify	4.0	Metformin HCl	52.0
7	Singulair	3.7	Lipitor	51.5
8	Actos	3.4	Amlodipine besylate	50.9
9	Enbrel	3.3	Amoxicillin	49.2
10	Epogen	3.2	Hydrochlorothiazide	47.1

HCl = hydrochloride.
Source: IMS Health, Natural Sales Perspectives™ 2009, 660 W. Germantown Pike, Plymouth Meeting, PA 19462-0905. Used with permission. Available at: http://www.imshealth.com. Accessed May 10, 2010.

in 2009 and identify the drugs that were sold and dispensed most often that year.)

The primary players in the pharmaceutical supply chain are[1]:

- Pharmaceutical manufacturers: A few large companies make up a majority of the brand pharmaceutical manufacturing industry today.
  - The 10 largest pharmaceutical corporations, as measured by U.S. revenue, are (1) Johnson & Johnson, (2) Pfizer, (3) Abbott Laboratories, (4) Merck & Co., (5) Wyeth, (6) Bristol-Myers Squibb, (7) Eli Lilly, (8) Schering-Plough, (9) Amgen, and (10) Gilead.[4]
  - Pharmaceutical manufacturers by far, have the most influence over pharmaceutical prices: They assess and anticipate expected demand, potential future competition, and evaluate and project marketing costs to establish the **wholesale acquisition cost**

(WAC), which is the baseline price at which wholesale distributors purchase drug products.[1]

■ Wholesale distributors: The wholesale distribution industry has consolidated in the last 30 years, with the number of wholesale distributors in the United States declining from approximately 200 in 1975 to fewer than 50 in 2000.[1] This consolidation trend has continued in the years following 2000.

● The top three wholesale distributors, ranked by revenue, account for almost 90% percent of the wholesale market: (1) McKesson, (2) Cardinal Health, and (3) AmerisourceBergen.[5]

● Automation and electronic processes make the business much more cost-effective and efficient. And, in recent years some wholesalers have diversified their businesses beyond "traditional" distribution services, offering more services and products.

■ Pharmacies: The type of pharmacy can range from hospital pharmacies to several types of outpatient pharmacies (e.g., independent pharmacies, chain drug stores, pharmacies in grocery stores, mail order pharmacies) to LTC or specialty pharmacies.

● Mail order pharmacies comprise a small overall percentage of total prescriptions filled (approximately 6% in 2004), but they are considered one of the fastest growing sectors of the U.S. prescription drug retail market.[1]

● Pharmacies may acquire drugs at lower costs by working with manufacturers or wholesalers to obtain discounts and/or rebates that are based on a drug's sales volume or market share. Similarly, pharmacies may ask to be included in the PBMs' network and to receive a reimbursement on each filled prescription that includes the drug's cost plus a dispensing fee.

■ Pharmacy benefit managers: It is estimated that approximately two-thirds of all prescriptions written in the United States are processed by a PBM.[1]

● These organizations help customers save money by negotiating with pharmaceutical manufacturers for discounted prices and by establishing programs that control the cost of drugs, such as using formularies, promoting and optimizing use of generic drugs, and implementing therapeutic interchange programs.

Delivery of Medications from Manufacturers to Patients

Pharmaceutical Manufacturers[1]

Brand-name and generic pharmaceutical companies manufacture and package prescription drugs. Some companies can manufacture branded as well as generic drugs. The primary difference between the two types of manufacturers is that most major brand-name manufacturers allot large sums of money to scientific research and development of new drugs. Generic drug manufacturers wait until the patent for a branded drug expires and then produce a drug containing the same ingredients, usually at a lower price to the consumer. These manufacturers usually do not develop new drugs and, therefore, spend much less money on research and development.

Drug wholesalers purchase drugs from manufacturers and are the largest volume customers for drug manufacturers. However, manufacturers sometimes sell and deliver drugs directly to pharmacies (i.e., community pharmacy chains, mail order pharmacies, and specialty pharmacies), hospitals, and some health plans. To educate and prevent prescribing errors, manufacturers produce informational labeling for prescribers and patients that conforms to the requirements of the U.S. Food and Drug Administration. In addition, manufacturers place electronic bar coding on drug packaging that can be used to track individual production lots of the drugs; this technology is important in ensuring safety in the pharmaceutical supply chain.

Pharmaceutical Wholesalers/Distributors[1]

Wholesale distributors purchase pharmaceuticals from manufacturers and distribute them to a wide range of customers, including hospital pharmacies, community pharmacies, mail order pharmacies, LTC facilities, as well as other medical practices (e.g., physician offices, clinics, and diagnostic laboratories). Some distributors sell to a broad range of pharmacy customers (e.g., hospital, specialty, LTC, community, and government entities), whereas other wholesale distributors focus on specialized or niche areas for either specific customer groups (e.g., nursing homes) or specialized products (e.g., biologics). In the past, distributors used traditional distribution functions that are sometimes referred to as "pick, pack, and ship."

Serving as the connection between the manufacturers and pharmacies remains an important cornerstone of the wholesale distributor business today. However, ongoing changes in the marketplace and patients' health care needs have prompted distributors to offer more comprehensive services, such as distribution of specialty drugs, repackaging of drugs, and the provision of other special services (electronic ordering, assistance with reimbursement, clinical support, consulting, and drug buy-back programs).

In the last three decades, the wholesale distribution industry has gone through significant change and consolidation. Because of this consolidation, the industry has changed its revenue model and has incorporated high-technology solutions to increase efficiencies and maximize economies of scale. The industry has expanded, and some distributors have added offerings such as automation, software, and information system solutions; specialty pharmacy services; sophisticated operational and clinical resources; access to experts in a variety of clinical, operational and financial areas; and medication adherence and disease management services. Some wholesalers have evolved to become much more than pick, pack, and ship, and some have become a "one-stop shop" for the entire portfolio of health care products and solutions.

Pharmacies[1]

Generally, the last step in the pharmaceutical supply chain—before the drug reaches the patient—is the pharmacy, which serves as the interface between the supply chain and the patient. Pharmacies purchase drugs from wholesalers; sometimes they purchase directly from manufacturers. Although there are variations in the flow of pharmaceuticals, the typical flow is as follows: The drug order is placed with the distributor and the drugs are delivered to the pharmacy. Once the drug is received by the pharmacy, the appropriate staff checks the medication received against the order and then places it in storage or in a filling area where the medication is either stored or selected and then prepared for the patient. Pharmacies assume responsibility for safe storage and dispensing of the product to patients. Pharmacies also have the responsibility to stock an appropriate amount of the drug and to provide counseling and drug information to patients to ensure safe and effective use of the drugs. Community pharmacies also process prescriptions for billing and payment on behalf of patients who have prescription insurance.

As mentioned previously, there are various types of outpatient pharmacies, for example, independent community pharmacies, chain community pharmacies, and mail order pharmacies. Most of these pharmacies purchase their drug supply from a wholesale distributor; however, in some cases, they order directly from a manufacturer or use a combination of the two sources.

In addition to outpatient pharmacies, there are LTC and specialty pharmacies. LTC pharmacies are known as a specialized type of outpatient pharmacy that caters to the unique needs of nursing homes. They provide packaging such as unit-dose supply or bubble packs as well as special access to expertise such as consultant pharmacists that specialize in LTC. In addition, LTC pharmacies provide other services such as emergency drug kits, medication carts, regular and emergency (24-hour-a-day) delivery services, and educational or in-service training programs for LTC staff.

Specialty pharmacies focus on dispensing high-cost drugs and more complex therapies such as injectable or biologic drugs used to treat either common diseases (e.g., rheumatoid arthritis) or rare diseases (e.g., blood disorders). The specialty pharmacy market has evolved rapidly and is expected to continue growing in the near future.

Mail order pharmacies have been one of the fastest growing segments in pharmacy in the past decade. These pharmacies receive prescriptions by phone, mail, fax, or Internet at a central location; process the prescription in large, automated centers; and mail the filled prescriptions back to the patient. Contributing factors to the rapid growth of mail order pharmacies are the aging population, patient convenience, and increased use of drugs for chronic conditions (i.e., depression) or maintenance therapy (i.e., high cholesterol).

The pharmacy industry has gone through significant changes over the last 10 to 15 years. Mergers of large chains have occurred as a way to increase purchasing power with manufacturers and distributors, resulting in much consolidation in the pharmacy industry. Services have changed too, with patients using more mail order pharmacies and specialty pharmacies. Rapid growth in these two segments is expected to continue in the near future.

Community pharmacies play a crucial role in relaying information between other members of the supply chain (pharmaceutical manufacturers, wholesale distributors, and PBMs). Compared with other health care sectors, members of the pharmaceutical supply chain, and pharmacies in particular, are highly automated and most submit claims electronically.

Pharmacy Benefit Managers (PBMs)

PBMs were once basic claims administrators. In the last three decades, however, PBMs have become complex organizations and offer comprehensive services (e.g., processing of claims, provision of tools for managing prescription drugs, and development of reporting programs tailored to the clients' needs). According to the National Association of Chain Drug Stores, PBMs process about two-thirds of all prescriptions written in the United States.[1] PBMs play an important role in most drug purchases by patients by working with third-party payers (e.g., private insurance plans, self-insured employers, and public health programs). PBMs also determine which drugs the third-party payer will pay for, how much of the reimbursement the pharmacy will receive, and how much the patient must pay for a filled prescription (co-pay).

PBMs offer services that pharmacists rely on to process prescriptions as well as advanced services for their patients and customers, including drug utilization review, disease management services, and consultative services. PBMs also help clients set up their benefit structure. A plan design can include[1]:

- Developing and maintaining a prescription drug formulary.
- Developing a network of pharmacy providers.
- Providing mail order fulfillment services.
- Negotiating rebates with manufacturers.

Because PBMs are a major player in the pharmaceutical supply chain, brief descriptions of their core services are described in the following sections.

Formularies[1]

PBMs compare the safety and efficacy of clinically similar drugs. If these properties are equivalent, PBMs consider the cost of each drug in building their formularies. This approach helps PBMs negotiate more favorable price discounts with manufacturers and encourages beneficiaries to use "preferred" or "formulary" drugs or lower cost medications.

Rebates[1]

PBMs develop a formulary and then negotiate with pharmaceutical manufacturers for rebates on products included in the formulary. As reimbursement for this service, PBMs usually retain a portion of the rebate.

Pharmacy Networks[1]

PBMs can also negotiate pharmacy networks on behalf of enrollees in a medical insurance or health plan. These networks comprise pharmacies that will dispense prescription drugs and provide pharmacy services to enrollees according to the negotiated terms and conditions. Because pharmacy networks can vary in size, PBMs can lower prescription drug prices by negotiating the reimbursement rate and dispensing fee with pharmacies.

Mail Order Pharmacy Service[1]

Many PBMs offer mail order pharmacy service. The best candidates for mail order prescriptions are patients who have chronic medical conditions and take maintenance medications. The medications are typically dispensed in a higher quantity (e.g., 90-day supply per prescription) compared with the typical 30-day supply per prescription dispensed by a community pharmacy. PBM mail order pharmacies reduce the cost of pharmaceutical drugs for patients and payers by:

- Using an automated dispensing process.
- Negotiating contracts with manufacturers to maximize use of formulary drugs, often in the form of therapeutic substitution and the conversion from brand to generic drugs.
- Driving market share for the formulary products.

Claims Adjudication[1]

PBMs use a real-time, point-of-sale system that is connected to retail and mail order pharmacies and distribution centers. This process provides verification of patient coverage, formulary restrictions or "preferred product" identification, drug interaction information, and individual patient co-pay information.

Quality-Focused Programs[1]

To promote the safe, effective use of drugs by patients, PBMs offer a variety of advanced programs to assist customers in managing diseases and developing methods to increase medication adherence. PBMs also participate and publish in outcomes research, and they often provide clinical information (e.g., drug and disease), tools, and resources, written by pharmacists, physicians, and nurses, to their members and sometimes to the public.

Pedigree

One recent hot topic concerning the pharmaceutical supply chain is pharmaceutical pedigrees. The term *e-pedigree,* as used in the pharmaceutical industry, means an auditable electronic record of every step taken by a retail package of prescription drugs as it moves from the factory to the final point of sale. This chain-of-custody record is used to ensure the integrity and safety of the nation's drug supply.[6] Technology plays a large role in the success of tracking pharmaceuticals. Radiofrequency identification (RFID), a technology that has been used in other industries for decades, is anticipated to play a predominant role in e-pedigree. RFID uses active and/or passive tags (affixed to the product or good of interest) to capture and transmit information about the product. This information can include product lot number, manufacturer's name, intended destination, temperatures to which the product has been exposed, and a variety of other information that is based on the product. In aggregate, this information may form an e-pedigree, which is intended to safeguard the public from counterfeiting and diversion of drugs, and it protects the public by tracing the drug from manufacturer to patient. e-Pedigree will likely remain a hot topic for years to come because of the logistical challenges and expense associated with its implementation.

Conclusion

Pharmaceuticals are a cornerstone of patient care, and their importance will continue to grow as the population ages and pharmaceutical innovation continues. Understanding the current pharmaceutical supply chain process requires knowledge of the various factors in the supply chain. Information technology plays a key role in managing the information about both the financial and the physical distribution aspects of the pharmaceutical supply chain. An understanding of the key players and the complex process involved is necessary for the background knowledge of health care professionals.

LEARNING ACTIVITIES

1. Determine all the different components in the supply chain where you work. What components were you not aware of?
2. Search the Internet and identify at least one technology that allows enhanced tracking of pharmaceuticals for pedigree requirements.
3. Identify the strengths and limitations of that technology identified in #2. How could the limitations or barriers to implementation be overcome?

References

1. The Henry J. Kaiser Family Foundation. Follow the pill: understanding the U.S. commercial pharmaceutical supply chain. March 2005. Available at: http://www.kff.org/rxdrugs/upload/Follow-The-Pill-Understanding-the-U-S-Commercial-Pharmaceutical-Supply-Chain-Report.pdf. Accessed July 15, 2009.
2. IMS Health. Top therapeutic classes by U.S. sales [table]. Available at: http://www.imshealth.com/deployedfiles/imshealth/Global/Content/StaticFile/Top_Line_Data/Top%20Therapy%20Classes%20by%20U.S.Sales.pdf. Accessed May 5, 2010.
3. IMS Health. IMS forecasts global pharmaceutical market growth of 5-8% annually through 2014; maintains expectations of 4-6% growth in 2010 [news release]. Available at: http://www.imshealth.com/portal/site/imshealth/menuitem.a46c6d4df3db4b3d88f611019418c22a/?vgnextoid=4b8c410b6c718210VgnVCM100000ed152ca2RCRD&vgnextchannel=41a67900b55a5110VgnVCM10000071812ca2RCRD&vgnextfmt=default. Accessed May 6, 2010.
4. Money Magazine. Fortune 500 rankings. Our annual ranking of America's largest corporations: pharmaceuticals. Available at: http://money.cnn.com/magazines/fortune/fortune500/2009/industries/21/index.html. Accessed October 9, 2009.
5. Money Magazine. Global 500 rankings. Our annual ranking of America's largest corporations: wholesalers: health care. Available at: http://money.cnn.com/magazines/fortune/global500/2009/industries/212/index.html. Accessed October 9, 2009
6. Messplay GC, Heisey C. Pharmaceutical pedigree requirements: implementing electronic track and trace. *Contract Pharma*. July/August 2006:18–20.

Automation of Acute Care Pharmacy Operations

Dennis A. Tribble

OBJECTIVES

1. Describe the role of the National Drug Code and other coding in automated drug identification.
2. Identify the types of automation available to automate medication distribution.
3. Identify steps in the fulfillment portion of the medication use process that can be automated.
4. Identify regulatory requirements around operation of medication distribution automation.
5. Describe non-technical implementation details for automation of operations.

One of the key benefits of pharmacy automation has been the advent of computer-controlled equipment to automate processes that were traditionally performed by pharmacists and technicians traversing the pharmacy, paper in hand, fulfilling requests for the dispensing and distribution of medications. Such automation now encompasses several aspects of the medication use process, including:

- Receiving and storing.
- Medication retrieval and assembly.
- Compounding of sterile doses.
- Labeling of doses for distribution.
- Pharmacist checking of completed doses.
- Distribution of completed doses to patient care areas.

All of these automated systems must:

- Be able to uniquely identify the products that they manage.
- Be able to receive and interpret medication orders sufficiently to deliver the appropriate drug products.
- Perform appropriate dose calculations as needed.
- Report transactions to other automated systems for billing and other purposes.

Therefore, a discussion of this automation must begin with a discussion of how drug products are marked, how systems recognize them, and how such systems account for them in the acute care hospital setting. This discussion must also address general considerations for the placement of automated technology, including installation, training, validation, and service.

Drug Product Identification

National Drug Code

Since April 2006, the Food and Drug Administration (FDA) has required that all prescription medication packaging be marked with the National Drug Code (NDC) assigned to the packaged product. The NDC is a three-part code consisting of:

- Labeler code: A 4- or 5-digit code that identifies the vendor responsible for the final package of the drug. This code is assigned by the FDA.
- Drug code: A 3- or 4-digit code that identifies the drug form and strength of the product. This code is assigned by the vendor.

■ Package code: A 1- or 2-digit code that identifies the packaging level being identified (e.g., unit, package, box, case, etc.).

The NDC is always 10 digits long; originally it always consisted of a 4-digit labeler code, a 4-digit drug code, and a 2-digit package code. More recently, with the growth of drug repackagers, the parts of the NDC may now contain various numbers of digits, yielding one of three different formats:

■ 4-4-2: The original format as described previously.
■ 5-4-1: A 5-digit labeler code is offset by a 1-digit package code.
■ 5-3-2: A 5-digit labeler code is offset by a 3-digit drug code.

Drug manufacturers must select which one of the three formats to use and then consistently use that format for all products they manufacture.

When viewed in human-readable format, the portions of the NDC are readily identified because they are separated by hyphens (1234-5678-90). However, when encoded in a bar code, the NDC is represented as a 10-digit unformatted number (1234567890) that could represent any of the three formats:

■ 1234-5678-90
■ 12345-6789-0
■ 12345-678-90

Further, because a drug code is defined by the manufacturer, there is no consistency in the use of the code. A review of the FDA database of assigned NDCs demonstrated more than 30 different drug codes used to represent a cefazolin sodium 1 gram vial for injection.[1]

Because only the labeler code is assigned by the FDA, there is no reliable central repository of currently extant NDC codes or their bar code representation. The manufacturer is required to report NDCs in use to the FDA, but approval is not required. There are, therefore, significant limitations to the ability to use the NDC code for anything other than identifying a specific drug product. It becomes incumbent on the pharmacy and its automated systems to maintain a current and accurate list of known NDC codes, and to ensure that all the dependent systems recognize each code accurately in terms of the product it represents.

Pharmacy information management systems (PIMS) must, therefore, become a repository of this information, and these systems must provide mechanisms to disseminate the information to other systems that may rely on the manufacturer's bar-coded NDC for proper drug identification and manipulation. PIMS are described in detail in Chapter 12; it is important, however, that a pharmacy consider when and how they will maintain up-to-date NDC listings during consideration of their use within the other applications that may depend on them. Any automated distribution application product that uses bar codes to verify proper product selection will require that the NDC lists be current, or the automated device will fail to properly identify medication products, leading to additional manual work for the pharmacy.

Because the pharmacy (especially in the acute care setting) may be responsible for compounding special preparations, which will require their own unique bar codes, it is especially important that these products also be encoded with a bar code. The pharmacy will need to establish a bar-coding methodology that ensures (1) the values used to encode these products do not conflict with manufacturers' NDC encoding, (2) the values are known and recognized by systems that will need to read the bar code, and (3) the values reliably identify the correct product.

Although it is unusual in the United States for a commercial product to lack a bar code, in some instances, the bar code may be difficult to read and the product may require re-labeling with an externally generated bar code. In this instance, the application of the new labeling must be a controlled process, preferably performed as a batch process during receiving or stocking, to ensure that subsequent use within automated systems reliably and correctly identifies each item. This process must include automated verification that the affixed bar code can be scanned, and that the scan results in proper identification of the drug product.

General Implementation Considerations for Automated Drug Distribution Systems

Policies, Procedures, and Training

Most of the automated systems that assist with drug preparation and distribution are a combination of computer software and the electro-mechanical mechanisms that they operate. These systems are designed to be operated in specific ways and under specific circumstances, so the decision to purchase and use such equipment requires a careful understanding of their intended use, as well as an understanding of their limitations. This process includes careful preparation of training materials, not only for use during initial implementation, but also for ongoing training of new employees and continued demonstration of competence to operate them. It also demands consideration and preparation of policies and procedures surrounding the use of such equipment so that:

- Individual roles are clear.
- Proper operation is clearly defined.
- Potential problems with operation are clearly identified, and resolution of those problems is properly prescribed.
- Any potential safety issues are anticipated with appropriate control procedures.

The performance of a Failure Mode and Effects Analysis (FMEA) around the proposed implementation and use of such technology is a good way to identify any weaknesses in the proposed uses that may require the creation of control procedures.[2,3]

Facilities Management

In addition to ensuring that the department is ready and trained to operate technology, it is also important to understand what physical changes, both in facilities and workflow, may be required. Facilities may require modification both in physical space and in availability of utilities (power, light, compressed air, etc.) to accommodate the technology. It is vital that equipment be housed in space sufficient for its operation, which may require careful consideration of whether or not technology can be physically placed in its intended location. Considerations may include weight, available power, availability of compressed air, heat generation, and sufficiency of heating, ventilating, and air conditioning (HVAC) support.

Change Management

Technology should change the way people work, for the better. Part of the consideration of any new technology must include how the adoption of that technology will change the workflow of the pharmacy, and whether or not such change is aligned with the goals and culture of the department. Technology should change the way work is done. If it does not, the implementer should question whether or not it will provide any benefits. However, change must provide some benefits to be worth the pain of the change.

One significant result of this reality is that both pharmacists and technicians are likely to need to learn new work habits around the use of new technology. The new skills and tasks associated with this use will hopefully be offset by the elimination of other skills and tasks. It takes time to develop productive habits around a new workflow, during which time pharmacists and technicians may feel uncomfortable, even incompetent. Leadership through this learning period is essential to the successful implementation of the technology.

Interfacing

The subject of interfacing is handled in other portions of this textbook, but it is important to realize that virtually all of these technologies are designed to receive critical operating information, either directly from the PIMS or from other distribution technology. Implementation and planning will require accounting for the costs of such interfaces, ensuring that the source systems can produce the expected interface transactions at the appropriate times, and ensuring that procedures and information are in place to ensure that the interfaces are properly maintained and operated.

Regulatory Considerations

With the exception of sterile compounding systems,[4] these automated dispensing devices are not considered medical devices and are therefore not regulated by the FDA. Most states, however, maintain regulations around their use, and some states demand registration of their use with the state board of pharmacy.

Products Used in Automated Drug Distribution Systems

The following sections describe families of products intended to automate portions of the drug distribution systems in acute care facilities. This is a rapidly growing and changing field, so photographs have not been included. They would be out of date shortly after they were printed. For information on specific products and photographs showing their use, please consult Table 16–1.

Automation of Inventory Management and Product Acquisition

A key form of automation seen within pharmacies is the use of automated storage facilities that both maintain inventory and facilitate acquisition of that inventory. These will generally take the form of carousel shelving, automated dispensing cabinets, and unit-dose robots.

Carousel Cabinets

Carousel cabinets are storage units that concentrate storage into shelving units in which the shelves are attached to a carousel that can cycle through the shelving and deliver the appropriate shelve(s) to the user,

TABLE 16–1

Manufacturers of Automated Pharmacy Equipment

Manufacturer	Web Site	Product(s)
B. Braun	www.bbraunusa.com	TPN compounders
Baxa	www.baxa.com	TPN compounders, pharmacy pumps, IV workflow management
CareFusion	www.carefusion.com	Automated storage devices, pharmacy workflow enhancement
Devon Robotics	www.devonrobotics.com	Automated chemotherapy preparation, automated IV admixtures
FHT, Inc.	www.fhtinc.com	Automated IV admixtures, automated IV workflow management, telepharmacy
Intelligent Hospital Systems	www.intelligenthospitals.com	Automated IV admixtures
McKesson	www.mckesson.com	Automated unit-dose cart filling
Omnicell	www.omnicell.com	Automated storage devices, pharmacy workflow enhancement
ScriptPro	www.scriptpro.com	Automated chemotherapy workflow management, telepharmacy
Talyst	www.talyst.com	Automated storage devices

IV = intravenous [admixtures]; TPN = total parenteral nutrition.
Source: Author.

rather than requiring the user to traverse fixed shelving to locate desired items. Typically, these units extend vertically into otherwise unused space up to, and even above, the ceiling of the department, permitting supplies to be stored in much less floor space than would be required for the same storage on fixed shelving.

Receiving of medications into such systems involves the use of a computer control panel application to inform the system of intended receipt of product and to present the appropriate storage location to the person performing the receiving. This process also may include bar code verification of the item being received and its actual storage in the correct location.

Subsequent distribution of products from these locations involves submitting a list of drugs required, either by entering product requests on the device control panel or by receiving interface transactions that queue up distribution requests. The user then initiates retrieval by commanding the device to fulfill an order, at which time the device rotates the appropriate shelve(s) to the user and uses indicators to point the user to the correct locations on those shelves from which to retrieve the desired items. In addition to freeing up floor space and reducing the walking associated with drug distribution, these kinds of units provide a more accurate method for accounting for inventory, better ensuring that items will be replaced as they are used.

Automated Dispensing Cabinets

Automated dispensing cabinets may be located either in the pharmacy or on patient care units. Similar to the carousels, these cabinets maintain inventory and prompt for inventory replacements according to usage and par levels. They do not, however, free up floor space.

These cabinets do require log-ins to maintain an audit trail of receiving and dispersal activity and also to automate charging of medication products as they are released for use by a patient. When placed in a patient care environment, these cabinets can be used to supply commonly used medications and can operate in a "profile mode" in which the cabinet keeps track of the medication administration schedule and controls access to appropriate medication supplies at appropriate times according to patient profiles maintained within the cabinet. This permits a nurse to request, for example, the 9 a.m. doses for a patient and have the cabinet system provide access to those medication supplies. The request is fulfilled as long as the supplies are in the cabinet and it is near enough to the administration time.

These cabinets may be configured with a variety of different drawers, including some that may open only a specific section in a drawer from which only the correct medications can be retrieved. More commonly, the cabinets will open a drawer subdivided into open compartments. In this case, the cabinet controls access by drawer but does not prevent retrieval of inappropriate drug products. None of these cabinets control the actual physical amount of product removed; there is nothing to prevent a user from opening the drawer that correlates with one patient's profile and taking more product than the prompted amount. Thus, these cabinets tend to require careful auditing to ensure that supplies are properly accounted for.

Because emergent medication needs may arise for which orders may not yet have been placed or approved, these cabinets permit override functions that allow the nurse to retrieve medications that are not currently on the patient's profile. This override capability has been associated with medication errors, and care must be taken to minimize its use.[5-7]

Some of these cabinets also come with bar code capabilities to ensure both that the cabinet was properly stocked and that the correct medications were actually retrieved.

Robotic Cart Filling Systems

A third type of automation for distribution of drug products is **robotic systems** that use bar coding to locate, obtain, package, label, and deliver medications for specific patients by filling unit-dose carts. These systems typically require significant amounts of floor space, and they will require both electricity and compressed air to operate. These systems will also likely require a significant repackaging effort to place the medication products into containers that can be manipulated by the device.

Many states permit these devices to operate with statistical checking; once the device has demonstrated its ability to operate accurately, the pharmacy is permitted to limit pharmacist checking of its output to a small percentage (typically 10%) of the work output by the device. A variant of these systems keeps oral solid drugs in bulk form and then unit-dose packages the doses on demand as they are to be distributed in unit-dose carts or as part of a first-dose distribution.

These devices use cassettes, each of which contains a specific tablet or capsule; a cassette must be specifically configured to the dimensions of the tablet or capsule that it contains. Substitution of one brand for another of the same drug or changes in the physical presentation of the same drug (diameter, shape, etc.) may require that the cassette be reconfigured, or

that a new cassette be configured and implemented for the changed supply. In some cases, this configuration may require return of the cassette to
the vendor.

Sterile Compounding Devices

Perhaps the newest and most rapidly growing segment of pharmacy automation involves the use of technology to automate the compounding of sterile
doses in a hospital pharmacy IV room. This segment is divisible into automated devices that physically prepare medication doses and software products that automate the workflow associated with manual dose preparation.
The latter group is the newest set of products in this environment.

Devices that Automate Physical Sterile Dose Preparation

Preparation of sterile doses in the pharmacy remains one of the most
labor-intensive and hazard-prone processes within the pharmacy operation. Preparing sterile doses requires:

- Knowledge of the chemistry of the medications involved.
- Ability to compute and measure dose amounts.
- Ability to manipulate sterile products without microbial contamination.
- Ability to observe the resulting admixture for signs of adulteration.
- Ability to prevent cross-contamination of drugs.
- Knowledge of special techniques for handling and disposing of
  potentially hazardous materials.

Devices that can automate the preparation of these doses significantly
address these concerns and can improve the reliability of the preparation
process.

The FDA treats devices that perform these functions as medical devices,
apparently because these devices perform manipulations for which errors
in product selection, reconstitution, or measurement cannot be directly
detected by pharmacist inspection at the end point. In a guidance document released in March 2001, the FDA classified these devices as pharmacy
compounding devices[4] and exempted them from the usual pre-market
approval process on the grounds that their risk is relatively low as long as
they are developed, designed, manufactured, installed, and serviced in
compliance with the medical device Quality System Regulations (21CFR §
820 and following).

FDA oversight of this technology places special constraints on devices that prepare sterile doses, which are primarily related to the kinds of computers that can be used for them, the software environment in which the control software operates, and the kinds of interventions that a hospital information technology organization is permitted to perform. These constraints do not apply to other pharmacy automation technologies.

Note that this category of devices does not include pharmacy pumps and other technologies whose function is simply to transfer the contents of one container into another. To be considered a pharmacy compounding device, the automation must physically alter commercial products, either by mixing or reconstitution, or must be a software component that drives a device that performs this function.

It is important to note that, because the FDA does not require pre-market approval of this technology, it is possible, and even likely, that vendors may enter this space and produce technology that has not yet been reviewed by the FDA. As a result, it is advisable to obtain clarification from the vendor regarding FDA status of both the vendor and the technology product, and to obtain contractual protections against FDA action if the vendor and/or the technology has not yet gone through FDA inspection.

This class of devices is called **total parenteral nutrition (TPN) compounders.** These devices perform the complex admixture processes of computing a TPN formulation from clinical requirements and then drive a machine to deliver the ingredients in the correct amounts and in the correct sequence. Subsequently, manufacturers have begun developing devices for preparation of some, or all kinds of, sterile doses. These include devices that produce syringes, prepare only chemotherapy, or prepare a variety of different sterile doses.

Workflow Automation in Sterile Product Preparation

Most recently, automation has arisen on the market that automates the flow of work through the sterile product preparation areas. This software stages work through various steps of product acquisition, preparation, checking, and distribution, and potentially all the way to patient care areas. The software receives individual requests for each dose to be prepared, uses bar code scanning to verify the selection of the correct products (both the actual drugs and any diluents or other adjuvant products), automates computation of dose amounts, captures pictures of key dose preparation activities, permits pharmacist checking from those pictures and the accumulated information from the bar code scanning, and then tracks doses through the distribution process, potentially all the way to the patient care area.

This kind of software may electronically "read" the labels printed from a PIMS or may take Health Level Seven transactions in a formal interface. Note that the software does not automate the actual preparation, but it maintains a significant amount of detail around the manual preparation process that is otherwise lost in its absence. Although it is unlikely that such software will reduce staffing, it can shift work from pharmacists to technicians, creating better opportunities for pharmacists to perform non-distributive activities.

Technology and the Pharmacy Staff

As previously described, the adoption of technology will change the way pharmacists and pharmacy technicians practice their roles. One goal in the adoption of this kind of technology is to provide avenues of control over the distributive portion of practice to permit it to be delegated to properly trained technicians.[8]

Technology must be managed; this implies the presence of someone on staff to fulfill this responsibility. This individual (or these individuals) need not be a pharmacist, but there will be maintenance issues that require the oversight of a pharmacist. Formulary decisions are an example, especially when the formulary drives processes that cannot be visually verified.[4] Note that simply being a pharmacist may not be sufficient for this role; the person taking responsibility for the formulary content must also be trained in the impact of specific formulary decisions on the way the technology will operate.

Increasingly, technology changes the way pharmacy technicians work. Technology can introduce in-process checks that up to now were unavailable, thereby substantially decreasing the number of errors that reach final pharmacist inspection and, perhaps, even obviating the need for such inspection.[8]

Pharmacy is now just learning what manufacturing has known for years: Quality cannot be inspected into a product (with end-process inspections); quality must be built into the process every step of the way. Technologies are now being introduced that do this, and such in-process checks virtually ensure that the resulting medication distribution is correct.

To this end, it is critical that technicians be trained in the reasons for what may appear to them to be additional, valueless tasks. Bar code-checking systems, for example, provide additional assurance that the technician selected the appropriate products. These systems can be subverted, however, if the technician scans the same item five times rather than scanning each of five items, or scans labels for containers without actually applying those labels to the containers for which they are intended. In these cases, the resulting scans are meaningless.

Note that this behavior is not confined to pharmacy technicians; Koppel et al. describe situations in which nurses applied copies of barcoded patient wristbands to the door jambs of patient rooms and scanned them rather than scanning the wrist bands actually worn by the patients in the rooms.[9]

Conclusion

A broad variety of automation is available to assist in the drug distribution role of the acute care inpatient pharmacy. Implementation of any of this technology requires careful consideration of its fit to the culture and goals of the pharmacy, significant planning, preparation of departmental procedures, staff training, resolution of any regulatory requirements, potential facilities work and expense, and ongoing management. Properly deployed, this technology can significantly relieve personnel requirements for distribution activities or shift those activities from pharmacists to technicians, freeing the pharmacists for clinical pursuits.

LEARNING ACTIVITIES

1. Visit each of the Web sites listed in Table 16–1. Create a brief report describing the various products that you observe on the sites. Many of the sites have short videos and/or animations depicting their products.
2. Interview the pharmacy informaticist (or automation manager) at a hospital that runs each of the types of equipment described in this chapter. List three benefits that this manager expected to achieve with the automation and how well those benefits were achieved.
3. During the interview in #2, identify two unexpected consequences of implementing the technology

References

1. U.S. Food and Drug Administration. National Drug Code Directory. October 30, 2009. Available at: http://www.accessdata.fda.gov/scripts/cder/ndc/default.cfm. Accessed November 4, 2009.

2. Young D. Six Sigma black-belt pharmacist improves patient safety. Am J Health Syst Pharm. 2004;61(19):1988, 1992, 1996.

3. Tosha B, Wetterneck KA, Skibinski TL, et al. Using failure mode and effects analysis to plan implementation of smart IV pump technology. Am J Health Syst Pharm. 2006;63(16):1528–38.

4. U.S. Department of Health and Human Services, Food and Drug Administration, Center for Devices and Radiological Health. Class II special controls guidance document: pharmacy compounding systems; final guidance for industry and FDA. March 12, 2001. Available at: http://www.fda.gov/downloads/medicaldevices/deviceregulationandguidance/guidancedocuments/ucm073589.pdf. Accessed October 1, 2009.

5. Oren E, Griffiths LP, Guglielmo BJ. Characteristics of antimicrobial overrides associated with automated dispensing machines. Am J Health Syst Pharm. 2002;59(15):1445–8.

6. Hicks RW, Sikirica V, Nelson W, et al. Medication errors involving patient-controlled analgesia. Am J Health Syst Pharm. 2008;65(5):429–40.

7. Oishi R. Current statues of preparation and distribution of medicines. Am J Health Syst Pharm. 2009; 66(5 Suppl 3):s35–s42.

8. ASHP Section of Pharmacy Informatics and Technology Executive Committee 2008–09. Technology-enabled practice: a vision statement by the ASHP Section of Pharmacy Informatics and Technology. Am J Health Syst Pharm. 2009;66(17):1573–7.

9. Koppel R, Wetterneck T, Telles J, et al. Workarounds in barcode medication administration systems: their occurrences, causes and threats to patient safety. J Am Med Inform Assoc. 2008;15(4):408–23.

CHAPTER 1

Automation of Ambulatory Care Pharmacy Operations

William A. Lockwood, III

OBJECTIVES

1. State three main areas in which technology can impact pharmacy operations and patients.
2. Describe the role of the pharmacy information management system.
3. Describe technologies that integrate with the pharmacy information management system.
4. Describe how technology can be applied to the flow of prescriptions through the dispensing process.
5. Describe two or three technologies that are new, but of increasing importance, in the ambulatory care pharmacy.

Editor's Note: Information in this chapter is based on the author's working knowledge of the topic acquired through his employment with ComputerTalk Associates, Inc. and his position as Assistant Executive Director of the American Society for Automation in Pharmacy.

A Short History of Technology in Ambulatory Care Pharmacy

On a national scale, pharmacy practice involves billions of annual sales. These transactions require careful attention to detail, making pharmacy practice an ideal environment for technology. In fact, pharmacy has long been a major user of computer-based products and services. Although computer use in pharmacy dates to the 1970s and is now pervasive, early on, pharmacists were leery of getting involved because they did not have any experience with computers and had concerns about their speed and reliability.

The early computers available in the 1970s were online systems that allowed users to access the processing power of mainframes using dial-up connections over phone lines. Companies then introduced stand-alone minicomputers, but these were expensive. The tipping point for accelerating adoption was the introduction in the early 1980s of the personal computer, which brought the price down to a more affordable level for a stand-alone system. The next big impetus came when pharmacy benefit managers introduced electronic adjudication of prescription claims. Pharmacists then needed a computer to bill prescriptions electronically and to receive a response confirming that the prescription would be paid and indicating the copay to charge the patient—all in real time.

Processing power and available memory increased, and the features and the range of tasks to which computers could be applied increased. As the pace of technology innovation picked up in the latter part of the 1990s, pharmacy began to see new software and hardware solutions—such as automated counting systems and robotics, interactive voice response (IVR) systems, electronic signature capture, bar code readers, and various services that increased the operating efficiency of the pharmacy while also addressing patient safety.

Current Status of Technology in Ambulatory Care Pharmacy

An extensive range of computer-based products and services is now available to support almost every aspect of ambulatory care pharmacy. Most pharmacies continue to invest in technology, which is a real driver for improvements in efficiency, accuracy, clinical care decision making, prevention of fraud and abuse, and regulatory compliance.

As part of its October 2009 *Cost Benefit Analysis on the Value of Technology*, the American Society for Automation in Pharmacy (ASAP) developed a grid that depicts the benefits of investing in pharmacy technology. Table 17–1 shows the areas of impact of different technologies on pharmacy operations and patients.

Technology Commonly Found in Ambulatory Care Pharmacy

Prescription-processing software is still the core—and is most likely the one piece—of technology that a pharmacy simply cannot do without. The role of the pharmacy information management system (PIMS) is to manage all the data associated with prescriptions, patients, and prescribers. This system contains key databases, such as drug files, Drug Enforcement Agency and national provider identifier numbers, physician contact information, prescription pricing tables, third-party plan details, and patient profiles. The PIMS is where data entry and claims submission happen for a new or refill prescription.

The PIMS offers the first opportunity for review of the appropriateness of the prescribed drug. The prospective drug utilization review activity looks for potential interactions with other drugs in the patient's profile and triggers a warning when there is a drug-drug interaction, duplicate therapy, drug allergy, and look-alike/sound-alike drug risk, among other types of warnings.

The PIMS can also be used to set minimum and maximum amounts of a particular drug that the pharmacy wants to keep on hand. When the stock reaches the minimum level, the PIMS can add the drug to an order to the wholesaler, but it will never order more than the preset maximum. The goal is to keep as lean an inventory as possible, which frees up cash for other purposes.

The PIMS software and related databases may be located in any of several places. It has been common for them to reside on a server in the pharmacy itself. Another option, potentially used in multi-location pharmacies, is to have the database on a central server that is accessed by clients running the PIMS software. Access to a common database means that each location is viewing current information, no matter where it was entered. A third option is to have both the data and the software hosted off-site in what is called a **"software as a service"** (SaaS) or an **"application**

TABLE 17–1

American Society for Automation in Pharmacy's Cost-Benefit Analysis on the Value of Technology Areas of Impact

Technology Used	Benefits Safety	Benefits Compliance	Prevents Fraud and Abuse
Pharmacy information management system	•	•	•
Prospective DUR module	•	•	
Warning labels	•	•	
Drug images	•		
Drug imprint information	•		
Consumer medication information	•	•	
Workflow system	•	•	•
Bar code scanning	•	•	
Document management	•		
Robotic dispensing	•		•
Automated counting	•		•
Counting scale	•		•
Interactive voice response	•	•	
Will-call bin management	•	•	
Compliance packaging		•	•
Electronic signature capture	•		•
Prescription monitoring program reporting	•		•
Pseudoephedrine tracking	•		•
Internet access*	•		
Electronic prescriptions	•	•	•
Printers	•		
Point-of-sale system	•		•

DUR = drug utilization review.
*Access to online drug information.
Source: American Society for Automation in Pharmacy. *Cost-Benefit Analysis on the Value of Technology.* Blue Bell, PA: American Society for Automation in Pharmacy; October 2009. © 2009 American Society for Automation in Pharmacy. Report also available at: http://www.asapnet.org/ASAP_Tech_Value_Report_v3-1.pdf.

service provider" (ASP) model. In addition to centralizing data, this model outsources server management and software maintenance.

The topic of storage raises the issue of data backup. These data are the lifeblood of a pharmacy. It is critical to have a mechanism that backs up data in a manner that makes the information readily accessible but also secure. If a copy of the data is kept at the pharmacy, a copy should also be kept off-site, perhaps by means of a remote backup service that offers professional-grade reliability and redundancy. Also vital is a solid disaster recovery plan that allows resumption of patient services as soon as possible after an event and with as complete access to the data as possible.

When it comes to the PIMS user interface, systems using a text-based, command-driven environment are still in use. However, the majority of systems now offer a graphical user interface that uses icons and menus that allow navigation with the keyboard, a mouse, or a touch screen.

Although the PIMS still remains the core platform, there is much to be gained by integrating an array of other technologies with it.

Handling of Incoming Prescriptions

New prescriptions are typically entered manually at a computer, although the increasing use of electronic prescribing is changing this. When it comes to refills, IVR and the World Wide Web (Web) are currently two common ways for prescriptions to be routed directly into the PIMS filling queue.

Patients and pharmacy staff can benefit from IVR and Web refills in several ways. For example, both can reduce the number of phone calls the pharmacy staff has to take during the day, while still allowing patients to opt out of the IVR when they need to speak to a person. This helps pharmacy staff prioritize time spent on the phone. Or, consider that patients can submit a refill request via IVR or the Web anytime, even after hours. Pharmacy staff can then process these refills before opening and get a jump on the day's work. The PIMS can also route refills received via IVR or the Web directly into the dispensing automation queue. There are other points of efficiency and convenience surrounding inbound calls. For example, the IVR can be set to offer special prompts for routing calls from physicians' offices or to departments in the pharmacy. And, the Web is not just an order entry tool for patients. It can also allow staff at long-term care (LTC) facilities to enter orders and review order status, saving more calls to the pharmacy.

IVR is increasingly being used to make automated outbound calls. These can be prescription pickup reminders, which offer the potential to improve prescription pickup rates. Or, outbound calls can inform patients of services available at the pharmacy, such as immunizations or disease-specific seminars. Text messages are another form of outbound contact now available to pharmacy. Any calls or texts can be targeted to specific, appropriate populations by age, gender, disease state, or medication use. Of course pharmacists have to consider privacy concerns when developing the content.

Electronic Prescribing

Electronic prescribing (e-prescribing) is another way in which new and refill prescriptions can enter the pharmacy-processing queue and is a feature of almost every PIMS. These prescriptions are routed through a national gateway, such as Surescripts, directly into the prescription-processing queue. Requests for refill authorizations can also be transmitted electronically from the pharmacy to prescribers. The volume of e-prescribing is growing, and increased adoption is a top priority of the federal government because e-prescribing is an important component of an interoperable electronic health record (EHR). An EHR allows health care providers to have access to a patient's medical records, including prescriptions. Eventually, paper prescriptions as they are known today will be eclipsed by electronic prescriptions. This transition will add still another level of efficiency in the pharmacy and accuracy in the filling process.

Document Scanning and Management

The simplest form of document scanning and management is scanning the paper prescription at intake. The digitized prescription will then be available for closer inspection at filling and at the final verification step. Other examples of items that may be scanned are patient's prescription benefit card or driver's license. More sophisticated document management systems are moving toward creating a paperless pharmacy by digitizing incoming fax transmissions and storing them in a database. These systems allow management of any form of inbound message by applying a bar code to it—tying it to specific patient, physician, and LTC facility records—and routing it to multiple points in the pharmacy as necessary. The key thing is that, because this document is electronic, it can go to multiple places at once and is very easy to retrieve at a later date.

Sophisticated document management systems can also improve outbound communications given that any paper form can be digitized, filled out on screen in standardized ways (using drop-down menus or other methods of selecting the appropriate data for the form), and sent out to the intended recipient, frequently as a fax. These communications can be organized and routed internally, just like incoming documents, and attached to other specific records. The broad idea of these systems is to both reduce the amount of paper handled in the pharmacy and provide a much faster way to file, index, share, and search information.

Workflow Systems

In community pharmacy, a **workflow system** is a PIMS that has multiple workstations with assigned specific tasks. For example, the workstation at intake lets the clerk scan in the paper prescription and enter the patient's insurance information. There is a workstation dedicated to processing these prescriptions, usually by a technician. Then, there is a workstation that is used by the pharmacist to verify that the prescription has been filled correctly. At this workstation, the pharmacist has access to the scanned copy of the paper prescription and an image of the drug that should be in the vial. A workstation can also be dedicated to troubleshooting and resubmitting insurance claims that are rejected for a variety of reasons or need a prior authorization to fill. Bar code scanning is an integral component of these systems from the point of processing the prescription to placement of the prescription in the will-call bin.

A workflow system allows tracking of every prescription through the filling queue so that at any given point in time, a pharmacist can see the status of a prescription at any workstation and even change the filling priority of prescriptions in the queue. The other advantage of workflow systems is that all the functions just described can be available through one or two workstations during off-peak hours. It is just a matter of turning off the access controls to provide the full range of software just as one would with a PIMS. Workflow systems are usually found in high-volume pharmacies because of the efficiency these systems provide.

Services

Another critical step in processing prescriptions in the ambulatory setting is submitting the prescription properly to payers and receiving payment for the correct amount. A **pre-edit** service can help; it reviews claims before their transmittal to the payer and offers the opportunity to correct any problems. The goal is to avoid rejects that require resubmission and an extra switching fee, as well as to manage reimbursement. **Post-edits** are reports that let you review all the prescriptions that were paid under circumstances that negatively impact pharmacy operations and reimbursement rates.

Both pre-edits and post-edits can also apply to the complexities of billing durable medical equipment claims to Medicare Part B and Medicaid programs. Each of these programs has very specific billing requirements, and pre-edits and post-edits can help a pharmacy receive maximum reimbursement.

These services can be performed both by the PIMS software and by a company offering **network switching services** that route claims for the pharmacy. These switches, in fact, are offering an increasing number of services that are based on the connectivity they have to the pharmacy and the transactions that pass through them.

Automation in the Dispensing Process

Dispensing automation reduces the need for pharmacy staff to spend time on the repetitive task of manually filling prescriptions. There are two types of automation: counting systems and robotics. **Counting systems** include countertop devices and stand-alone cabinets. **Robotic dispensing** fills and labels vials and can also automate compliance packaging. It is possible to automate more than 60% of a pharmacy's dispensing volume using counting systems or robotics. These systems also factor into a structured workflow by using bar codes to ensure that the right stock bottle is used to refill the dispensing cells and by using biometrics or bar code scanning of identification tags to record identities of the staff servicing the dispensers.

Printers

The printers used in the pharmacy have changed substantially over the years. Although dot matrix printers may still be in use, the majority of pharmacies have made the move to laser printers and, to a degree, to thermal printers. Laser printers are still the primary means of printing prescription labels, usually on a single sheet that also includes warning stickers, information for the patient on the drug dispensed, and the receipt. Double-drawer laser printers can hold both label stock and plain paper. Using plain paper in a double-drawer printer allows printing of drug-related information that requires more space than is available on the prescription label stock. Duplex printers allow printing on both sides of the page. Of course, laser printers require toner, which is perhaps the main cost of using them. Although color laser printers are available, they are not used often in pharmacies. The cost per page is significantly higher than that for black-and-white printers.

Thermal printers use a special print head that uses heat to create text and images, generally in black and white, although it is technically possible to add a second color by heating specially coated paper. Thermal printers have a smaller footprint than laser printers, and the only consumable is the paper itself. Some pharmacies will use a thermal printer for labels, warning stickers, and receipts, and a laser printer for consumer medication information.

Will-Call Bin Management

The will-call bin can still be viewed as perhaps the second-to-last step in the workflow, and its management is certainly amenable to the application of technology. Poorly managed will-call can mean that prescriptions sit for long periods when they could be returned to stock, the status (whether a prescription has made it into or out of will-call) cannot be determined, or all the prescriptions filled for one patient are not checked out because they are not grouped together. One of the most common ways to tie will-call into the technology-driven workflow is through bar code scanning that checks each prescription into and out of the will-call bin. This provides one more searchable data point about a given prescription, allowing the pharmacist to look up a specific prescription or run reports that show, for example, all prescriptions that have been in will-call for a certain length of time. Such a report can be the basis for making reminder calls to patients and determining when to return prescriptions to stock.

A variety of other systems are designed to better manage the will-call bin in busy pharmacies. One example is using storage units that automatically assign a location for prescriptions on the basis of a specific logic. To retrieve the prescription, the pharmacist can enter patient details or the prescription number into the PIMS or a workflow station and receive the prescription location in return. There are also patient-facing will-call units that allow for pickup outside of pharmacy hours or in circumstances when a patient prefers to retrieve a prescription this way, such as when there is a line at the pharmacy counter. This technology operates much like an automated teller machine.

Point-of-Sale Systems

Perhaps the very last point at which technology can come into play in the ambulatory care pharmacy is at checkout. Point-of-sale (POS) systems are increasingly found at this step. These systems can manage front-store retail activities such as pricing, inventory, and processing of credit and debit card payments. But, POS also allows a pharmacy to close the loop on the prescription-dispensing process. Not only does the PIMS record the date the prescription was filled; the POS system also records the date the prescription was actually picked up and paid for. When the POS system is integrated with the PIMS, the fact that a prescription has been successfully delivered to the patient and paid for is available throughout the pharmacy.

POS systems use electronic signature capture devices to record patient signatures not only for credit card payments, but also for third-party signature logs and signatures required for regulatory compliance with programs such as the program for pseudoephedrine sales. The electronic signature can also acknowledge receipt of the pharmacy's privacy protection policy, which is a federal requirement. Electronic signatures, which are easily searched, can be very useful when a pharmacy is audited.

POS can also be a billing management system that plays a role both in securely storing credit card numbers and in streamlining house charge accounts. Storing credit card numbers to facilitate mail order or delivery, for example, must comply with the payment card industry's data security standards. Generally speaking, this means that data are secured from improper use, something many POS systems can do. To streamline the management of house charge accounts, the pharmacist can, for example, use POS to charge purchases to subaccounts that are then collected on a single monthly statement. Or, POS can charge to one address and bill to another, which is particularly useful for deliveries to residents of LTC facilities whose guardians are paying the bills.

POS also offers the ability to ensure that your pharmacy's business protocols are being properly followed, which eliminates the need to rely on pharmacy staff to remember each important step during checkout, including steps that are required for regulatory compliance. Staff are guided through the transaction by the prompts on the screen. Using POS to run these protocols can also reduce the opportunity for unauthorized discounts or returns. If anything unusual does happen, appropriate staff can search the transaction record and review the circumstances, as well as identify the staff involved.

MTM Documentation and Billing

One of the new opportunities in pharmacy is medication therapy management (MTM) and, not surprisingly, technology is being used here to record the patient encounter and to bill. Tools may exist in the PIMS to support tracking and billing for MTM services. Also, companies that manage MTM networks are offering Web-based services for these tasks.

The Future of Technology in Pharmacy

That technology will continue to play a major role in ambulatory care pharmacy is certain. Perhaps a greater variety of choices will evolve, making it easier to find the technology that is the right fit for a particular pharmacy. Development of options that reduce investment cost and the time needed to deploy a new technology is likely. And, every pharmacist will want to keep abreast of all the ways that the technology in pharmacy can be integrated into the broader health care technology continuum. This will mean establishing connectivity and data exchange with repositories of health information available to other health care professionals. It will also mean allowing patients to tie their pharmacy records into their personal health records. What is certain is that ambulatory care pharmacy will continue a long history of putting innovative technology to work to serve patients better.

LEARNING ACTIVITIES

1. Review the technology you are using in your pharmacy operations. Which features do you use most? Which features would you like to use more? Which features do you consider most important for ensuring safety and compliance and for preventing fraud and abuse?
2. Diagram the workflow in your pharmacy. How does a prescription travel through your dispensing process? Can you identify bottlenecks in the dispensing process? How do the different systems integrate with each other? Where does your pharmacy data flow?
3. Pick a technology that you would like to use in your pharmacy. How would it impact your operations? What benefits would it offer? What issues do you see? What are the barriers that have prevented you from implementing this technology? Have you encountered similar barriers when you considered new technology?

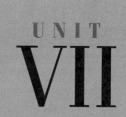

UNIT

VII

Medication Use Process IV: Electronic Systems for Medication Verification, Administration, and Documentation

CHAPTER 18. Enterprise Clinical Systems for Acute Care

CHAPTER 19. Ambulatory Electronic Medical Records and Medication Reconciliation

UNIT COMPETENCIES

- Discuss the benefits and limitations of systematically processing data, information, and knowledge in health care.
- Discuss the impact of data quality on health outcomes.
- Describe the structure and key elements of an electronic health record.
- Discuss key issues affecting human-computer interaction.
- Differentiate between spreadsheets, databases, and user interfaces.
- Describe the role of information systems in health care management.

UNIT DESCRIPTION

The fourth step in the medication use process is medication administration. Pharmacists are not normally directly involved with the administration of medications (except for some activities such as vaccinations). However, the electronic systems that communicate and capture medication administration data to and from nurses are critical sources of information for pharmacists' clinical activities. These systems include much more information than medication administration-related activities. Because of their use as the central repository of health care information, these electronic systems are the core of health care information management. These systems are discussed in this unit.

Enterprise Clinical Systems for Acute Care

Allen J. Flynn

OBJECTIVES

1. Define what an enterprise clinical system is and distinguish between the various types.
2. Describe the functional components of an acute care computerized patient record system.
3. Explain how to conduct a conversation about improving an electronic clinical system within your organization or directly with an enterprise clinical system vendor.
4. Discuss why properly managing an enterprise clinical system requires a structured approach to system change management.
5. List integrated and peripheral components of an electronic clinical system that are associated with the medication use process.

An **enterprise clinical system** is a system engineered to be highly reliable and to handle large volumes of data while supporting many concurrent clinician users throughout a large health care enterprise.

Unfortunately, the terms used to describe enterprise clinical systems are numerous and confusing. Clinicians in all health care disciplines today are likely to learn and use a number of enterprise clinical systems during their careers as health care providers. The enterprise clinical system is becoming the principal information system tool used by many clinicians in their daily patient care practices. One of the most important facts to know about these systems is that they cannot be managed like consumer or personal software applications used at home or in the office. Because of their size and the risks associated with information system errors or failures in health care, enterprise clinical systems require an extraordinary level of testing before configuration and functionality changes can be safely implemented. These systems are very carefully monitored and managed, often by sizable teams of health care information technology (IT) professionals.

Types of Enterprise Clinical Systems

Enterprise clinical systems may include computerized patient records (CPRs), electronic medical records (EMRs), electronic health record systems (EHRS), and clinical data repositories (CDRs). Yet, this is only a small sampling of the types and names of the "enterprise clinicals." Other terms for this type of system include the following: clinical information systems, acute care information systems, ambulatory care information systems, clinical documentation systems, patient care information systems, and so on. Even more confusing, enterprise clinical systems are complex combinations of known components and functions, but their various names and acronyms do not indicate precisely the components and functions that are included in any particular enterprise clinical system! Worse, subsets of the data and functionality of the enterprise clinicals must also be distinguished. For example, a subset of data managed by patients and caregivers together is the **personal health record** (PHR), whereas a subset of data intended to be easily shared between health care organizations across state and international borders is the **continuity of care record.** To keep up and understand, one must be ready for health care IT's unique recipe for alphabet soup!

Acute Care CPRS versus Ambulatory Care EMRs

It is important to bring some clarity and consistency to the naming of enterprise clinical systems. A distinction is commonly made between enterprise clinical systems used in acute care settings (e.g., hospitals) and those used in ambulatory care settings (e.g., outpatient clinics). This distinction is important because both the vendors and the software used to support acute care and ambulatory care processes can be different. Many health care provider organizations have chosen to purchase, implement, and use different acute care and ambulatory care enterprise clinical systems.

Acute care enterprise clinical systems are referred to as **computerized patient record systems** (CPRS). The term *electronic medical record* (EMR) is also used to describe acute care enterprise clinical systems, as well as ambulatory systems found in clinics and physicians' offices. To distinguish inpatient systems from other systems, this chapter uses the term CPRS for acute care systems. However, throughout this book, the term EMRs denotes both acute and ambulatory systems. Expect to find CPRS within hospitals. These systems include software for managing clinical data in databases and are composed of online functions and views of patient information. CPRS functions support inpatient workflow and include computerized provider order entry (CPOE) for ordering, clinical decision support (CDS) for assisting with decision making, electronic medication administration records (eMARs) for charting, online flow sheets for temporal data capture, structured documentation tools for planning and documenting care, and clinician-to-clinician messaging. CPRS views of patient data include demographic data, laboratory results, medication order lists, and overviews of medical information along with online medical images, notes, and reports.

Ambulatory enterprise clinical systems are referred to as EMRs (see following paragraph). Outpatient clinics, individual physician offices, and group practices purchase and implement EMRs as they migrate from paper charts to online patient records. Often, EMRs are combined with physician practice management software solutions, enabling the clinical and business processes of a physician practice to be managed in one information system. Furthermore, EMRs have sometimes been created to support the unique information management needs of specific medical disciplines, such as oncology. More general EMRs can also be customized to meet the needs of specialty practices through unique configuration. Unlike inpatient-oriented CPRS implementations, which generally support many hospital-based clinicians simultaneously, not all EMR implementations qualify as enterprise clinical application implementations. Some EMRs are implemented and used in small medical practices for which the term *enterprise* does not apply.

Electronic medical records are software applications that also manage clinical data in databases and are composed of functions and views needed to support care workflows. Common EMR functions include electronic pre-scribing, CDS, structured documentation, immunization documentation, scheduling, communication, care plan management, and billing. EMR views of patient information include demographic data, laboratory result views, medication lists, and overviews of medical information along with online medical images, notes, and reports, including records from con-sultations with other caregivers.

The Electronic Health Record

The **electronic health record** (EHR) is presently as much a concept as a working information system. The EHR refers to a summary aggregation of individual patient data from a variety of CPRs and EMRs. The larger EHR is intended to receive patient data from multiple sources and to share patient data nationally and internationally. It is safe to say that the EHR is still in development and that it will be for a long time to come. To achieve the vision of the EHR as it is described by the Healthcare Information and Management Systems Society,[1] care delivery organizations of all types and sizes will need to send and receive highly standardized (see Chapter 7) subsets of patient medical information through regional intermediaries over a proposed National Health Information Network (see Chapters 7 and 8). One important goal of the EHR is to empower patients and caregivers with the information they need at the point of care. In our highly mobile society, this goal may seem reasonable, even critical to those in the health care industry. However, EHR privacy and security concerns are also real, reasonable, and deserving of consider-able attention. As it is built and becomes operable, the EHR is certain to be an enterprise clinical system, and perhaps it will become one of the largest enterprise clinicals. Figure 18–1 depicts the relationships between the enterprise clinical system terminologies.

Anticipate Convergence of Patient Record Systems

As helpful as it is to distinguish between the CPR, EMR, and EHR, it is important to remember that what is most difficult about distinguishing between these names and concepts is that the systems they describe are continuously evolving! The convergence of the inpatient CPRS with the outpatient EMRs is already happening in some provider organizations.

FIGURE 18-1

Diagram of enterprise clinical system taxonomy.

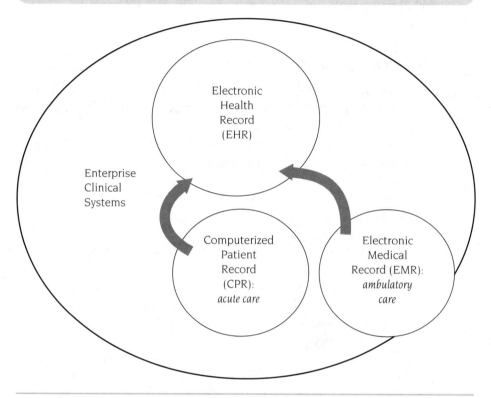

Source: Author.

Some vendors sell CPR and EMR systems with the same "look and feel" for clinician users. Some functions of the inpatient CPRS and outpatient EMRs are analogous, such as CPOE and electronic prescribing. As the convergence of systems continues, it may not be possible to distinguish the CPRS from the EMRs.

Acute Care CPRS

An enterprise clinical information system used in a hospital, surgery center, or anywhere else acute patient care is provided by caregiver teams is a computerized patient record system. CPRS are not as new or novel as they may seem. In fact, several exemplar CPRS were conceived and implemented in the 1960s and 1970s. However, the anticipated wave of CPRS adoption presaged during those years failed to materialize for many reasons, including cost and usability. Today widespread CPRS adoption is finally happening.

Functional Components of the CPRS

Hospitals are purchasing and implementing enterprise CPRS with many integrated components. An integrated component is defined as a portion of the enterprise CPRS platform that exists directly within the enterprise software and relies on the same database. Contrast integrated components with interfaced components, which exist outside of the CPRS and must rely on electronic messaging to and from the system for their functions. Interfaced components may not be provided by the CPRS platform vendor. Whether CPRS components are integrated or interfaced, typically hospitals are implementing the enterprise CPRS component by component instead of all at once. From the point of view of clinician users, the most common functional components of the acute care CPRS are listed in Table 18–1. The sequence of activation for the functional components of this system is varied. Still, it is clear that most hospitals will eventually implement most functional components of the CPRS.

The list of CPRS components in Table 18–1 may seem exhaustive, but it is not. Other specialized components exist, for example, online tumor registries used in oncology, patient care provider assignment management software, and total parenteral nutrition management components. Other components are likely to be needed; for example, some pharmacists and nurses envision an integrated IV line management component of the CPRS that would help manage IV flush protocols, drug compatibility information, and other IV access information. In light of the many components of the acute care CPRS, it is no wonder that only enterprise-wide platforms can provide the necessary information architecture to support them. It is important to remember that CPRS are highly complex systems that require continuous, collaborative, active management by health care and IT professionals.

The Pharmacist and the CPRS

Pharmacists practicing in acute care venues will find themselves using a number of integrated and interfaced functional components of the CPRS.

TABLE 18-1

Most Common Functional Components of CPRS for Clinician Users

Anesthesia management and documentation	Information security
Bar coding at the point of care	Knowledge management with online references
Bed management	
Care planning tools	Laboratory information system
Charge capture with revenue cycle management	Longitudinal health records
	Obstetric documentation and fetal monitoring
Clinical decision support	
Clinical documentation	Order reconciliation
Clinical nutrition information	Patient medical education tools
Computerized provider order entry	Patient retrieval, identification and tracking
Communication and messaging	Pharmacy information management system
Continuity of care document	Picture archiving and communication system
Electronic medication administration record	Radiology information system
Device integration	Registration system
Discharge and depart management	Reporting and clinical analytics
Electronic flow sheets	Scheduling system
Emergency department visit management and documentation	Surgery management and documentation
	Tracking boards

CPRS = computerized patient record systems.
Source: Author.

Pharmacists will also be presented with various other pharmacy information technologies for supply chain management, formulary management, pharmaco-surveillance, diversion surveillance, drug knowledge management (see Chapters 11 and 14), and other functions of the pharmacy (e.g., packaging and labeling).

In part, because the number of pharmacists is small relative to the number of physicians and nurses using the CPRS, the development of CPRS components often does not directly account for the unique roles and specific information needs of the health-system pharmacist. Instead, the pharmacist will frequently utilize common functional CPRS components such as CPOE, CDS, eMAR, and documentation tools that have been designed to support the workflow of various other clinicians.

One exception to this general rule is the pharmacy information management system (PIMS). The PIMS is a key component of the CPRS. Whether integrated or interfaced, the PIMS is the principal CPRS component used most frequently by pharmacists. PIMS generally include patient-specific information such as age, gender, height, and weight, along with allergy information, laboratory results, and comprehensive, individual patient lists of all drug orders and drug products dispensed during a patient visit. Within the PIMS, an ordered drug item, or "orderable," is matched to an available drug product, or "dispensable." The difference between an orderable and a dispensable is shown in Figure 18–2. With most integrated and interfaced CPRS, drug product selection has been automated to a large degree; however, there are times when automated product selection will not suffice and a pharmacist is needed to select the best product among available alternatives.

The pharmacist is a frequent CPRS user. As the CPRS continues to evolve and expand, it will be important for pharmacists to participate in the conception, planning, development, configuration, and deployment of system components. For the health-system pharmacist, the CPRS represents an excellent opportunity to become further established in the patient care environment. At the same time, for pharmacists, the import of the CPRS represents a major collaborative challenge to guarantee that the unique role and information needs of the pharmacist are accounted for within the system's functional components.

FIGURE 18–2

Difference between an orderable and a dispensable in CPRS.

Difference between an orderable and dispensable in CPRS.

Orderable: A named drug entity with a specified route of administration. Examples include:

aspirin oral
vancomycin intravenous

Dispensable: A specific drug product matched to the specified orderable with a defined unit of use. Examples include:

aspirin tablet 325 mg
vancomycin 1 gram in 250 mL dextrose 5%

CPRS = computerized patient record systems.
Source: Author.

CPRS Platform Architecture

The integrated functional components of the CPRS rely on the system's IT platform, as do connected devices and interfaced systems. The information architecture of the CPRS platform is quite important to all CPRS users because it ultimately determines the system's capability and performance. As important as the IT platform architecture is to CPRS capability and performance, platform architecture is often not considered directly by clinician users of the system. In fact, even when considered, little is known about how the IT platforms used to construct various CPRS govern system utility.

The architecture of the CPRS can be broadly considered in terms of seven layers, which, from top to bottom, are functions, views, databases, interfaces, networks, hardware, and the physical environment.

The highest layer of the CPRS architecture is the functional layer. The functional layer is governed by software code. The programming language used to create and adapt the software code of the CPRS platform is a key part of the system's architecture. Once programmed, CPRS software includes many things such as configuration tools, CDR rules engines, hyperlink support, data filters, and search capability. These functions are familiar to all computer users. Generally, to make functional changes to the CPRS requires the software vendors to make code changes. Vendors upgrade their CPR software periodically to add functionality and improve the user experience. Hospitals put resources into sharing their unmet functional needs with CPRS vendors and keeping CPR software updated to take advantage of new functions when they become available.

The second layer of CPRS architecture is the information retrieval and viewing layer. This layer is directly governed by CPR software code just as with the functional layer. It is important, however, to distinguish between performing functions and simply viewing information onscreen or retrieving information by printing reports. Information retrieval and presentation to support decision making are important capabilities of CPR software. Physicians, nurses, and other CPRS users are still developing the best methods for online presentation of information to support clinical workflow and medical decision making. Some information is historical, whereas other information is temporal and still other information is only of immediate import. Information in free-text format may simultaneously be richer in content and less functional for software manipulation and online presentation.

In terms of CPRS architecture, a common user complaint is that the viewing layer of the system is not functional: It permits data to be read only—not acted on. For example, when physicians are presented with view-only summary lists of medications within the CPRS, they expect to be able to modify, suspend, discontinue, or otherwise act on the medication orders provided in the summary view, although these functions are not available in a view-only mode. Over time, the viewing layer and the higher functional layer may become one within the architecture of the CPRS.

The third layer in the architecture of the CPRS is the database layer. Users do not experience this layer directly, but the database layer directly influences the user experience in myriad ways. Databases are customized data structures used to store both the CPRS configuration and the individual patient information within the system. CPRS databases are complex: They include a model of all data that will be stored within the system. CPRS data models are generally constructed by defining all data elements and their fields, then by organizing related data elements into data tables and, finally, by specifying explicit relationships between disparate data elements and data tables.

To make a custom data request, called a "query," from a CPRS, a database analyst who knows the data model is often required to construct the query. For example, if a pharmacist wants to know how many times intravenous levofloxacin was ordered from a community-acquired pneumonia order set within the last 6 months for female patients older than 59 years without any documented drug allergies, a query can be created to poll the necessary table or tables in the CPRS database and retrieve the information.

Databases interact with the higher functional layer of software and sometimes inadvertently govern functionality. For example, a CPRS must provide lists of open nursing units to users. If a new nursing unit is opened, a conceptually simple update to all user profiles to add the new nursing unit to the users' onscreen lists may not be as simple as it seems. Depending on the structure of the database tables and fields (i.e., the data model of the database), the IT staff may have no way to automate the addition of a new unit to the online lists of open nursing units used by clinicians. Instead, each clinician user may have to perform a manual update to his or her list of open nursing units. This is an example of how the structure of a database may impact users' experience of the system.

Databases in enterprise clinical systems also directly determine system performance and reliability. For this reason, database architecture accounts for different types of uses. Databases that are intended to be used simultaneously by hundreds of users with similar data needs have different architectures and data models than those intended to be used by a few simultaneous users with uncharacteristic data needs. Databases now have sophisticated backup and error detection schemes that help to provide a downtime-free CPRS platform for the health care environment. (See Chapter 6 for more information on data management in pharmacy.)

The fourth layer of CPRS architecture is the interface layer. Even the most integrated CPRS will still have many interfaces that shuttle data to and from other systems and established CPRS components. In pharmacy, interfaces often exist between the enterprise CPRS and PIMS, automated dispensing cabinet (ADC) systems, pharmaco-surveillance systems, bar coding at the point-of-care systems, and smart infusion device systems. **Health Level 7 standard** is an interface data standard that is commonly used in health care. This human-readable messaging standard exists to move patient information between disparate information systems. (See Chapter 7 for more information on data communication standards.)

Although interfaces and their messages are not directly experienced by clinician users of CPRS, as with databases, interfaces ultimately govern aspects of functionality and the end user experience. Because each interface can share only a predefined subset of patient or drug order data, some medical context and order context information is inevitably lost during deployment of interfaced systems. Furthermore, interfaces themselves rely on separate hardware and software sub-components, which become part of the architecture of the overall CPRS. For end users, this means that a failure at the level of an interface or a failure at the level of an interfaced component is likely to have a direct, negative impact on some of the functions of the CPRS. For example, if allergy information is entered into an interfaced system and then sent to the enterprise CPRS platform via an interface, a failure in the component that gathers disparate allergy data can interrupt medication management in the CPRS and other interfaced medication management systems. This disruption can eventually reach the patient and potentially lead to patient harm.

The fifth layer of the CPRS platform is the network layer. CPRS require networks to function. Enterprise CPRS are highly distributed systems, and users require access in all areas of the hospital as well as remote access from clinics, offices, and homes. The CPRS architecture includes a layer of networking hardware and software. The CPRS user experience relies on a stable, secure, and reliable networking layer. Catastrophic power failures and natural disasters have disrupted hospital networks in the past, making CPRS unavailable for use. Hospitals and health systems continue to invest in redundant networking hardware and software to preclude network outages that impact the enterprise CPRS. (Chapters 4 and 5 provide more information on networks, hardware, and software.)

The sixth layer of the CPRS platform is the system's hardware. CPRS rely on many high-powered computers, called servers, for their operations. These multiple servers must be continuously monitored, updated, protected from viruses, and actively managed. IT professionals provide this vital service to health care organizations. The speed, reliability, and redundancy of the CPRS' servers determine, in part, the user experience with regard to the speed and availability of the enterprise CPRS. As CPRS grow and server technology improves simultaneously, a substantial work effort is required to update the CPRS hardware. Often, users experience server updates indirectly as system downtime—downtime that is usually planned and typically occurs during the hours of least activity at the hospital.

The seventh and final layer of the CPRS architecture is the physical environment layer. For the server hardware and network hardware to function properly, highly secured, protected, environmentally stable data rooms and data centers are required. A data center is typically a secure room or rooms with many racks of servers, enormous power and cooling equipment, and substantial network bandwidth. The IT resources used to support the enterprise CPRS are connected and protected in the confines of a hospital data center or centers.

The architecture of the CPRS platform is much different than the information system architecture used in the typical home, which often includes only a personal computer, locally managed software for home use, a modem, and a printer. The CPRS architecture is much more robust and reliable, but it also requires much more time and effort to manage and maintain. All CPRS rely on large teams of IT professionals and health care professionals for their successful operation.

Importance of Best Practice Change Management

Enterprise CPRS have great architectural and functional complexity. CPRS configuration errors or software faults can have severe consequences in health care; therefore, several best practices have been developed for managing enterprise CPRS changes.

Both extraordinary and routine changes to the configuration of the enterprise CPRS carry real risks. For example, adding a new drug orderable to a CPOE component—a common change—exposes risks that the online dosing, routes, and ordering information added to the CPOE system could be inaccurate. If that happens, potential drug errors have been systematized so that multiple errors could result. To manage such risks, the health care IT industry has adopted best practices for managing CPRS configuration, hardware, software, interface, database, and other changes.

The most important best practice change-management processes include (1) establishing a defined, standardized process for instituting change in the CPRS; (2) documenting all changes made to the CPRS so that changes can be planned for, monitored, and reviewed; and (3) adopting safe configuration practices, which may include independent quality assurance and confirmation of correct configuration by clinical experts, who are sometimes referred to as "CPR content gatekeepers."

CPRS Vendor Marketplace

A health care IT vendor is a for-profit corporation in the business of creating, selling, and supporting health care IT solutions, including enterprise clinical systems. However, before discussing the vendor marketplace for CPRS, consider first a common conundrum in IT: whether it is better to build or buy an information system.

Build versus Buy a CPRS

In light of the long list of components required to create an enterprise CPRS, the costs of building such a system are enormous. Therefore, in some cases it makes sense to have software vendors (whose primary business is software development) create and sell CPRS to hospitals. However, because many of the CPRS components are relatively new and in need of substantial refinement—whereas other components have yet to be developed—building a CPRS has been a viable alternative for several leading health care organizations.

The dilemma of whether to build or buy a CPRS is often stated too simply. In reality, hospitals and health systems that choose to purchase components of a CPRS from a vendor may add their own locally developed components and extensions to the CPRS at their locations. Further, health care organizations that elect to build their own CPRS must still rely heavily on IT solution vendors for the underlying technologies of their homegrown CPRS, namely databases, programming environments, and hardware. For these reasons, all CPRS are hybrid systems on a continuum between "built and bought."

Know Your CPRS Vendor

In the U.S. market, the vendors listed in Table 18–2 sell and support the majority of CPRS used by health care practitioners.[2] The names, capabilities, and histories of the common CPRS vendors are often referred to in hospitals and health systems. It is important for health care practitioners

TABLE 18–2

Some Common Vendors for CPRS Certified by CCHIT in 2007

Vendor	System(s)	Version Certified
Cerner	Millennium Powerchart	2007
CPSI	CPSI System	16
Eclipsys	Sunrise Acute Care, Sunrise Clinical Manager	4.5 sp 4
Epic	EpicCare Inpatient	Spring 2007
GE Healthcare	Centricity Enterprise	6.7
Healthcare Management Systems	Healthcare Management Systems	7.0
Healthland	Clinical Information Systems	9.0.0
Meditech	Advanced Clinical Systems, Magic	5.6
McKesson	Horizon Clinicals Suite	ER 7.8.2
Siemens Healthcare	Soarian Clinicals	2.0C6

CCHIT = Certification Commission for Health Information Technology; CPRS = computerized patient record systems.
Source: Reference 2.

to know some basic details of the vendor of the CPRS at their workplace, starting with the name of the company and its CPRS. The core strengths and economic health of these vendors influence clinical practices at the hospitals where their CPRS are in use.

Furthermore, hospitals employ teams of specialists with clinical, IT, and hybrid backgrounds to manage CPRS provided by the common vendors. An important career path exists for pharmacists and pharmacy specialists in health care IT (pharmacy informaticians). Hospital IT and pharmacy departments have growing groups of information systems experts working alongside other health system pharmacy personnel in the exciting field of pharmacy informatics.

Enhancement Requests

Pharmacists and pharmacy specialists working in the hospital often have great ideas to improve or enhance the functions and features of CPRS components. The best ideas for enhancements to existing system components typically come from clinician users of CPR software. Such ideas are often critical to creating safer, more functional, and easier to use CPRS components. Nevertheless, it can be difficult to know with whom to share great ideas for improving the system, and it can be frustrating when suggested improvements cannot be quickly adopted.

As part of the health care team, pharmacists and pharmacy specialists should seek a forum or forums to share their experiences with and ideas for enhancing CPRS. Typically, health systems create and prioritize lists of good enhancement requests to be taken to the vendor community for action. As CPRS users, pharmacists should seek out leaders and decision makers who are managing the system and ask about the process for submitting enhancement requests. The scale and complexity of the CPRS require stringent change management, and many of its components are relatively new and subject to ongoing enhancement over periods of many years. Therefore, pharmacists should not give up or become frustrated if their great ideas are not immediately implemented. Although there is no substitute for user enhancement requests, there are real cost and technological constraints that can forestall innovation at times. The best advice for sharing enhancement requests is to identify those in the organization charged with managing CPRS enhancements and to build collaborative working relationships with them.

Partnering for Success

Here is one final note about the work of developing and deploying CPRS components. Experience demonstrates that partnerships between health care providers and health care IT vendors are paramount to achieving success with an enterprise CPRS. The power and promise of this system have yet to be fully achieved. An enormous work effort remains. The most effective and efficient approach to the remaining work effort will likely include strong, sustained customer-vendor partnerships. Health care vendor leaders, including chief executive officers and others, readily admit that market success is very difficult to sustain in health care given the prevailing risk and complexities. Hospitals and health systems have high expectations for successful use of CPRS but often underestimate the costs in capital, time, and effort required to deploy the system. However, through sustained partnership, successful business models and better care have already been achieved. A climate of mutual respect and appreciation between vendor and customer is an important goal.

Medication Use Process Components of the CPRS

Interfaced Medication Use Process Components

The medication use process in the hospital includes five main steps: ordering of medications, medication order review by pharmacists, dispensing of medications, administering of medications, and monitoring of ongoing medication therapies. Chapter 1 provides a closer look at the medication use process.

When two disparate information systems share standardized information over a network, they are said to be interfaced one to the other. Currently, CPRS components associated with the medication use process are frequently interfaced. Medication use process systems such as the PIMS, pharmaco-surveillance systems, ADCs, drug-compounding robots, and smart infusion pump systems have mostly been developed separately from the CPRS by various, competing health care IT vendors. Interfaces that permit disparate systems to send and receive patient data make data sharing between these medication use process systems and the enterprise CPRS possible. In this way, interfaces are vital to the current operations of medication use process information systems. Without data-sharing interfaces, written medication order information would have to be entered into multiple systems, increasing the likelihood of order transcription errors.

The most typical interface types used to support medication use process systems are admission, discharge, and transfer (ADT) interfaces, which keep all systems updated with (1) patient location and status information, (2) allergy interfaces that share updates to patient allergy histories, (3) medication order interfaces that share the facts of medication orders, (4) verification interfaces that send signals from the pharmacy system to indicate which orders have been reviewed by a pharmacist and, finally (5) charting interfaces that send messages from the eMAR to share which medications have been administered to patients over time.

Interfaced systems provide unique challenges and benefits. Challenges include managing multiple potential points of communication failure between systems and properly mapping data fields between disparate system databases. Interfaced system benefits include the ability to utilize legacy and best-of-breed systems in conjunction with the CPRS and the ability for disparate systems to remain operational when the CPRS is experiencing downtime.

Integrated Medication Use Process Components

Unlike disparate systems that share patient data via interfaces, integrated CPRS components are those components that utilize the same platform, especially the same database. Over time, there is a trend to incorporate more medication use process components into the CPRS as fully integrated components.

PIMS systems are being integrated directly into CPRS. This can be helpful to pharmacists and can improve pharmaceutical care. Integrated PIMS provide the same "look and feel" to users as the rest of the CPRS. Integrated pharmacy systems offer enhanced features such as the ability to edit orders in the pharmacy system without returning to the CPOE system to do so. Integrated pharmacy systems also may provide advantages in the area of CDRs by making use of the CPRS' decision support functionality.

At least one CPRS vendor, Cerner, has chosen to integrate ADCs within its CPRS software and hardware architecture. An ADC platform, which shares its database with the CPRS, may offer unique opportunities for utilizing decision support and for coordinating eMAR and ADC workflow. Chapter 16 provides a more thorough description of ADCs and other automation technologies.

As with disparate, interfaced systems, medication use process components integrated into the CPRS offer unique challenges and benefits. The rationale for integration is increased effectiveness through significantly greater sharing of more timely information between physicians, pharmacists, and nurses. When physicians and nurses are able to review online documented interventions by pharmacists, communication is improved. Similarly, pharmacists' effectiveness is improved, in the context of providing pharmaceutical care, when they are able to review online information about medical decision making, patient care plans, and documented care.

One challenge associated with software components of integrated medication use processes includes relinquishing control of the change to slower, enterprise-level change-management practices. Another challenge is the downtime that occurs any time the CPRS is unavailable for use.

Peripheral Medication Use Process Components

Some computer peripherals are used in conjunction with both interfaced and integrated CPRS components of the medication use process.

The most common peripheral used in pharmacy is the pharmacy label printer. In light of the importance of safe labeling, reliable printers are required by pharmacies. Although printer brands and technologies vary, the label printer must always be considered a necessary part of the pharmacy's IT infrastructure. Some printers provide software that allows the printers to add value by manipulating the print data stream to enhance label output with pictures, easy-to-read fonts, color printing, and other features.

Another peripheral used in the medication use process is the personal data assistant (PDA). PDAs with on-board bar code scanners can be used to support medication administration safety system workflows related to mobile bar codes. PDAs are also used for patient data retrieval, communications, online drug libraries, and other services. Some PDAs have been combined with phones to become smart phones. Expect PDA and smartphone devices to be increasingly used to support the information needs of highly mobile, busy health care workers.

Medical devices associated with the medication use process are a third type of peripheral. The most common devices integrated with the CPRS are smart infusion pump devices. These devices can be used to infuse medications from syringes or IV bags. Smart pumps include drug error reduction software to prevent pump programming errors. Typically, the caregiver programming the smart pump will select the drug to be infused from a menu displayed on the pump itself. Next, during programming of parameters for the infusion, the pump's resident drug library of information will guide the caregiver in programming the pump to avoid mistaken data entry during programming that could result in a medication error and harm to the patient. Smart pumps have become wireless network devices, capable of sharing information with dedicated computer servers as part of a networked smart pump information system. Anticipate smart pump data sharing through interfacing and integration between the smart pump servers and the CPRS.

Conclusion

Enterprise clinical systems are complex computing environments that are designed to support the information needs of a broad user base. Pharmacists should understand the differences between the various terms and acronyms surrounding enterprise clinical systems—in acute and ambulatory care environments. Just as importantly, pharmacists should recognize that the enterprise clinical systems environment is continuously evolving and is an important area to closely follow.

The PIMS is the core application that supports pharmacists' clinical and administrative activities in all practice environments. There are many considerations for managing the PIMS, including how to acquire it, how to keep databases up to date, and how to interface with the vendor for enhancements and modifications. The ongoing, appropriate functioning of interfaced and integrated components also requires considerable oversight by pharmacy staff.

It is inconceivable to envision a future pharmacy practice environment that is not fully supported by health information technology (HIT), including the technologies discussed in the present chapter. Pharmacists must be aware of the relationship of their PIMS to other system components. This understanding will enable the pharmacist to judiciously and efficiently utilize all HIT to ensure optimal medication-related patient outcomes.

LEARNING ACTIVITIES

1. Establish a relationship with the pharmacy department in a local hospital. Identify the institution's approach to clinical enterprise computing. What do they call their system—EMR, EHR, CPR, or something else? What access rights do pharmacists have for reading and writing to the record? Where are pharmacists providing the most input into the record?

2. With regard to the hospital in question 1, does it rely on interfaced or integrated components of its CPRS? What components are integrated versus interfaced? What benefits does the hospital describe for its approach? What limitations does the hospital describe for its approach? What role does pharmacy play in the communication of medication-related electronic information across components?

3. Visit two local community pharmacies—an independent and a chain. Describe their PIMS. Was it developed in-house or did they purchase it from a vendor? What database components are utilized? Can pharmacists at one location access patient records from other pharmacies? Does the pharmacy electronically communicate with hospitals or physician clinics? If yes, what information is shared?

4. At both pharmacy locations in #3, determine each pharmacy's involvement with its vendor's enhancement request process. What type of enhancements have the pharmacies submitted? What is the general time frame for their requests being addressed? How would they change the enhancement request process to make it better?

References

1. Garets D, Davis M. Electronic medical records vs. electronic health records: yes, there is a difference. January 26, 2006. Available at: http://www.himssanalytics.org/docs/WP_EMR_EHR.pdf. Accessed November 1, 2009.
2. Certification Commission for Healthcare Information Technology. Inpatient EHR products. Available at: http://www.cchit.org/products/inpatient. Accessed November 1, 2009.

Ambulatory Electronic Medical Records and Medication Reconciliation

Bill G. Felkey

OBJECTIVES

1. Distinguish between the focus of the electronic medical record (EMR) and the electronic health record (EHR).
2. Describe the historical relationship between pharmacy management information systems and pharmacy-specific EMRs.
3. Discuss how EMRs can help facilitate clinical research.
4. List at least three considerations for selecting an EMR for a specific practice application.
5. Describe the importance of interoperability in a collaborative environment.
6. Define the parameters of medication reconciliation as required by the Joint Commission.

The United States health care system is under pressure to transform its industry to become safer, less costly, and more effective. The pressure to make these changes comes from major stakeholders such as the federal government, employers who pay a tremendous percentage of the costs associated with health care, the media, and the public. A growing number of patients would like to enjoy the same kind of connectivity they have with their banks and airlines. The expected benefits that will be accrued from transforming health care into a digital field include decreased overall costs and a reduction in errors. These benefits are anticipated even though the cost to implement electronic systems will be substantial in the beginning. Other expected benefits focus on the reduction of waste such as unnecessary and redundant testing by health care providers, as well as the ability to share the results of laboratory tests and other important information. Access time and accuracy are also expected to improve as information can be readily retrieved when and where it is required.

There is a lot of excitement about the prospects of anytime, anywhere access to patient-specific health information because it will eventually be possible to retrieve the information needed to reduce uncertainty when making clinical decisions. A focus of these efforts is to use devices as small as smartphones and ultra-mobile personal computers to access desired information. This focus further implies that real-time connectivity to both patients and providers will make collaborative care more possible and will allow for a multidisciplinary team approach to health care. In this team approach, with full connectivity between providers, the right provider should be able to provide the right intervention for the right patient in the appropriate facility at the right time. Streamlining the information so that it is packaged in the manner that an ambulatory care provider wants to see it is one of the driving factors for specialized electronic medical records (EMRs). The National Alliance for Health Information Technology defines an **electronic medical record** as "an electronic record of health-related information on an individual that can be created, gathered, managed, and consulted by authorized clinicians and staff within one health care organization."[1] EMRs are not synonymous with **electronic health records** (EHRs), which aggregate all of the data being generated by individual EMRs.

Typically, EMRs have two other components whose functions are commonly used by practice staff members rather than clinicians. The two components are commonly labeled "front-office" and "back-office" software, with the clinical application positioned in the middle. The front-office components of the application manage processes such as scheduling of appointments for patients. The ideal scheduling application provides patients with online access through a Web browser that is synchronized in real time to the office-based application.

When patients are connected electronically to a practice, appointment reminders can occur through channels such as text messaging and e-mail. The actual episode of care for the patient is managed in the EMR component of the application and allows, in the best circumstances, electronic prescription processing, management of digital images from radiologists, and connectivity with laboratories for immediate posting of results to the EMR when available. The back-office component of an EMR application handles functions for reimbursement claims processing and reporting requirements for regulatory bodies.

Because EMRs must be able to communicate data within the health system, interoperability is an important factor for determining which EMR will be selected to support a practice, regardless of the discipline or specialty of that practice. (Chapters 7 and 8 discusses interoperability.) At the national level, the Centers for Medicare and Medicaid Services has published[2] and the Office of the National Coordinator for Health Information Technology is updating[3] meaningful use regulations that describe certain functionality that must be achieved through the use of the EMR/EHR. These functionalities include the ability for computerized order entry, drug interaction checking, the maintenance of an updated problem list specific to each patient, and the ability for the generation of transmissible prescriptions. Of course, a pharmacy EMR would use a specialized form of these meaningful use criteria to support its practice. Although pharmacists might create orders necessary for patients' treatments, perform drug interaction checking, and maintain medication-related problem lists for patients, the pharmacist EMR would need to be interoperable in such a way that it could receive and process transmissible prescriptions instead of having the capability to generate them.

Interoperability between multiple EMR systems will be facilitated further by health information exchange processes. For example, a pharmacist performs a medication therapy management (MTM) session with a patient and documents the patient's level of medication regimen adherence. These data will not only become available to prescribers during electronic prescription entry but will also populate an active problem list in the EMR of every other health care provider that is caring for the patient. Other entities receiving the data could include pharmacy benefit managers and the patient's personal health record (PHR). These exchanges of information can either take place through a central data repository that supports an EHR or through a federated model whereby patient data are extracted from their native systems on demand. Today, this fully functioning interoperable model of health information exchange across locations of care does not exist across the United States. It is, however, a major focus of considerable efforts. These efforts are described further in Chapter 8.

Interoperability is so important that a certification process is being developed to ensure that meaningful use functions are operating in such a way that the standardized sharing of information is possible. Pharmacy management systems adhere to certain standards to support activities such as claims processing, but these systems are not currently using certification processes that are used by other health care providers. It may be necessary for pharmacists to pursue certification to show that their ability to share information and work with other systems is occurring according to industry standards. Without this certification, the data coming out of pharmacy systems may be considered suspect. Certified EMRs that are functioning properly can participate in patient care coordination that reflects factors such as timeliness and convenience, accuracy, efficiency, and the ability to respond to emergency situations.

Ambulatory EMRs also have the potential to accelerate clinical research initiatives. When initiating a new research study, it should be possible to query the EMR database to determine how many potential study candidates reside in a given community. During the study enrollment phase, screening parameters will help further refine selection of study participants. During the actual study, data can be gathered as a byproduct of clinical visits. Adverse reactions experienced in the study would be documented and be retrievable from the EMR database. When studies involve protocol-driven research, EMRs can be fed the protocols needed by clinicians so that they can be inserted appropriately into the normal workflow of the practice.

EMR developers face several challenges for getting the best benefit in any practice that utilizes their applications. The usability and design of an EMR have to be sensitive to the workflow used in every practice in which it is installed. The typical experience with EMRs is that a loss of productivity occurs during the initial implementation of the application. Usually, unscheduled downtime requires new procedures that do not mimic the previous operation because any clinical work done when the EMR is down will have to be input when the system returns to normal functionality. Care must be taken in the selection of the EMR to make sure that it communicates with other systems such as inpatient-based EMRs. Again, ongoing certification processes are taking place to help ensure interoperability and other functionality needed for collaboration.

History of Pharmacist-Specific EMRs

Historically, pharmacists have operated their practices using pharmacy information management systems (PIMS) that are not categorized as EMRs. Each management system provided a means for processing orders and prescriptions in the support of dispensing operations specific to a type of practice. For example, community pharmacy systems, long-term care (nursing home) systems, and departmental solutions for hospital pharmacy practices represented separate and distinct products that were designed to provide practice-specific features and benefits.

In community pharmacy, during the introduction of the pharmaceutical care movement in the United States in the mid-1990s, a new class of pharmacy software was developed. Many of the pharmaceutical care software products were stand-alone, patient-focused, cognitive service (non-dispensing) applications. These products did much of the same work as an EMR in that they provided a place to document laboratory results, vital signs, review of systems, and SOAP (subjective objective assessment plan) notes. Some dispensing systems added these pharmaceutical care components to their products. Later some pharmaceutical care products added dispensing to their functionality.

A similar kind of innovation has taken place to respond to the need for software that supports the provision of MTM services detailed by Medicare Part D legislation passed in 2003 and enacted in 2005. Pharmacy dispensing systems and stand-alone software developers prepared their products to support this service provision. When pharmacists who operated in a clinic environment where patient services may not include the dispensing of medications looked for software support, they attempted to adopt and modify EMRs that were designed for physician use. These physician-oriented applications typically work better when pharmacists and physicians work together as a team in the same facility. If the clinic is operated only by pharmacists, the application's orientation to physicians and a variety of problems with a lack of support for the specialized needs of a pharmacist quickly surface. Small items such as user authorization levels, words selected for reporting purposes, the robustness of the medication profile, and many other deficits quickly reveal that, just like any other medical discipline or specialty, pharmacists require specialized products that are sensitive to their workflow.

EMR Selection Considerations

A systematic process usually works best for making the important decision of which application to use as an EMR for a specific practice. A team approach is usually recommended so that the insights of the stakeholders who will be impacted by the adoption of the EMR will be garnered and the ownership of the final decision will be shared. A commitment is required by this team to sort through the potential hundreds of options available. This decision is important enough to consider site visits to users of installed applications. A total cost projection for all operating expenses beyond the acquisition cost should also be performed.

Because the EMR should eventually connect with an EHR, it is important to find out what other pharmacies, local hospitals, ambulatory physician practices, and regional information exchange initiatives are established or are being planned. Some, if not all, of these parties will be surprised that a pharmacist is actively pursuing participation in the EHR planning process. Many of these acute care and ambulatory providers believe that the medication-related data they require can be solicited from pharmacy benefit managers. The providers may also need to be educated on a pharmacist's impact on health outcomes.

Plan on starting the pharmacist EMR selection process with the stakeholder team, headed by a project manager, and establish goals and expectations for how an EMR will ideally impact the pharmacy practice. Next, discuss definitions and priorities for requirements of the EMR. Armed with goals and requirements, a vendor search can take place, and the short list of those most closely matching selection criteria can be scheduled for product demonstrations. Due diligence in this process requires verifying references for each vendor and conducting site visits to practices that have adopted the application. Ideally, a practice can be located for visits in your community or to a community with similar interoperability requirements. Once all of the costs have been calculated for each product that still remains in the "viable" category, a finalist is selected and the contract for the product can then be negotiated. (See Chapter 27 for more information on management of information technology projects.)

Bear in mind that selecting an EMR for a practice will always impact the workflow in that practice. Start by mapping out current processes and workflows; then consider where in the workflow the new clinical functionality of the EMR will be placed; and, finally, attempt to anticipate the impact of that placement on current daily activities in the practice. The idea is not to simply automate a manual process but to look for opportunities to integrate the process so that it supports optimal achievement of the established goals for the practice. Also, consider the ripple effect of adding new services to the existing workload of all personnel and any opportunity for integration of ancillary systems in the practice to the new EMR. Consider, for example, how the delegation of additional duties for dispensing will be necessary to cover a pharmacist's distribution duties when he or she is conducting a 15-minute, one-on-one patient session.

When considering the ideal future state for the operation of the EMR in the practice, make sure that internal and external communication factors are covered for both systems and personnel. Determine how organization of data will need to change, what charting standard and follow-up reminders will be utilized for patient handoffs between pharmacists, and how the status of each patient will be posted in the work queue for clinicians and staff. Determine how clinical references and clinical decision support system alerts will provide a safety net for decision making. Describe the specific methods, tools, and update process that will be performed at predetermined intervals and by predetermined personnel. Finally, ensure successful initiation of new clinical services in the practice by operating the new EMR on a hardware system that allows scalability to handle increased workloads, and that contains the interfaces necessary to send and receive data between collaborating systems.

Case Study of a Pharmacist EMR

A pharmacist-focused EMR is an option to utilizing a primary care, generic EMR and settling for a workflow and/or a design that anticipates the end user would be a physician and/or a nurse.

Auburn University's Harrison School of Pharmacy has been using a pharmacist EMR for the last 2 years for both educational purposes for Doctor of Pharmacy students and for patient care in its in-house clinic operations. The product is named Medication Pathfinder (www.medication pathfinder.com), and it would be accurately classified as a clinical product only (dispensing is not supported) that is specifically designed to support the rendering of MTM services.

The product is workflow sensitive upon log-in because it presents collaborative communication and the status of all active patients who require workup by the pharmacist responsible for their care. Initiation of new patients prompts queries for the entry of the patient's name, Social Security number, medical record numbers, date of birth, blood type, sexual orientation, race, and marital status. The product displays whether any potential patients who have already been included in the patient census could match the new entry.

Adding a new patient into the charting database then provides tabs to collect address, provider, and insurance information. Attachment of scanned reports or other documents to the newly created chart is also allowed. A "Claims" tab collects the prescribed medications, filled medications, and patient procedures and conditions, including the American Medical Association Current Procedural Terminology (CPT) codes. A "Patient Registry" tab allows documentation of the patient's medical history, preventive health, social/family history, laboratories, diagnostics, vitals, and additional medication profile notes. This section also captures documentation on patient allergies and intolerance data, as well as provides an opportunity for pharmacist-performed patient evaluations to be conducted and documented.

A library of pharmacist-specific patient assessment tools is then offered in the workflow. These include follow-up and function assessments, cognition, proton pump inhibitor, angina, Parkinson's disease, and SOAP assessment tools, as well as tools that assess lifestyle, cardiovascular, respiratory, and psychiatric patient status. Pain assessment and medication-related issues to include in a complete drug regimen review are also structured in the pharmacist EMR. New procedures and assessments can be added at the request of pharmacist end users.

Medication Pathfinder software supports the generation of pharmacist recommendations to both physicians and patients. Summary reports that are generated directly from the medical record help eliminate the tedious job of pharmacists retyping their findings into correspondence. Back-office functions of creating and tracking billing of services are also included in the application. This billing function can either prepare invoices for direct billing of patients or collect the necessary data for third-party billing using standardized forms.

The Medication Pathfinder application is classified as an **Application Service Provider** product, which means that it is operated entirely by using an Internet-connected Web browser. Data are redundantly stored off-site, which means that a local event affecting the pharmacy end user, such as a tornado or hurricane, will not place the practice's data storage needs at risk. **Redundant data storage** by the service provider ensures that data are backed up regularly, and that the data are housed in geographically dispersed computer data storage facilities for additional security. Purchasing services from this type of product line is usually done on a cost-per-pharmacist basis.

Medication Reconciliation

Medication errors continue to be one of the most frequent causes of preventable harm in health care.[4] Medication reconciliation is the process of comparing a patient's historical and current medications to determine the accurate, current medication list. In 2005, the Joint Commission, which is an accrediting body for U.S. health systems, published its National Patient Safety Goals, in which goal number 8 required medication reconciliation for patients as they were admitted to, transferred within, and discharged from accredited U.S. hospitals. Since this requirement was instituted, hospitals have been struggling to comply with this goal. The goal was subsequently relaxed for 2009, with refinement and reinstatement planned for 2010.[5] Despite the relaxing of this patient safety requirement, many hospitals and partner facilities continue their efforts to develop and implement an effective medication reconciliation process.

Although the focus of this accreditation goal is hospital-based care, compiling an accurate list of active medications and supplements that the patient is taking creates problems throughout the continuum of care. For example, when patients present a new prescription at a community pharmacy, it is frequently unknown if they have filled other prescriptions in other pharmacies. When medical specialists write prescriptions, they frequently rely on the self-report of patients for their active drug list.

At the time of admission into a hospital, reconciliation must take place to determine what medication patients have been taking at home so that it can be compared with the medication that is about to be prescribed upon admission. In some cases, medications taken at home will be maintained and additional medications will be ordered. In other cases, therapeutic alternatives will be used to replace existing drug regimens. Medication reconciliation is done to avoid medication errors that could include the omission of necessary drugs, duplication of therapies within the same class, and potential drug interactions. Additional benefits of medication reconciliation include the ability to help facilitate communication between providers across the care continuum.

It is important to note that the definition of the types of medications subject to reconciliation is fairly broad. Although prescription drugs (including sample medications that the patient is taking) are usual priorities, a comprehensive medication reconciliation will identify herbal remedies, vitamins, nutraceuticals, over-the-counter medications, vaccines, diagnostic agents, and other Food and Drug Administration products designated as drugs.

Medication reconciliation will usually involve a multidisciplinary team. These teams commonly comprise nurses, physicians, pharmacists, and dietitians. Interestingly, in many instances, pharmacists leave much of this duty to nurses, even though it would be easy to assume that pharmacists might play a primary role in the reconciliation process. Physicians, by policy, are usually required to review and make final adjustments on patient medication regimens within 24 hours of admission. This will include addressing any discrepancies that are identified at admission.

Identification of discrepancies usually occurs when the individual charged with gathering data to create a complete and accurate medication list identifies, through a variety of sources, what was prescribed for the patient and how the patient is actually taking his or her medication. Details that are captured include the medication name, strength, route, frequency, and storage conditions; indication; date and time of last dose; and adherence details. Methods to gather these data include patient interviews, brown-bag reviews of medications brought to the hospital, and requests for information from pharmacies and prescribers. Some data gathering occurs by electronic polling of prescription gateways and insurance company sources to determine what claims have been processed. These electronic tools (Table 19–1) can identify as much as 60% to 80% of the active medications, but these tools frequently have missing data fields (such as dosing frequency) that require further investigation.

Additional data might be available on a given patient from prior admissions. Usually the method for gathering accurate medication data will depend on the patient's type of admission. For example, admission

TABLE 19-1

Representative Commercial Applications for Electronic Medication Reconciliation*

Vendor	Application Name	Web Site
Design Clinicals	MedsTracker	www.designclinicals.com
DrFirst	Rcopia AC	www.drfirst.com
Healthcare Systems	Medication Reconciliation	www.hcsinc.net
RelayHealth	IntegrateRx	www.relayhealth.com
Thomson Reuters	Clinical Xpert Medication Reconciliation	www.micromedex.com

*These applications are added onto existing clinical systems. Medication reconciliation applications are also available through clinical information system vendors who provide complete enterprise-wide systems. *Source:* Author.

through an emergency department after a motor vehicle accident will preclude the actual medications being available at the time of admission. Scheduled admissions for non-emergent surgical procedures will typically allow data gathering with the actual medications being available at admission. Interestingly, electronic data-gathering methods will frequently reveal active medications that patients fail to report during an interview, or that they fail to classify as a medication when bringing their medications from home. For example, male patients who are about to receive a dose of nitrates in the emergency department may fail to report that they have consumed a medication to treat erectile dysfunction such as Cialis prior to their admission.

Once the data are gathered for the patient's medication list, it is necessary to determine the status of each of the medications. Active medications are usually classified as those from home sources or as those prescribed since the patient's arrival at the hospital. Some medications are classified as a reorder when home therapies are continued. The remaining medications are classified as either being inactive or discontinued depending on who made the determination for the patient to stop taking the medication. One role of the pharmacist in reviewing this medication list would be to try to determine whether the patient's admission to an acute care facility is actually caused by a drug-related problem.

In some health systems, a medical specialist commonly called a "hospitalist" is heavily involved in reconciliation. Ambulatory physicians can, in this scenario, choose to "hand off" a patient into the care of the hospitalist, who oversees the acute care episode of that patient until the patient is discharged back into the care of the ambulatory physician. Within the hospital, primary care responsibility can be managed by another specialist, called an "intensivist," who provides specialized care, specifically diagnostic and monitoring procedures, for critically ill patients.[6] During each of these transfers of responsibility for patients, an additional medication reconciliation requirement is made. When patients are discharged, a final medication reconciliation must be done as the handoff to ambulatory care takes place. In addition, many hospitals provide discharge education sessions to make sure patients are equipped with the knowledge and skills necessary to manage their self-care behaviors upon discharge. When software programs oversee this process, it is possible to use clinical decision support systems such as a prospective drug utilization review that identifies conflicts such as drug interactions, duplicate therapies, and the potential for drug allergies in the patient.

Another consideration in the medication reconciliation process is that of the criteria-based involvement of the pharmacist under certain conditions, such as the age of the patient being 75 or greater. Other criteria could include a situation in which a polypharmacy review would be indicated. This need for a pharmacist consult could be triggered when the patient is taking 10 or more medications because, under these circumstances, the likelihood of a drug-related problem is increased. Other criteria include medication doses that are out of normal ranges, laboratory results out of normal ranges, medications unfamiliar to the nurse, and occurrence of early readmission (recidivism issues), all of which indicate a potential drug-related problem.

Conclusion

Electronic medical and health records will change the practice of pharmacy and medicine. Historically, few electronic record applications existed to support the clinical services that pharmacists provided. Applications that functioned similarly to EMRs did emerge in the 1990s in conjunction with the pharmaceutical care movement. Those applications lacked interoperability, which is the key enabling factor that will allow exchange of health-related information across providers, clinical laboratories, and health care institutions.

Today, pharmacists should carefully examine their practice and the potential role of their PIMS as a tool to connect with other providers to share clinical information. Many considerations should be addressed when examining a practice and when evaluating potential applications for incorporation into that practice.

A key component of all pharmacy practice environments will be the ability to effectively and accurately exchange medication-related information to satisfy medication reconciliation requirements. Although the Joint Commission accredits hospitals (and not community pharmacies), its requirement for medication reconciliation cuts across all pharmacy practice environments. Any transfer of a patient's care into, within, and out of a hospital will require an accurate reconciliation. This includes reconciling the medications the patient took while in the community. Pharmacy is closely watching the refinement of the medication reconciliation goal to determine the exact impact it will have on practice.

LEARNING ACTIVITIES

1. Go to RxInsider's Virtual Tradeshow (www.rxshowcase.com), and look at the medication therapy management link. Examine the various vendor products, and compare the applications for their ability to address the evaluation characteristics discussed above.

2. Go to www.scholar.google.com and www.pubmed.gov, and search for the phrase "medication reconciliation" utilizing the quotation marks in the search. Examine the first several articles on each site. What do they describe as the current challenges, successes, and initiatives related to medication reconciliation?

3. Read the description of products and services offered for a pharmacist EMR at the Medication Pathfinder Web site (www.medication-pathfinder.com). Do these features fit your needs (real or potential)? What features are missing?

4. Visit the ComputerTalk Web site (www.computertalk.com), and look at the PIMS features currently offered by vendors (by accessing the Buyers Guide edition). What features predominate? Are the features focused on the business or clinical side of pharmacy? What features are missing?

References

1. Minnesota e-Health Initiative Advisory Committee and the Minnesota Department of Health. Glossary of selected terms and acronyms. Available at: http://www.health.state.mn.us/divs/orhpc/hit/terms.pdf. Accessed March 22, 2010.
2. Centers for Medicare and Medicaid Services. CMS information related to the economic recovery act of 2009, health information technology. Available at: http://www.cms.hhs.gov/Recovery/11_HealthIT.asp. Accessed March 22, 2010.
3. Health Information Technology. Standards and certification. Available at: http://healthit.hhs.gov/portal/server.pt?open=512&objID=1153&mode=2. Accessed March 22, 2010.
4. The Joint Commission. National Patient Safety Goals. Medication reconciliation national patient safety goal to be reviewed, refined. March 11, 2009. Available at: http://www.joint commission.org/PatientSafety/NationalPatientSafetyGoals/npsg8_review.htm. Accessed September 25, 2009.
5. Joint Commission Perspectives. Approved: will not score medication reconciliation in 2009. March 2009. Available at: http://www.jcrinc.com/common/PDFs/fpdfs/pubs/pdfs/JCReqs/JCP-03-09-S1.pdf. Accessed October 26, 2009.
6. Bagley, B. The hospitalist movement and family practice—an uneasy fit [commentary]. J *Fam Pract.* 2002;51(2):1028–9. Available at: http://www.jfponline.com/Pages.asp?AID=1349&issue=December%202002&UID=. Accessed March 18, 2010.

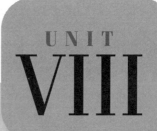
Medication Use Process V: Medication-Related Monitoring and Outcomes Measurement

UNIT COMPETENCIES

- Discuss the impact of data quality on health outcomes.
- Discuss standards for interoperability related to medications, diagnoses, communication, and electronic data interchange.
- Differentiate between spreadsheets, databases, and user interfaces.

- Demonstrate efficient and responsible use of clinical decision support tools to solve patient-related problems.
- Identify common clinical decision support tools.
- Document and report health care quality benchmarks.

UNIT DESCRIPTION

Monitoring and follow-up comprise the final step of the medication use process. The activities that pharmacists perform in this step are highly dependent on their practice setting. Chapters in this unit address the tools available to pharmacists to manage the growing amount of medication-related information that they must sort through in their efforts to ensure safe and efficacious medication therapy. This unit also addresses the patient-centered medical home, which presents a significant opportunity for pharmacists to collaborate with other providers. Finally, this unit addresses the growing emphasis on health care quality improvement and the implications for pharmacy practice.

Clinical Surveillance Systems

Christian Hartman

OBJECTIVES

1. Define clinical surveillance.
2. Describe the components of a clinical surveillance system.
3. Describe the methodology for a basic rules algorithm.
4. Describe the differences between active and passive surveillance.
5. Describe the application of clinical surveillance to health care.

Lean resources, difficult-to-implement regulatory requirements, segregated information systems, and increasingly complex disease management constantly challenge health care productivity. Missed clinical opportunities and drug-related events contribute to delayed therapy, patient harm, and missed or incorrect diagnosis. Specifically, experts suggest that nearly 50% of specific antimicrobial usage is inappropriate, resulting in a high number of health care-associated infections, increased microbial resistance, increased toxicity, and increased cost.[1-3] Further, studies suggest that adverse drug events (ADEs; i.e., harm caused by a drug) occur 2.4 to 6.1 times per 100 hospital admissions.[4,5] The annual national cost of preventable ADEs is estimated to be $2 billion.[6]

With the growing amount of clinical information available to health care practitioners, the sheer amount of data is overwhelming. Internalizing these data and making clinical decisions are time-consuming processes that require (1) readily available information, (2) ability to competently interpret the information, (3) clinical knowledge to make decisions, and (4) expertise to apply the decision to patient care.

Clinical decision support tools have been developed to address these challenges. These tools assist health care practitioners in interpreting data and providing advice at the time of order or prescription entry of the medication use process. As discussed in previous chapters, each major step of the medication use process (ordering, dispensing, transcribing, administering, monitoring) relies on specific technology to improve medication management. **Clinical surveillance** in health care refers to active surveillance or a "watchful waiting" that includes collection and/or analysis of specific patient or disease information that can then be used to drive decisions.

Clinical surveillance—when applied to clinical decision support—can be described as a computer system that provides watchful waiting, interprets data into knowledge, and provides advice to health care practitioners. A key distinction between clinical decision support systems and clinical decision support surveillance is the *time* at which the data are interpreted and presented to the health care practitioner. With surveillance, the data are continuously monitored in the background versus during a specific task such as entering a prescription into a pharmacy information system. Thus, very helpful clinical decisions can be made during the entire process of medication delivery.

Basic Components of Clinical Surveillance Systems

The following components provide the basis for clinical surveillance systems and are presented in Figure 20–1:

- **Medication database:** A database in an integrated health information system or module-based pharmacy information management system that contains current and, in some cases, historical, patient-specific medication information.
- **Laboratory database:** A database in an integrated health information system or module-based laboratory information system that contains current and historical patient-specific laboratory information.

FIGURE 20-1

Graphic depiction of the components of a clinical surveillance system.

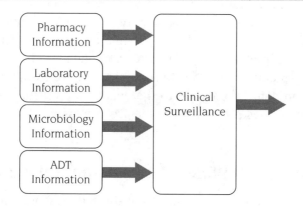

ADT = admission, discharge, and transfer.
Source: Author.

- **Admissions/discharge/transfer database:** A database in an integrated health information system or module-based system that contains patient-specific demographic information and the patient's current location within the health system.
- **Microbiology database:** A database in an integrated health information system or module-based laboratory information system that contains current and historical patient-specific microbiology information. Specific details for culture source (e.g., sputum, blood, etc.), organism type (e.g., cocci), and sensitivity analysis are usually provided.
- **Health Level 7 (HL7) interface:** Health care industry standard interface for clinical and administrative data that moves patient information between disparate information systems.
- **Knowledge base:** A database in a clinical surveillance system that collates various interface feeds and sends the data through a preset algorithm.
- **User interface:** The mechanism utilized by the health care practitioner to access information in the clinical surveillance system, usually either an electronic dashboard or an electronically generated report.

The greatest challenge encountered is the general disconnect and segregation of the various data, such as medication and laboratory data. Although such information may have been provided at the time of order and prescription entry, changing patient conditions provide additional information that could be helpful when providing care. A clinical surveillance system internalizes the basic components of health information technology databases, filters the data through a rules algorithm, and presents pertinent information to the health care practitioner during the monitoring phase of the medication use process.

Clinical Surveillance Design and Rules Logic

The basic design of most clinical surveillance systems includes an interface engine, knowledge base, and user interface. As previously described, an HL7 interface is the health care industry standard for communication and exchange of clinical and administrative information between software systems. These interfaces provide functional interoperability between the source databases (i.e., medications/laboratory/microbiology) and the clinical surveillance system. Messaging is sent to the clinical surveillance system in a standard format utilized in health care. In addition, semantic interoperability may be needed if the message crosses over different computer systems. Semantic interoperability standardizes the taxonomy and nomenclature that gives meaning to the messages across computer systems. An example of semantic interoperability for clinical terminology is the Systemized Nomenclature of Medicine (SNOMED). Without interoperability, the clinical surveillance system could not process the messages into useful information.

The knowledge base is the clinical surveillance system that compiles the individual data interfaces and filters the messages through the rules algorithm. Depending on the type of clinical surveillance system used, the knowledge base may reside with the health-system information technology (IT) data center or may be hosted by the vendor. Vendor-hosted systems require an additional feature to address the Health Insurance Portability and Accountability Act (HIPAA) security requirements (see Chapter 26). Data sent outside of a health-system network require the development of a secure, encrypted virtual private network line to transmit protected health information.

Once the data are compiled in the clinical surveillance system, the knowledge base system then utilizes some form of if-then rules logic to isolate pertinent information. An example rule used for warfarin (Coumadin) monitoring can be found in Figure 20–2. Most readers are probably familiar with similar rules logic found in certain formulas in spreadsheet software such as Microsoft Excel. The algorithm contained within the rules logic allows for isolation of pertinent information and elimination of unimportant data. The rules utilized in the knowledge base algorithm may be developed by the health system and/or by the vendor following expert opinion and clinical practice guidelines.

The end user (i.e., health care practitioner) interacts with the clinical surveillance system through the user interface by one of two distinct methods. The first is a real-time dashboard or electronically generated report intended to be used for prospective clinical intervention. The real-time dashboard may or may not contain clinical decision support assistance depending on the design of the system. Clinical surveillance with real-time clinical decision support provides a list of patients who have satisfied the preset rules with suggested clinical action.

The second method of presenting the clinical surveillance system information is an aggregate retrospective report showing trends across a set period of time, location, and so on. Such information provides high-level analysis typically utilized by the health system's infection control or quality department. Either method presents the end user with the decision to provide patient care intervention or broad system/process improvements.

FIGURE 20–2

An example of clinical surveillance rule logic.

All patients **Not Located in an ICU**[1] older than **18 years**[1] on **Warfarin**[2] for more than 3 days with an **INR greater than 6.**[3]

1: Admissions/discharge/transfer database

2: Medication database

3: Laboratory database

Note: Superscript numbers denote the appropriate database for the boldface information.
ICU = intensive care unit; INR = international normalized ratio.
Source: Author.

Active versus Passive Surveillance

Active clinical surveillance processes data through a knowledge base and alerts a health care practitioner when criteria for clinical intervention are met. This type of surveillance system provides clinical decision support based on expert guidelines to assist with the final decision making. These alerts and notifications can be very helpful when a pharmacist is taking care of several patients and has limited time to prioritize the work. An active surveillance system provides the most useful results because the most important information is presented to the practitioner with suggested actions. When this system is used, the practitioner spends less time seeking patient information and clinical knowledge, and more time making decisions that can improve the care of patients.

A **passive surveillance system** requires the end user to recognize that the information presented in the clinical surveillance system warrants action. Further, a passive system does not provide robust clinical decision support, leaving the health care practitioner with the responsibility of seeking clinical knowledge from secondary resources. As one would expect, a passive system requires more effort from the end user and has the potential for misinterpretation of information. Although a passive system might not be the ideal approach, well-designed rules within a passive system can be superior to the traditional manual identification of clinical intervention.

Application of Clinical Surveillance to Health Care

During the past 20 years, several studies have been completed that evaluate the impact of clinical surveillance and its utility when integrated with clinical decision support. Literature has, for the most part, focused on identifying opportunities for clinical intervention, ADE detection and mitigation, appropriate antimicrobial use, and the reliability of computer-assisted decision support.

The traditional manual method of identifying ADEs through chart review and an organization's risk management reporting has been shown to grossly underestimate the true incidence of ADEs. In 1991, researchers from the University of Utah actively monitored more than 36,000 patients over an 18-month period for evidence of harm caused by a medication. They compared traditional methods, such as human real-time review (not computer assisted) and incident reporting, with an automated computer-assisted surveillance system. During the study period, 731 ADEs were identified; of which, nine were detected by the traditional method, 90 were reported via incident reporting, and 641 were detected by the computer system (Figure 20–3).[7]

To further explore the use of computer-assisted ADE detection, researchers from Harvard University compared the identification of ADEs by a computer-monitoring system and by a manual chart review over an 8-month period in nine units. The computer surveillance system identified 275 ADEs, the manual chart review method identified 398 ADEs, and voluntary reporting identified 23 events. Of the total ADEs detected in the study period (n = 617), only 76 were detected by both the clinical surveillance system and chart review. ADEs detected by clinical surveillance were also noted to be more severe than those detected by chart review, suggesting that clinical surveillance is more effective at identifying severe ADEs not traditionally found using the gold standard. Additional analysis found that the manual chart review method required a mean of 55 person hours/week compared with the 11 person hours/week that was required for the clinical surveillance method (Figure 20–4).[8]

FIGURE 20–3

Comparison of adverse drug event (ADE) rates across three methods of identification.

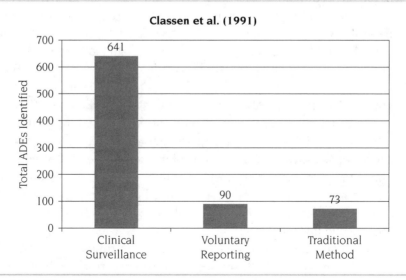

Classen et al. (1991)

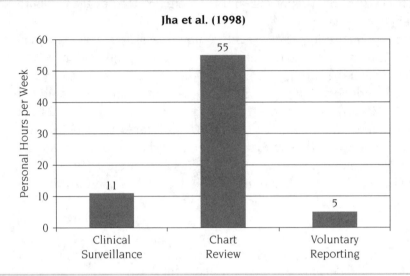

FIGURE 20–4

Comparison of time requirements for three methods of detecting adverse drug events.

Source: Adapted from Reference 8.

With the use of clinical surveillance, there is a possibility of false positives: that is, the clinical surveillance system may highlight certain patients for additional attention when in fact nothing is wrong. An example would be a rule that is triggered by an opiate reversal agent such as naloxone in a patient's profile, when naloxone was part of a standard order set but was not actually administered. A study completed by researchers at Brigham and Women's Hospital examined the accuracy of a clinical surveillance program at detecting true ADEs that resulted in a clinical intervention. A 15% increase in the number of clinical interventions was noted after implementation of the clinical surveillance system; however, researchers also noted a wide range of accuracy for the individual rules (0%–60%).[9] Although such a wide range of accuracy is most likely unique to each organization, it provides a reminder that continuous refinement and improvement in rules development are needed for a clinical surveillance system to provide the most useful information.

Clinical surveillance—when applied to antimicrobial stewardship research—has yielded positive results with antibiotic prescribing, antibiotic selection, and microbial resistance (Table 20–1). A study published in

TABLE 20-1

TABLE 20-1

The Impact of Clinical Surveillance on Antimicrobial Stewardship

Variable	Pre-intervention (n = 766)	Intervention, Surveillance Followed (n = 203)	Intervention, Surveillance Not Followed (n = 195)	Overall *p* Value
No. of different anti-infectives ordered	2.0	1.5	2.7	<0.001
Duration of therapy (hours)	214	103	330	<0.001
No. of anti-infective agent doses	23.6	11.4	27.6	<0.001
Day of excess anti-infective dosage	5.4	1.4	3.6	<0.001
Cost of anti-infective agents ($)	340	102	427	<0.001
No. of microbiology cultures	6.8	3.2	10.6	<0.001
Length of ICU stay (days)	4.9	2.7	8.3	<0.001
Total cost of hospitalization ($)	35,283	26,315	44,865	<0.001

ICU = intensive care unit.
Source: Adapted from Reference 10.

the *New England Journal of Medicine* examined the use of clinical surveillance and its ability to improve antimicrobial management in the critical care setting. Use of the clinical surveillance program led to significant reductions in the duration of use of anti-infective agents from 214 hours to 103 hours. The mean number of days of excessive antimicrobial dosage was reduced from 5.4 days prior to clinical surveillance to 1.4 days during the intervention period. Total hospitalization cost was reported to decrease from $35,283 to $26,315 after implementation of clinical surveillance targeted at improving the use of anti-infective agents.[10]

Clinical surveillance in the community hospital setting was described in a study published in the *American Journal of Health-System Pharmacy*. In the study, pharmacists' use of clinical surveillance to monitor antibiotic use in 1384 patients was reviewed during a 6-month intervention period. Of the study population, 348 interventions were performed with 289 accepted by physicians. For the group with accepted interventions, 280 infections subsided subsequent to the clinical surveillance-directed recommendations. Further analysis of cost avoidance was shown to be $32,000 as a result of the targeted antimicrobial interventions.[11]

Although ADE detection and antimicrobial stewardship represent the majority of clinical surveillance data published in the literature, the application of clinical surveillance to other clinical programs seems probable. The most promising application appears to be its use with the improvement of publicly reported quality measures such as the Joint Commission core measures related to medication use (acute myocardial infarction, community acquired pneumonia, etc.).

Conclusion

With the evolution of advanced clinical information technology in health care, the major steps in the medication use process have been addressed with targeted technology. The use of clinical surveillance in the monitoring step provides an added tool to improve the management of patients. By eliminating manual retrieval of information and augmenting clinical programs, clinical surveillance has been shown to provide a valuable tool for health care practitioners, especially for the medication-management activities of pharmacists.

LEARNING ACTIVITIES

1. Go to www.sentri7.com and www.theradoc.com, and review the key differences between their clinical surveillance systems. How are the rules developed? Do the vendors use standard vocabulary such as SNOMED? Is clinical decision support integrated in the system?
2. Utilizing basic if-then logic, develop a clinical surveillance rule to identify patients who may be experiencing an adverse drug event. What medication and/or laboratory information is needed?

References

1. Gerding DN. The search for good antimicrobial stewardship. *Jt Comm J Qual Improv.* 2001; 27(8):403–4.
2. Avorn J, Solomon DH. Cultural and economic factors that (mis)shape antibiotic use: the non-pharmacologic basis of therapeutics. *Ann Intern Med.* 2000;133(2):128–35.
3. Classen DC, Evans RS, Pestotnik SL, et al. The timing of prophylactic administration of antibiotics and the risk of surgical-wound infections. *N Engl J Med.* 1992;326(5):281–6.
4. Bates DW, Cullen DJ, Laird N, et al. Incidence of adverse drug events and potential adverse drug events. Implications for prevention. ADE prevention study group. *JAMA.* 1995;274(1): 29–34.

5. Thomas EJ, Brennan TA. Incidence and types of preventable adverse events in elderly patients: population based review of medical records. BMJ. 2000;320(7237):741–4.

6. Bates DW, Spell N, Cullen DJ, et al. The costs of adverse drug events in hospitalized patients. JAMA. 1997;277(4):307 11.

7. Classen DC, Pestotnik SL, Evans RS, et al. Computerized surveillance of adverse drug events in hospital patients. JAMA. 1991;266(20):2847–51.

8. Jha AK, Kuperman GJ, Teich JM, et al. Identifying adverse drug events: development of a computer-based monitor and comparison with chart review and stimulated voluntary report. J Am Med Inform Assoc. 1998;5(3):305–14.

9. Silverman JB, Stapinski CD, Huber C, et al. Computer-based system for preventing adverse drug events. Am J Health Syst Pharm. 2004;61(15):1599–1603.

10. Evans RS, Pestotnik SL, Classen DC, et al. A computer-assisted management program for antibiotics and other antiinfective agents. N Engl J Med. 1998;338(4):232–8.

11. Jozefiak ET, Lewicki JE, Kozinn WP. Computer-assisted antimicrobial surveillance in a community teaching hospital. Am J Health Syst Pharm. 1995;52(14):1536–40.

Documentation of Clinical Interventions

Charles W. Westergard and Steve Pickette

OBJECTIVES

1. Describe a pharmacy clinical intervention.
2. Describe why the documentation of interventions has value.
3. List four reasons to document interventions.
4. Define the elements of a good documentation system for clinical interventions.
5. List the various ways that pharmacists document interventions today, and describe the pros and cons of each method.

The profession of pharmacy has undergone widespread change over the last few decades.[1-3] Pharmacy is unique in health care professions in that it has both a distributional aspect (processes to physically deliver drug product safely to the patient) as well as a clinical aspect (services to ensure appropriateness, safety, and cost-effectiveness of the selected therapy). Historically, clinical or cognitive pharmacy services were generally provided free of charge. The costs of providing these services were embedded in the medication-dispensing process. As part of the physical preparation and delivery of a pharmaceutical product, a pharmacist would review the prescription for appropriateness of the drug to the condition being treated, ensure the dose was correct for the patient, and ensure there were no allergies or interactions between other drugs the patient was taking.

With the advent of automated dispensing technology, the pharmacist's direct role in drug delivery was minimized. Simultaneously, the number of medications available for use was skyrocketing. The complexity of use and monitoring of these medications were increasing as well. Pharmacists were being asked to step into more and more clinical roles—not just dispensing medications, but managing the whole medication use process from patient assessment and diagnosis to prescribing and dosing appropriate medications to performing clinical monitoring. Clinical services were quickly becoming the desired future role for pharmacists.[1]

This chapter primarily addresses clinical intervention documentation within hospitals and health systems. In community practice, intervention documentation is often less structured, primarily because of the inability to electronically communicate across pharmacies and from pharmacies to physician offices and hospitals. Additionally, the financial drivers discussed below for intervention documentation in the institutional environment are not found in the community pharmacy setting. However, drivers have been and still are pushing community pharmacy toward a focus on documentation of services and their outcomes. Several of these drivers and associated topics are addressed in Chapter 19.

The firmly established, growing change toward focusing on clinical services just described was dramatic and caught many health care administrators off guard. The perception of pharmacy remains entrenched in many administrators' minds as "distributional." Clinical pharmacy managers knew that a time would come when they would be asked to justify the clinical programs and staff they had. But, without a mechanism to bill for the clinical services, this was going to be difficult. The first step was to identify the clinical activities. What services were pharmacists delivering? These activities fell into three broad categories:

- Activities that promote safety: Medications are inherently dangerous when not used properly. Pharmacists were stepping in to ensure that medications were being used safely.
  - An example of this is a pharmacist questioning and stopping a drug order for a patient who is allergic to a therapeutically similar medication.

- Activities that promote quality: The fact that many patients are seen by more than one physician can lead to a "too many cooks in the kitchen" syndrome.
  - Pharmacists perform profile review to ensure that medication use is following best practice standards and to minimize duplication of therapy.
- Activities that promote efficiency and cost-effectiveness: Medications can be very expensive. Pharmacists can identify when generic or other appropriate alternatives may exist to minimize the cost of care.
  - Converting patients from expensive intravenous medications to less expensive oral alternatives can reduce overall cost and also minimize the incidence of infection due to IV catheters being in place too long.

What are Clinical Interventions?

So, what is a clinical pharmacy intervention? The word *intervene* comes from the Latin *intervenire*, which means "to come between." In pharmacy, an **intervention** is the act of interceding with the intent of modifying the medication use process to make it safer or more cost-effective.

Think of the medication use process (see Chapter 1) as a river starting high in the mountains with the prescriber assessing the patient and selecting a therapy. The process flows downhill to order generation and transcribing, to preparation and compounding, to delivery to the patient, and finally flows to administration. But, the process does not stop there. The river continues to flow as clinicians review the impact of the therapy and continue to monitor its effectiveness, modifying the drug order as needed for changes in the patient's clinical condition. At any stage in the process, the river may "jump its banks." Think of clinical interventions as the sandbags and levees set up to keep the medication use process gently flowing from beginning to end. Levees are set up in advance where dangerous conditions in the river exist. Formulary management, standardized order sets, and drug use policies are the levees in our metaphor. Enforcement of these policies is an essential clinical activity. But, there are times when the river breaks through and you need sandbags: intercepting medication orders for which allergies or interactions exist, identifying that a drug dose is too high for the patient's renal function, catching a drug transcription error . . . the list goes on and on. These events just happen, and a pharmacist needs to be vigilant to apply his or her knowledge and skills as needed to keep the river flowing smoothly in its banks.

Intervention opportunities are identified through profile review, order review and entry, rounds, target drug systems, and automated clinical surveillance systems. Profile review is the process of holistically reviewing each medication on a patient's profile for possible need for intervention. A pharmacist uses his or her full experience and knowledge to look for medication problems such as duplication of therapy, interactions, and opportunities for improvement in medication use. Profile review includes comparing a patient's medications with current laboratory values and demographics to ensure that the medication regimen is optimal. Target drug systems are usually computer-generated reports that identify all patients on the drug in question. Pharmacists then use this report to ensure that the drug in question is being used according to internal policies. An example of a target drug system is the intravenous (IV) to oral conversion (IV/PO) list. Patients on certain IV target medications are identified in a report that is usually run nightly by the pharmacy technology team. Patients on the list are reviewed by pharmacists throughout the day and converted to oral therapy if deemed appropriate.

Clinical surveillance systems are tools that automate the identification of patients with clinical intervention opportunities that are identified across data systems. Rather than just identifying all patients on a target drug, logical rules can be set up to identify patients on a specific drug (or class of drugs) whose laboratory values are outside of a certain range and whose demographic features are present. Most of these systems analyze data in near real time, giving the pharmacist an up-to-the-minute view of patients who require attention. Clinical surveillance systems are discussed in more detail in Chapter 21. Common systematic problems may warrant that policies be adopted by various organizational bodies (primarily the pharmacy and therapeutics committee) to institutionalize the intervention in standard order sets or policies.

An old mantra in quality improvement circles says "not documented, not done." Documentation of pharmacists' clinical activities is the essential step in demonstrating to people outside the profession the value of the services that pharmacists provide as clinicians. The next section will look at the various reasons to document interventions.

Purpose of Clinical Intervention Documentation

Demonstrate the Cost and Quality Impact of Clinical Pharmacy Programs

When considering the purpose of documenting interventions, most think first that it is to justify the value of the clinical pharmacist. Although there are a number of reasons to document, this is indeed one of the primary purposes for this activity. The value of pharmacist involvement in the medication use process is intuitive, but financial constraints force administrators to make tough choices about where to apply limited resources. As a result, funding for clinical programs is often limited to those that are able to demonstrate a significant impact on financial and/or quality indicators.

Measuring the financial impact of the clinical pharmacist is not a simple process. Ideally, the impact of a pharmacist's interventions on patient therapy would be measured by tracking the actual change in financial and/or clinical outcome for each patient that results from the particular intervention. Sometimes this can be done, for example, when use of a less expensive medication is based on a pharmacist's recommendation or on therapeutic substitution. In situations such as this, the cost difference between the two medications can be calculated and the reduction in direct costs measured. These types of values are often referred to as "hard dollar" savings. Some examples of hard dollar savings are when a pharmacist switches an intravenous medication to a less expensive oral form and when a medication is switched to a less expensive formulary alternative.

In most situations, however, this type of value is not practical. In many cases, we are trying to measure what did NOT happen as a result of the pharmacist's intervention, such as an adverse drug event that was prevented. First, recognize that it is very difficult to predict what effect an intervention may or may not have on the clinical course of a patient. Second, there are too many variables in the course of caring for a patient to say with certainty what effect any single change has on the direct costs associated with that patient. Therefore, most intervention documentation programs assign values to interventions that are based on estimates derived from predictive modeling. These values are often referred to as "soft dollar" or "cost avoidance" savings.[4–10] Table 21–1 shows some common intervention types and the typical method of associating cost savings with them.

One example of this type of savings estimate is the value of a reduction of the gentamicin dose by the pharmacist per recommendation or by

TABLE 21-1

Intervention Examples and Their Predominant Cost Impact

Intervention Type	Typical Cost Justification
Allergy information clarified	Soft, avoidance of cost intervention
Allergy prevented	Soft, avoidance of cost intervention
Antibiotic recommendations	Hard cost savings
Chemotherapy dose changed	Soft, avoidance of cost intervention
Chemotherapy dose evaluation	Soft, avoidance of cost intervention
Clarification of orders	Soft, avoidance of cost intervention
Committee time/preparation	Soft, avoidance of cost intervention
CPR/code attended	Soft, avoidance of cost intervention
Dose evaluation	Soft, avoidance of cost intervention
Drug information	Soft, avoidance of cost intervention
Drug levels avoided	Hard cost savings
Drug therapy consultation	Soft, avoidance of cost intervention
Drug-laboratory interaction	Soft, avoidance of cost intervention
Drug-drug interaction	Soft, avoidance of cost intervention
Drug-food interaction	Soft, avoidance of cost intervention
Heparin dosed	Soft, avoidance of cost intervention
Inpatient counseled	Soft, avoidance of cost intervention
In-service done	Soft, avoidance of cost intervention
In-service preparation	Soft, avoidance of cost intervention
IV drug compatibility	Soft, avoidance of cost intervention
IV-to-PO done	Hard cost savings
IV-to-PO recommended	Soft, avoidance of cost intervention
Laboratory evaluation	Soft, avoidance of cost intervention
MUE review	Soft, avoidance of cost intervention
Newsletter article	Soft, avoidance of cost intervention
Non-form processed	Soft, avoidance of cost intervention
Other dosage evaluation	Soft, avoidance of cost intervention
Other pharmacy intervention	Soft, avoidance of cost intervention
Outpatient counseled	Soft, avoidance of cost intervention
Patient medication Hx	Soft, avoidance of cost intervention
PK evaluation: AG	Soft, avoidance of cost intervention
PK evaluation: digoxin	Soft, avoidance of cost intervention

TABLE 21-1

Intervention Examples and Their Predominant Cost Impact (*Continued*)

Intervention Type	Typical Cost Justification
PK evaluation: other	Soft, avoidance of cost intervention
PK evaluation: theophylline	Soft, avoidance of cost intervention
PK evaluation: vancomycin	Soft, avoidance of cost intervention
Poison information	Soft, avoidance of cost intervention
POM evaluation	Soft, avoidance of cost intervention
Renal dose change	Soft, avoidance of cost intervention
Renal dose evaluation	Soft, avoidance of cost intervention
Renal dose recommended	Soft, avoidance of cost intervention
Therapeutic duplication avoided	Soft, avoidance of cost intervention
Therapeutic interchange done	Hard cost savings
Therapeutic interchange recommended	Soft, avoidance of cost intervention
TPN adjustment	Soft, avoidance of cost intervention
TPN evaluation	Soft, avoidance of cost intervention
TPN monitoring	Soft, avoidance of cost intervention
Warfarin dosed	Soft, avoidance of cost intervention
Weight evaluation	Soft, avoidance of cost intervention

AG = aminoglycoside; CPR, cardiopulmonary resuscitation; Hx = history; IV = intravenous; MUE = medication use evaluation; PK = pharmacokinetic; PO = oral; POM = patient's own medication; TPN = total parenteral nutrition.
Source: Quantifi® Intervention Cost Model. Pharmacy OneSource, Bellevue, Washington. Used with permission.

protocol. According to evidence published in the biomedical literature, the incidence of renal toxicity is much greater when the dose is not appropriate for a patient's renal function. Therefore, the reduced risk will result in one fewer instance of renal toxicity for approximately X patients for whom the dose has been adjusted. The average additional cost of a patient experiencing renal toxicity as a complication in the course of therapy is $$, so each intervention made by a pharmacist to adjust the dose of gentamicin for a patient is estimated to be $ ($$ divided by X).[11]

Another example is the management of warfarin therapy by the pharmacist. Studies have shown that anticoagulation therapy managed by a pharmacist reduces the instance of significant bleeding by approximately

5% compared with management by a primary care physician.[12] Therefore, a calculation similar to the previous example can be made to determine the estimated value for each instance when a pharmacist doses warfarin. Figure 21–1 demonstrates a model for determining the cost savings associated with cost avoidance interventions.[13–19]

Because the values associated with documented interventions are primarily the result of estimates, they often will not stand for much when used alone to demonstrate the value of pharmacy clinical services. A hospital administrator may wonder if there was a real financial or quality impact as a result of the increased number of pharmacist's documented interventions or if the pharmacist had simply documented more aggressively than in the past. The intervention data can be paired with trends in other metrics such as pharmaceutical supply expense, adverse drug events, length of stay, readmissions, and patient satisfaction.[6,11,20] If a correlation can be shown between the clinical intervention documentation and these other financial and quality metrics, then it can usually be concluded that they are connected. Without the clinical intervention documentation, the hospital administrator may not associate the other metrics with pharmacy clinical activity.

Staff Performance Improvement

One of the key activities of management is evaluating the performance of pharmacy staff and improving that performance through staff development and training. Without adequate documentation of what clinical staff members are doing, it is very difficult to provide constructive help in improving their efforts.

Documentation of clinical activities provides clinical managers with the data they need to work with their clinicians. Documentation can identify areas of strength and weakness in a clinician's clinical performance. Armed with this information, a valuable and constructive conversation can then ensue that will help the clinician provide better care for patients. Collected documentation of clinical activities can provide excellent case presentations for staff meetings. "Good catches" as well as "opportunities for improvement" can be identified from the documented actions of all staff. Using real-world case examples in staff meetings gives managers a way of modeling best practice care by providing practical examples.

FIGURE 21–1

A model to calculate the avoided costs per intervention.

Step 1: Establish a health care inflation rate factor: 4.5% per year

Literature-Supported Range	
Study	Inflation Rate
Bergstrom et al.	11%
Kaiser	9.8%
Strunk et al.	5%
AVERAGE	**8.6%**

Note: Approximately half the average rate is used to be conservative.

Step 2: Establish the cost of a preventable ADE: $5896.13

Literature-Supported Range				
Study	Year	No. of Years Ago (from 2009)	Cost per ADE	Cost per ADE ($2009)
Suh et al.	1999	10	$5483	$8514.93
Classen et al.	1993	16	$2262	$4574.60
Bates et al.	1996	13	$2595	$4598.85
AVERAGE			**$3447**	**$5896.13**

Step 3: Establish preventable ADE rate: 2.6%, or 1 ADE per 38 patient interventions

Literature-Supported Range	
Study	Rate
Lazarou et al.	6.70%
Classen et al.	2.43%
Bates et al.	6.5%
AVERAGE	**5.21%**

Note: Half the average rate is used to be conservative.

Costs Avoided per Pharmacy Intervention = $5896.13 × 0.026 = $153.30

ADE = adverse drug event.
Source: Author; calculations are based on References 13–19.

Quality Improvement Activities

Important quality improvement initiatives rely on documentation of clinical activities.[21] Physician credentialing criteria often include a measure of the number of recommendations made for medication therapy changes along with the percentage of acceptance or rejection of those recommendations. It is also common to document instances of noncompliance with prescribing standards, such as the use of unaccepted abbreviations as defined by the Joint Commission (e.g., use of "QD" instead of "daily" as a frequency). This important quality improvement information potentially has significant consequences; therefore, it must be complete and accurate. This type of documentation may be done periodically or on an ongoing basis.

Another important quality improvement initiative that relies on reliable clinical documentation is ensuring and measuring compliance with medication-related quality indicators and core measures set by the Centers for Medicare and Medicaid Services.[22] The medication quality indicators (e.g., myocardial infarction patients receiving aspirin) were chosen because of the overwhelming evidence that relates compliance with improved outcomes for patients. For this reason, great efforts are made to track and follow up on the therapy for each patient meeting the clinical criteria to ensure that the appropriate medication is prescribed or that a contraindication is documented in the patient record by the physician.

One final opportunity for using a system to document interventions is to run medication use evaluations (MUEs). An MUE is a targeted data collection activity involving a specific drug or drug class to identify if the drugs are being used in compliance with internal or external policies. Typically, drugs that are MUE candidates are designated as such by the pharmacy and therapeutics committee at a hospital. The drug in question may be particularly costly or have safety issues, and there may be specific guidelines for its appropriate use. The pharmacy would identify patients taking this medication and collect data defined in the policies to determine whether the drug is being used appropriately. The collected data in the MUE would be evaluated to drive additional policy measures to ensure appropriate use.

Workflow

Aside from any link to financial and quality improvement measures, clinical documentation plays a fundamental role in the daily workflow of the pharmacist. Whether the pharmacist is simply processing orders, or performing patient rounds or chart review, medication-related issues requiring some sort of follow-up action will be identified. A process is necessary to communicate medication-related issues that need to be addressed in an efficient and organized manner. For example, a pharmacist processing new medication orders in the main pharmacy may identify a potential medication-related issue that needs to be communicated to the clinical pharmacist who is responsible for addressing issues for patients in the patient care area. The clinical pharmacist performing rounds or chart review also needs a process to track issues for follow-up throughout the day or at a future date such as when laboratory or test results are pending. It is also common that clinical information related to medication therapy might be relevant to a future admit for that patient. Written notes, on a copy of the prescription or a piece of paper, that describe the issue and the necessary steps to be taken are not reliable or efficient processes. This is especially true in the acute care setting where patients transfer to different nursing units frequently, and pharmacy staff providing care for the patient may be doing so from different locations.

Another purpose of clinical documentation of workflow is to track activities and gather data that allow evaluation of new processes and the required labor resources. This could be as basic as recording each time the pharmacist performs an activity such as answering the phone or checking a medication to evaluate the time it requires during a shift, to something as complex as tracking the number of times a new protocol is used to evaluate its impact on the daily workflow of the pharmacist.

Elements of a Good Documentation System

Many methods are available to document clinical interventions. These include paper systems, home-grown systems in Excel or Access, building of documentation in the pharmacy ordering system, or use of a third-party solution designed specifically for the task. Any system selected should be easy for the pharmacists to use and fit into their workflow. The system should allow for quick documentation of clinical events with enough detail to facilitate understanding of the issue by staff members who will be following up on the event. The documentation should be searchable and should provide an easily accessible complete record of all clinical activities related to the patient. Ultimately, the collected data will be a repository of clinical performance that clinical managers will use to develop management reporting to justify programs, develop performance evaluations, and accomplish the other activities discussed above. The data elements critical to a usable documentation system are summarized in Table 21–2.

Customization

Customization is an important feature of a good documentation system. Clinical practices vary across the nation. It is important that the systems

TABLE 21–2

Types of Intervention Documentation Data

Field Name/Description	Field Type	Related Data
Patient name	Demographic	
Medical record number	Demographic	
Account or visit number	Demographic	
Age	Demographic	Age units (years, months, days)
Weight	Demographic	Weight units (pounds, kilograms)
Gender	Demographic	
Medication allergies	Demographic	
Service area	Demographic	Service class
Location/bed number	Demographic	
Event date/time	Event	
Drug(s) involved	Event	Drug class
Intervention(s) type	Event	Cost savings, relative value units
Significance	Event	
Notes	Event	
Time taken	Event	
Pharmacist	Event	
Follow-up status	Follow-up	
Follow-up note	Follow-up	
Follow-up due date	Follow-up	
Outcome: accepted/rejected	Outcome	
Physician	Outcome	
Outcome: other	Outcome	
Outcome note	Outcome	

Source: Quantifi®. Pharmacy OneSource, Bellevue, Washington. Used with permission.

used to document clinical activities be able to adapt to the various practice models in clinical pharmacy. The system should have the capability to modify or add additional interventions for staff to document, adjust service locations to match the organization's format, and manage drug and prescriber databases. Security settings should be able to mirror the organization's security policies

Notification by e-mail, pager, or text message of when events have been documented is an invaluable feature. Certain interventions may warrant immediate notification to risk management personnel or other administrative staff. Specialist staff (e.g., in pediatrics) might like to be notified when interventions related to their specialty are documented by non-specialist staff.

Reporting

Reporting is the critical output of the pharmacy intervention documentation system. Clinical managers should be able to quickly and easily generate, in real time, reporting on any combination of the documented fields in the system. Reporting should easily answer questions such as:

- How many interventions did our department do last week, month, quarter, year?
- Can I break out total interventions by person? By service location? By prescriber?
- Can I identify which of my department's interventions were accepted by the prescriber?
- Can I assign a hard and soft cost dollar amount to each intervention and create summary reports of savings?
- Can I generate high-level overview reporting and drill down to the individual interventions that make up the report?
- Can I incorporate workload statistics (such as average patient-days, discharges, or admits) and run reporting ratios that are adjusted for overall workload?

Benchmarking

Another critical aspect of reporting is benchmarking. **Benchmarking** is a term used to compare a defined metric with a representative group to gauge performance. This information is a very important piece of the performance improvement process. There are two forms of benchmarking: internal and external. **Internal benchmarking** compares a hospital's performance at two periods of time for the same interventions. So, for example, comparisons might include the number of renal dosing changes the staff performed in the first quarter of last year to the first quarter of this year. Internal benchmarking allows for pre- and post-comparative analytics of a significant change in clinical productivity to determine the impact of the change on prevailing documentation patterns.

External benchmarking is a type of reporting that compares one organization with another in terms of the number of interventions documented. This type of benchmarking is much more challenging. The key problem is one of data standardization and definitions. Two hospitals that use the same documentation system and intervention definitions may interpret the definitions slightly differently, leading to numbers that cannot be readily compared.

Conclusion

As the profession of pharmacy moves from a practice focused on distribution of medication to one in which the provision of clinical services dominates, it is imperative that documentation of clinical interventions takes place. Clinical informatics tools can make the burden of collecting this information less onerous on the workflow of the clinician. Documentation systems that integrate with the ongoing communication of clinical issues between staff members will be more readily accepted by staff; therefore, staff will do a better job of collecting the essential data to make better clinical management decisions.

LEARNING ACTIVITIES

1. Examine the current processes of intervention documentation at a local health care organization. What data elements are being collected? How much time does it take to collect these data?
2. Talk to the clinical manager at a local health care organization. What types of reporting does he or she generate? At what frequency are these reports generated? Who are the ultimate recipients?

3. Discuss the current documentation system with a member of the clinical staff at a local health care organization. What value does the clinician derive from the system? Does the clinician understand the overall need for good documentation of clinical activities? Does the clinical documentation system facilitate the clinician's workflow?

References

1. American Society of Hospital Pharmacists. ASHP statement on pharmaceutical care. *Am J Hosp Pharm.* 1993;50:1720–3.
2. Directions for clinical practice in pharmacy. Proceedings of an invitational conference conducted by the ASHP Research and Education Foundation and the American Society of Hospital Pharmacists. *Am J Health Syst Pharm.* 1985;42(6):1287–342.
3. Hepler CD, Strand LM. Opportunities and responsibilities in pharmaceutical care. *Am J Hosp Pharm.* 1990;47(3):533–43.
4. Kane SL, Weber RJ, Dasta JF. The impact of critical care pharmacists on enhancing patient outcomes. *Intensive Care Med.* 2003;29(5):691–8 [Epub ahead of print March 29, 2003].
5. Gandhi PJ, Smith BS, Tataronis GR, et al. Impact of a pharmacist on drug costs in a coronary care unit. *Am J Health Syst Pharm.* 2001;58(6):497–503.
6. Crows K, Collette D, Dang M, et al. Transformation of pharmacy department: impact of pharmacist interventions, error prevention and cost. *Jt Comm J Qual Improv.* 2002;28(6):324–30.
7. Chuang LC, Sutton JD, Henderson GT. Impact of a clinical pharmacist on cost saving and cost avoidance in drug therapy in an intensive care unit. *Hosp Pharm.* 1994;29(3):215–8, 221.
8. Nesbit TW, Shermock KM, Bobek MB, et al. Implementation and pharmacoeconomic analysis of a clinical staff pharmacist practice model. *Am J Health Syst Pharm.* 2001;58(9):784–90.
9. Perez A, Doloresco F, Hoffman JM, et al. Economic evaluations of clinical pharmacy services: 2001–2005. *Pharmacotherapy.* 2008;28(11):285c–323c.
10. Hatoum HT, Hutchinson RA, Witte KW, et al. Evaluation of the contribution of clinical pharmacists: inpatient care and cost reduction. *Drug Intell Clin Pharm.* 1988;22(3):252–9.
11. Kopp BJ, Mrsan M, Erstad BL, et al. Cost implications of and potential adverse events prevented by interventions of a critical care pharmacist. *Am J Health Syst Pharm.* 2007; 64(23):2483–7.
12. Dager WE, Branch JM, King JH, et al. Optimization of inpatient warfarin therapy: impact of daily consultation by a pharmacist-managed anticoagulation service. *Ann Pharmacother.* 2000; 34(5)567–72.
13. Bergstrom RJ, Mclaughlin EJ, Fleming PD, et al. Financial planning for the risk of long life; how to cope with the rising cost of getting old. *J Accountancy.* September 1, 1991:172.
14. Kaiser Family Foundation. Trends in healthcare costs and spending. September 2007. Available at: http://www.kff.org/insurance/upload/7692.pdf. Accessed October 22, 2009.
15. Strunk BC, Ginsburg PB, Gabel JR. Tracking health care costs. September 2001. Health Affairs. Available at: http://content.healthaffairs.org/cgi/content/full/hlthaff.w1.39v1/DC1. Accessed October 10, 2009.

16. Suh DC, Woodall BS, Shin SK, et al. Clinical and economic impact of adverse drug reactions in hospitalized patients. *Ann Pharmacother.* 2000;34(12):1373–9.

17. Classen DC, Pestotnik SL, Evans RS, et al. Adverse drug events in hospitalized patients. Excess length of stay, extra costs, and attributable mortality. JAMA. 1997;277(4):301–6.

18. Bates DW, Spell N, Cullen DJ, et al. The costs of adverse drug events in hospitalized patients. Adverse Drug Events Prevention Study Group. JAMA. 1997;277(4):307–11.

19. Lazarou J, Pomeranz BH, Corey PN. Incidence of adverse drug reactions in hospitalized patients: a meta-analysis of prospective studies. JAMA. 1998;279(15):1200–5.

20. Bond CA, Raehl CL. Clinical pharmacy services, pharmacy staffing, and hospital mortality rates. *Pharmacotherapy.* 2007;27(4):481–93.

21. Kohn LT, Corrigan JM, Donaldson MS, eds. *To Err Is Human: Building a Safer Health System.* Washington, DC: National Academies of Science; 2000.

22. U.S. Department of Health and Human Services, Centers for Medicare and Medicaid Services. Process of care measures. July 30, 2009. Available at: http://www.cms.hhs.gov/Hospital QualityInits/18_HospitalProcessOfCareMeasures.asp. Accessed October 12, 2009.

The Patient-Centered Medical Home

Helen L. Figge

OBJECTIVES

1. Describe the key elements of a patient-centered medical home.
2. Discuss criteria used to credential patient-centered medical homes.
3. Discuss meaningful use of an electronic medical record as it pertains to the patient-centered medical home.
4. Describe implementation of electronic prescribing in the context of a patient-centered medical home.
5. Describe the role of pharmacists with respect to the patient-centered medical home.

The United States currently faces a crisis in the delivery of primary, preventive, and chronic care. At the same time that the population is aging, fewer medical students are entering the field of primary care. The burden of managing chronically ill patients has been shifted to specialty care providers. Such care is often more expensive and less well coordinated than the care provided in the primary care setting. The lack of adequate primary care capacity in the United States has likely contributed to the increasing cost of care, as well as the fact that the outcomes achieved in the United States with regard to preventive services are some of the worst among developed countries.[1] These circumstances have pointed to the need for new strategies for managing chronic care and for delivering primary and preventive care services.

The **patient-centered medical home,** sometimes called the "advanced medical home," has been introduced as a model to improve the delivery of primary and preventive care services.[2] Grounded in the Wagner Chronic Care Model[3] (CCM), the patient-centered medical home provides enhanced care for all patients, with or without a chronic condition. The patient-centered medical home builds on the Wagner CCM and generalizes the model's key features to encompass the delivery of all primary, preventive, and chronic care. A number of practice management principles needed to create a patient-centered medical home have been articulated by practitioner organizations including the American College of Physicians, American Academy of Family Physicians, American Academy of Pediatrics, and American Osteopathic Association.[2]

As envisioned by these organizations, the patient-centered medical home features a personal clinician who leads a health care team that takes responsibility for ongoing care of the patient. The personal clinician provides for all of the patient's health care needs or arranges for appropriate care with other professionals. All care is coordinated across the continuum of the health care system. Care coordination is facilitated by patient registries, information technology such as electronic medical records (EMRs), health information exchange (HIE), and electronic prescribing (e-prescribing). Decision making is guided by evidence-based medicine and clinical decision support (CDS) tools.

Clinicians are engaged in continuous quality improvement activities including quality performance measurement: Quality metrics are measured and reported. Information technology occupies an important role as a tool to support optimal patient care, performance measurement, patient education, quality improvement, and communication. A patient-centered medical home must deploy and use an EMR, exchange clinical data using HIE, and adopt e-prescribing to achieve full functionality.[4] Major features of the patient-centered medical home are listed in Table 22–1. Major advantages to the patient include better coordination of care between the primary care clinician and specialists, 24-hour access to care, patient education and engagement in preventive measures, improved safety associated with e-prescribing, and patient reminder systems.

In general, the patient-centered medical home functions best with enhanced reimbursement models that do not rely exclusively on fee-for-

> ### TABLE 22–1
> Major Features of the Patient-Centered Medical Home

Personal clinician	Quality and safety
Clinician-directed medical practice	Enhanced access
Team-based care	Meaningful use of HIT tools
Whole-person orientation	Monitoring and measurement of outcomes
Coordinated and integrated care	Electronic prescribing

HIT = health information technology.
Source: Reference 2.

service payments. For example, some models feature care coordination fees paid on a per-member, per-month basis, in addition to fees paid specifically for discrete services. These mixed reimbursement models provide the enhanced funding to encourage the flexibility that is required to implement coordinated care services in the patient-centered medical home. If third-party payers are considering payment of enhanced rates to medical homes, then it is necessary to implement an objective standardized tool to credential practices as a medical home. The next section describes one such recognition program.

Medical Home Recognition

The National Committee for Quality Assurance (NCQA)[4] has designed a **medical home recognition** program to objectively measure the degree to which a primary care practice meets the operational principles of a patient-centered medical home.[2] The NCQA program features three tiers of recognition. Achievement of a given tier is dependent on a point-scoring system in which points are awarded if the practice has achieved competency in a given business/practice management process. Level 1 is the most basic tier and can be achieved without deploying EMRs. Level 2 requires some electronic functions, and level 3 requires a fully functional EMR. In addition to the point-scoring system, 10 "must-pass" elements are required to achieve level 2 or 3. NCQA uses nine different standards to score practices, focusing on critical practice management processes. These standards are illustrated in Table 22–2. To achieve level 1, a practice must achieve at least 25 of 100 points and must achieve 5 of the 10 must-pass elements. To achieve level 2, a practice must score at least 50 points and

TABLE 22–2

Practice Management Processes Scored by NCQA

Access and communication	Test tracking
Patient tracking and registry	Referral tracking
Care management	Performance reporting and improvement
Patient self-management support	Advance electronic communications
Electronic prescribing	

NCQA = National Committee for Quality Assurance.
Source: Reference 4.

must achieve all 10 must-pass criteria. Similarly, for level 3, the practice must score at least 75 points and must achieve all 10 must-pass criteria.

Meaningful Use of an EMR

To achieve recognition as a medical home at the highest level, a practice must successfully reengineer its workflow to meet the basic definition of **meaningful use:** demonstration of meaningful use of electronic patient records by eligible providers (institutions and physicians) to be eligible for financial incentives and to avoid financial penalties. Incorporating the use of an EMR technology into everyday activities satisfies the definition and becomes one of the distinguishing criteria of a medical home. The definition of *meaningful use* has taken on great significance under the American Recovery and Reinvestment Act of 2009 (ARRA).[5] Within ARRA is the Health Information Technology for Economic and Clinical Health Act (HITECH Act), which provides incentive funds for meaningful use of certified EMR technology by eligible clinicians and hospitals in the Medicare and Medicaid programs. The goal of ARRA is to incentivize the use of electronic tools to improve care quality and coordination. Hence, this legislation synergizes nicely with the conceptual basis behind the patient-centered medical home. ARRA defines three components of meaningful use in the statute and allows the full definition to be articulated by the Health and Human Services Secretary. The three components of meaningful use as defined in ARRA are[5]:

- e-Prescribing.
- Engaging in HIE to improve care coordination.
- Reporting quality metrics.

All three of these core activities will also count toward NCQA certification of a primary care practice as a medical home.

In addition, the Office of the National Coordinator for Health Information Technology has convened a policy committee as required under the HITECH Act, the purpose of which is to advise on policy issues related to implementation of national standards for health information technology. The HIT Policy Committee has developed a draft document[6] outlining additional key aspects of meaningful use for an EMR. These are classified under five categories of health outcomes priorities, as shown in Table 22–3.

Under the first major category, recommended activities for 2011 include:

- Use of CPOE (computerized provider order entry).
- Implementation of drug-drug, drug-allergy, and formulary checks.
- Maintenance of problem lists and active diagnoses.
- e-Prescribing.
- Maintenance of active medication lists.
- Maintenance of active allergy lists.
- A record of demographics.
- A record of advance directives.
- A record of vital signs.
- A flag for smoking status.
- A record of laboratory results as structured data.
- A list of patient-specific conditions.
- The ability to report ambulatory quality measures, send patient reminders, implement one clinical decision rule, document a progress note for each encounter, and check insurance eligibility.

TABLE 22–3

Major Categories of Health Outcomes Priorities for Meaningful Use of an EMR, as Proposed by the HIT Policy Committee

- Improve quality, safety, and efficiency, and reduce health disparities.
- Engage patients and families.
- Improve care coordination.
- Improve population and public health.
- Ensure adequate privacy and security protections for personal health information.

EMR = electronic medical record; HIT = health information technology.
Source: Reference 6.

These activities represent core practice management activities that would also help a primary care practice develop into a patient-centered medical home. In light of the synergies between meaningful use under ARRA and the NCQA credentialing criteria for a patient-centered medical home, it is expected that incentive payments under ARRA will help drive the development of new medical homes.

e-Prescribing

e-Prescribing represents one of the core components of meaningful use of an EMR under the ARRA HITECH Act and is one of the standards employed by NCQA for recognition of a patient-centered medical home. e-Prescribing offers great potential to reduce medication errors. It is also an important tool in the medical home tool kit because it contributes toward improvements in quality and patient safety. Two major elements of e-prescribing contribute toward a reduction in medication errors. The first is the elimination of errors related to poor penmanship and illegible handwriting. Second, information available in an EMR, including medication history, allergies, and laboratory results, can be used in conjunction with point-of-care CDS software to flag potential drug allergies, adverse drug interactions, therapeutic duplication, contraindications based on laboratory results, and other clinical issues.[7]

When properly implemented, CDS alerts can improve patient safety and help eliminate errors. It is important that these alerts be clinically relevant to avoid the phenomenon of "alert fatigue." When combined with HIE capabilities, CDS and electronic prescribing can be powerful tools. Use of HIE allows downloading of the patient's medication history from many sources, including retail pharmacy, pharmacy benefit managers, and some state Medicaid programs. The downloaded medication history can be reconciled, de-duplicated, and then loaded into the e-prescribing software to enhance the performance of the CDS module.

Role of Pharmacists in the Medical Home

Interventions by pharmacists have been demonstrated in many studies to improve clinical care,[8] one classic example being a community pharmacy diabetes program.[9] In the hospital, rates of adverse drug events are reduced when pharmacists attend rounds in the intensive care unit.[10,11] Pharmacists, as participants of the medical home team, can play a variety of important roles. For example, pharmacists can contact patients shortly after hospital discharge to ensure that the medication regimen has properly transitioned to the outpatient setting. One study demonstrated that this intervention can significantly reduce adverse drug events.[12]

Pharmacists can play a role in the ambulatory management of chronic illnesses (e.g., diabetes and hypertension), particularly with reference to medication adherence. Pharmacists can educate patients about their chronic medication regimen and oversee evidence-based protocols to improve adherence. For example, one study based at Kaiser Permanente of Colorado demonstrated that "a pharmacist-managed, physician-supervised population-management approach in patients with coronary artery disease significantly improved blood pressure control. Clinically meaningful reductions in blood pressure were achieved by using evidence-based, cost-effective drug regimens."[13]

Formal medication therapy management (MTM) programs offer a setting in which the pharmacist can perform a comprehensive review of all the patient's medications, including over-the-counter and herbal preparations. The pharmacist can then develop a fully annotated and reconciled personal medication record (PMR), a detailed assessment of medication-related problems, and a set of recommendations for review by the primary care clinician. Comprehensive patient education is included in the visit. Ideally, the reconciled PMR, assessment, and recommendations can be submitted electronically by the pharmacist directly to the EMR system in the medical home. Data standards for interoperable transmission of MTM data have not yet been developed and should be a priority for standards development organizations.[14]

The institutional MTM pharmacist can play a key role in facilitating coordination of care when patients transition from the ambulatory to inpatient setting, and again when patients transition to a subacute, long-term care, or outpatient setting. These transitions are often associated with significant changes in the medication regimen, and they present unique opportunities to educate patients about their medications. Reconciliation of the PMR at such key transitions is critical to provide continuity of care and avoid medication errors. Electronic communication between the institutional MTM pharmacist and the medical home can ensure continuity of care and patient safety. For example, plans for appropriate monitoring of medications and necessary follow-up laboratory tests can be confirmed with the medical home at the time of the transition.

These and other examples illustrate the emerging role of the pharmacist in the patient-centered medical home. In all of these models, pharmacists will rely on HIT to monitor and manage medication-related medical outcomes.

Conclusion

The patient-centered medical home offers a structured framework of practice management principles that holds great promise in improving the quality and safety of medical care while simultaneously reducing costs. The successful implementation of the patient-centered medical home requires the adoption and meaningful use of EMRs and e-prescribing tools. Pharmacists can fill an integral role in the team-based care of patients in the medical home. Many studies have demonstrated that interventions by pharmacists can improve patient care in ambulatory and inpatient settings, and during the transition between these settings. Health information technology tools, used in conjunction with MTM protocols, can help to integrate the pharmacist with the patient-centered medical home.

LEARNING ACTIVITIES

1. Compare the NCQA criteria for a level 3 medical home (found at www.ncqa.org/tabid/631/Default.aspx) against the proposed elements of meaningful use of an EMR under ARRA. What are the synergies and gaps between the two sets of criteria?
2. Obtain and read Reference 8. Discuss with a colleague the implications for pharmacy in general and the specific implications for your career.
3. Review the features of the medical home in Table 22–1. (Consult Reference 2 for additional details.) What challenges do you see to full achievement of these features? What enablers do you envision that could facilitate achieving these features?

References

1. The Commonwealth Fund Commission on a High Performance Health System. Why not the best? Results from the national scorecard on U.S. health system performance, 2008. Available

at: http://www.commonwealthfund.org/usr_doc/Why_Not_the_Best_national_scorecard_2008. pdf. Accessed October 4, 2009.

2. American Academy of Family Physicians (AAFP), American Academy of Pediatrics (AAP), American College of Physicians (ACP), American Osteopathic Association (AOA). Joint principles of the patient-centered medical home. March, 2007. Available at: http://www. medicalhomeinfo.org/downloads/pdfs/JointStatement.pdf. Accessed October 4, 2009.

3. Von Korff M, Gruman J, Schafer J, et al. Collaborative management of chronic illness. *Ann Intern Med.* 1997;127(12):1097–102.

4. National Committee for Quality Assurance (NCQA). NCQA program to evaluate patient-centered medical homes [news release]. January 8, 2008. Available at: http://www.ncqa.org/ tabid/641/Default.aspx. Accessed October 4, 2009.

5. The American Recovery and Reinvestment Act of 2009. The 111th Congress. Public Law 111-5. Available at: http://frwebgate.access.gpo.gov/cgi-bin/getdoc.cgi?dbname=111_cong_bills& docid=f:hlenr.pdf. Accessed October 4, 2009.

6. Department of Health and Human Services. Health IT policy council recommendations to national coordinator for defining meaningful use. Final—August, 2009. Available at: http://healthit.hhs.gov/portal/server.pt/gateway/PTARGS_0_10741_888532_0_0_18/FINAL%20 MU%20RECOMMENDATIONS%20TABLE.pdf. Accessed October 4, 2009.

7. Figge H. Electronic prescribing in the ambulatory setting. *Am J Health Syst Pharm.* 2009; 66(1): 16–8.

8. Bates DW. Role of pharmacists in the medical home. *Am J Health Syst Pharm.* 2009; 66(12): 1116–8.

9. Cranor CW, Bunting BA, Christensen DB. The Asheville Project: long-term clinical and economic outcomes of a community pharmacy diabetes care program. *J Am Pharm Assoc* (Wash). 2003;43(2):173–84.

10. Leape LL, Cullen DJ, Clapp MD, et al. Pharmacist participation on physician rounds and adverse drug events in the intensive care unit. *JAMA.* 1999;282(3):267–70.

11. Kaushal R, Bates DW, Abramson EL, et al. Unit-based clinical pharmacists' prevention of serious medication errors in pediatric inpatients. *Am J Health Syst Pharm.* 2008;65(13): 1254–60.

12. Schnipper JL, Kirwin JL, Cotugno MC, et al. Role of pharmacist counseling in preventing adverse drug events after hospitalization. *Arch Intern Med.* 2006;166(5):565–71.

13. McConnell KJ, Zadvorny EB, Hardy AM, et al. Clinical Pharmacy Cardiac Risk Service Study Group. Coronary artery disease and hypertension: outcomes of a pharmacist-managed blood pressure program. *Pharmacotherapy.* 2006;26(9):1333–41.

14. Figge H. Collaborative MTM—medical home model. *Am J Health Syst Pharm.* 2011; 67:190–1.

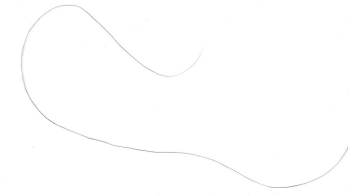

Quality Improvement in Health Care

Margaret R. Thrower

OBJECTIVES

1. Define quality improvement in health care.
2. Identify key organizations that are dedicated to quality improvement in health care.
3. Discuss the impact of data quality on health outcomes.

The Institute of Medicine (IOM) defines **quality** as "the degree to which health services for individuals and populations increase the likelihood of desired health outcomes and are consistent with current professional knowledge."[1] Despite significant advances in medical technology and science, there are still overwhelming challenges in American health care, such as unequal distribution of health care and suboptimal quality, to overcome.[2] Treatment of chronic diseases (e.g., asthma, cardiovascular disease, and diabetes) is especially burdensome.[3] In most communities, health care is delivered through dysfunctional systems; even though health care providers know many of the best practices that will improve the quality of treatment, difficult barriers prevent these practices from being adopted and transforming health care across the United States.[2]

In addition to these burdens, health care costs are growing at a rate that places an even greater financial burden on the U.S. economy.[2] Therefore, better ways are needed to determine if all participants in the U.S. health care system (patients, physicians, nurses, hospitals, health plans, businesses, and government) receive value that is equivalent to the money and other investments allotted to the system.[2] Health care in America represents one of the biggest expenditures by the federal government, and people are still not getting the right care when they need it. One example is illustrated in the *Dartmouth Atlas*, a report on an ongoing research project that produces data on regional differences in the delivery of health care services.[2] This report highlighted huge variations in Medicare spending for end-of-life care in hospitals. One region showed an average of $20,000 of Medicare expenditures in seriously ill patients, whereas another region showed approximately $50,000. Of note, these differences in Medicare spending were not directly related to how many patients were treated, how severely ill the patients were, or even whether patients experienced better outcomes as a result of the higher spending. The bottom line here is that the more costly care did not equal better care.[2]

Problems with the U.S. health care system are not limited to just quality and value issues; research shows that certain groups (e.g., those of specific racial, ethnic, cultural, and socioeconomic backgrounds) commonly receive the lowest quality care.[2] These differences in quality of care between minority and non-minority patients remain even when other factors, such as insurance status and income level, are taken out of the picture.[2] In recent years, national organizations and the U.S. government have started collaborating on concepts of value and public reporting of quality and cost information.[1,2] These concepts are based on the belief that it is important to make health care information (e.g., cost and quality of care) more available to consumers.[1,2] Access to this information is expected to create a better understanding of what high-quality care looks like and how to demand and achieve it.[1,2]

Evidence to Support That Technology Can Improve Quality of Health Care

American health care has been criticized as expensive, dysfunctional, unfair, and even unsafe.[1] Health information technologies including electronic medical records, computerized provider order entry (CPOE) systems, and clinical decision support systems have offered benefits by reducing errors and waste, improving communication among health care providers, increasing quality of care, and providing automated performance measurement.[4,5] However, studies that examine the impact of these technologies are not generally applicable beyond the study site, given that currently published studies are limited to single-site studies performed by academic institutions that have developed their systems internally and over a long period of time (i.e., 10 years or more).[5]

In reality, most hospitals must consider purchasing a commercially available clinical information system. Lack of available data contributes to the challenge because few studies have been performed across multiple hospitals to understand the effect of these technologies in these settings. One study published in 2009 used a cross-sectional survey of physicians in urban hospitals in Texas; the authors used a clinical information technology assessment tool that measured a hospital's level of automation on the basis of physician interactions with the information system. Study results indicated lower rates of mortality and complications, as well as lower costs in hospitals with automated notes and records, CPOE, and clinical decision support.[6] This study highlights an important breakthrough in available data to reflect "real-world" application of clinical information technologies and how they impact the quality of health care.

Passage of the American Recovery and Reinvestment Act of 2009 provided substantial financial incentives for physicians and hospitals to adopt and use electronic medical records (EMRs). This Act also charged the Department of Health and Human Services (HHS) with development of uniform electronic standards that allow communication between various health information technologies (HITs), which is another challenge for successful adoption of HIT. Organizations are nervous about these goals. There is also a great deal of uncertainty about the details of how the money will be distributed, whether all practices will choose good systems, and how sustainable the changes will be. A report from Bridges to Excellence shows that widespread use of EMRs is being successfully implemented in some communities across the country, and that these systems are also helping to support performance measurement and quality improvement programs.[7] The authors discuss case studies of implementation of EMRs in New York City, Cincinnati, and Cleveland. As participants in the Robert Wood Johnson Foundation's Aligning Forces for Quality initiative, Cincinnati and Cleveland are great examples of how local stakeholder partnerships can effectively connect HIT with efforts to improve and share information on the quality of care. The report offers a refreshingly optimistic view of adoption of HIT and concludes that EMRs can help achieve the following in health care:

- Enable physicians to have the information they need to improve the quality of care that they deliver.
- Allow employers and health plans to access information on physician performance so that they can create meaningful incentives for excellence.
- Inform consumers which physicians deliver quality care.

Adoption of Quality Improvement Practices

In a recently published study, it was demonstrated that incentives do have a significant effect on physician behavior. More specifically, physician participation in quality improvement and pay for performance programs (P4P programs) is *directly* related to the amount of incentives offered.[8] A paper from deBrantes and colleagues predict that most physicians will adopt EMRs as a result of the incentives offered.[9]

In June of 2008, an article based on many years of research was published; it outlined the results of cost-benefit studies related to certain performance measures. The publication highlighted that intermediate outcomes and other measures that are highly predictive of positive clinical results in the management of patients also produce the highest returns for patients and payers.[10] A recently published paper has highlighted that a significant cost is associated with potentially avoidable complications that have and can occur in patients with chronic conditions; these studies also show that better management resulted in lower cost of care.[11] Another study has brought attention to the significant amount of hospitalizations and re-hospitalizations of Medicare patients.[12]

These studies represent an important departure from the "traditional" practice of trying to equate quality of care by measuring whether a test or preventive care screening has been completed or delivered, given that this practice is not the best way to measure quality in inpatient and outpatient settings. These studies prompted development of programs called CareLinks, which measure how well a patient is being managed either in a physician practice and/or across practice settings. These programs collect data to measure quality automatically and in a systematic fashion from various EMRs that are installed in physician practices.[2]

Organizations Devoted to Quality in Health Care

The Institute for Healthcare Improvement

No chapter about quality in health care could be complete without mention of the Institute for Healthcare Improvement (IHI). This independent, nonprofit organization has a global mission to improve health care worldwide by focusing on education, best practices, and the development and dissemination of new ideas. IHI is based in Cambridge, Massachusetts, and works with provider organizations in a collaborative learning environment that focuses on the organizations' members learning from each other to ultimately improve health care for patients.[13]

Agency for Healthcare Research and Quality

The mission of the Agency for Healthcare Research and Quality (AHRQ) is to improve the quality, safety, efficiency, and effectiveness of health care for all Americans. The agency is part of HHS. Information from AHRQ's research helps people make more informed decisions and improve the quality of health care services. (AHRQ was formerly known as the Agency for Health Care Policy and Research).[14]

Institute of Medicine

The Institute of Medicine (IOM) launched a well-known effort in 1996 that focused on assessing and improving the nation's quality of care. This ongoing initiative, called Crossing the Quality Chasm, is currently in its third phase. The first phase of the initiative discussed the severity of the challenges for providing quality health care in the United States; the authors concluded that "the burden of harm conveyed by the collective impact of all of our health care quality problems is staggering."[1] During the second phase, from 1999 to 2001, the Committee on Quality of Health Care in America communicated a vision for how the health care system and related policy environment must be transformed to close the chasm between what is known to be good quality care and what actually exists in practice. The reports released during this phase—*To Err Is Human: Building a Safer Health System* (1999)[15] and *Crossing the Quality Chasm: A New Health System for the 21st Century* (2001)[1] emphasize that reform needs to be comprehensive and thorough to truly fix the system.

Phase three of the IOM's quality initiative focuses on implementing the vision of the future health system described in the *Crossing the Quality Chasm* report.[1] In addition to the IOM, many others are working to create a more patient-responsive 21st-century health system, including clinicians/health care organizations, employers/consumers, foundations/research organizations, government agencies, and quality organizations.[16] (Table 23–1 lists specific organizations involved in this effort.) This collaborative effort focuses reform at three different levels of the system that overlap: the environmental level, the health care organization level, and the interface between clinicians and patients.

TABLE 23–1
Quality-Focused Web Resources

Resource	Web Site
Clinicians and Health Care Organizations	
Alliance of Community Health Plans	www.achp.org
American Academy of Pediatrics	www.aap.org
American College of Physicians	www.acponline.org
Association of Academic Health Centers	www.aahcdc.org/index.php
Association of American Medical Colleges	www.aamc.org
Patient Safety First (Association of periOperative Registered Nurses)	www.aorn.org
Employers and Consumers	
Center for Medical Consumers	www.medicalconsumers.org
Kaiser Family Foundation 2006 Report on Employers Health Benefits	www.kff.org/insurance/7527/index.cfm
The Leapfrog Group	www.leapfroggroup.org
National Chronic Care Consortium	www.nccconline.org/index.htm

TABLE 23-1

Quality-Focused Web Resources (*Continued*)

Resource	Web Site
Foundations and Research Organizations	
California Health Care Foundation	www.chcf.org
The Commonwealth Fund	www.commonwealthfund.org
Kaiser Permanente Institute for Health Policy	www.kpihp.org
W. K. Kellogg Foundation	www.wkkf.org
Markle Foundation—Connecting for Health Initiative	www.connectingforhealth.org
Robert Wood Johnson Foundation	www.rwjf.org/qualityequality
Government Agencies	
Agency for Healthcare Research and Quality	www.ahrq.gov
Medical Errors and Patient Safety	www.ahrq.gov/qual/errorsix.htm
Quality & Patient Safety	www.ahrq.gov/qual
Centers for Medicare and Medicaid Services: Hospital Quality Initiatives	www.cms.hhs.gov/HospitalQualityInits
Council on Graduate Medical Education	www.cogme.gov/jointmtg.htm
National Academy for State Health Policy	www.nashp.org
Quality Interagency Coordination Task Force	www.quic.gov
Veterans Affairs National Center for Patient Safety	www.patientsafety.gov/
Quality Organizations	
American Health Quality Association	www.ahqa.org/pub/quality/161_684_2440.CFM
Institute for Healthcare Improvement	www.ihi.org/IHI/Topics/PatientSafety
Institute for Safe Medication Practices	www.ismp.org
The Joint Commission	www.jointcommission.org/PatientSafety
National Center for Healthcare Leadership	www.nchl.org
National Coalition on Health Care	www.nchc.org
National Committee for Quality Assurance	www.ncqa.org
National Quality Forum	www.qualityforum.org
URAC	www.urac.org
Publication Guidelines for Quality Improvement in Health Care	www.rwjf.org/pr/product.jsp?id=35700

Source: Author.

Quality Improvement Initiatives Specific to Pharmacy

What does quality improvement look like in pharmacy? Quality improvement initiatives are found across all types of pharmacy practice, with much of the current attention focusing on acute care because the majority of data related to quality originate in this practice setting. Efforts generally focus on the appropriate utilization of medications in specific disease states or conditions, as described in clinical practice guidelines. "Appropriateness" can include using appropriate dosing, using corollary medications, and monitoring for safety and efficacy. Pharmacists frequently use the tools described in Chapter 20 to identify potential quality needs to address. After determining the appropriate course of action, pharmacists then use the documentation tools addressed in Chapter 21 to record their activities and the associated outcomes.

A key characteristic of pharmacists' involvement in quality improvement initiatives within acute care settings is that their involvement is prospective in nature. This allows pharmacists to share their knowledge with other providers in the development of drug therapy plans. The next step is to be involved in the longitudinal management of a patient's medication regimen. Pharmacists are also involved in the continuous monitoring of patients' response (or absence of response) to medication therapy to ensure that desired outcomes are achieved.

One last topic of pharmacy practice in the acute setting is the instrumental role of pharmacists in developing institutional policies and procedures that direct medication management across the entire institution. This seemingly administrative role has a profound impact on the clinical use of medications. These policies and procedures are developed according to clinically driven guidelines that are often established through a consensus process. The decisions made regarding institution-wide use of medications clearly impact all patients.

In the community setting, pharmacists are also involved in quality improvement initiatives. One of the more focused initiatives is described by the Alliance for Patient Medication Safety (APMS), a federally certified patient safety organization. APMS focuses on development of a culture within pharmacy that strives to achieve quality medication care through continuous assessment and improvement of medication use. The alliance includes on-line tools for reporting patient safety issues related to compounding and to the use of electronic prescriptions.[17]

Pharmacy Quality Commitment, a service of APMS, uses anonymous, voluntary reporting to identify medication-related patient safety issues.[18] The ability to anonymously report medication errors has consistently been identified as a critical factor to pharmacists' reporting of errors. Pharmacies participating in any of the alliance's services receive best practice and work-flow recommendations that are based on the data collected. This culture of non-punitive reporting of data—which is then used to educate others on how to improve medication use—is the cornerstone of the alliance's approach to quality improvement.

Conclusion

Many organizations and initiatives are attempting to create higher quality in health care. As health care professionals, it is important for pharmacists to be familiar with leading quality initiatives and organizations. As described in previous text, quality improvement is found throughout pharmacy practice, with pharmacists playing a critical role in acute and community quality initiatives. Quality improvement can be found in every practice.

Quality in health care is a vast topic involving many important organizations; therefore, Table 23–1 provides Web links to organizations that focus on and promote high quality in health care. A good place to learn more about quality improvement is to become familiar with these organizations and the resources they offer.

LEARNING ACTIVITIES

1. Identify five quality-focused organizations or Web sites in addition to those listed in Table 23–1. What are their primary areas of focus? What role do they indicate for the pharmacist in quality initiatives?
2. For each site or organization identified in #1, list the resources or information produced by the organization that could help you as a pharmacist.
3. Identify a leader in quality improvement (organization, facility, or individual) that is geographically close to you and schedule a tour or meeting. Make note of the practices or technologies that might be applicable to your organization or work.
4. Obtain and read Reference 15. Discuss the publication with a colleague. What are the major points of emphasis? What can you apply to your current or future practice?

References

1. Committee on Quality of Health Care in America, Institute of Medicine. *Crossing the Quality Chasm: A New Health System for the 21st Century.* Washington, DC: National Academies of Science; 2001. Available at: http://www.iom.edu/Reports/2001/Crossing-the-Quality-Chasm-A-New-Health-System-for-the-21st-Century.aspx. Accessed October 4, 2009.

2. Robert Johnson Wood Foundation. The quality challenge. Available at: http://www.rwjf.org/qualityequality/challenge.jsp. Accessed October 4, 2009.

3. The Darmouth Institute. The Darthmouth atlas of health care. Available at: http://www.dartmouthatlas.org. Accessed October 4, 2009.

4. Bates DW, Gawande AA. Improving safety with information technology. N Engl J Med. 2003;348(25):2526–34.

5. Chaudhry B, Wang J, Wu S, et al. Systematic review: impact of health information technology on quality, efficiency, and cost of medical care. Ann Intern Med. 2006;144(10):742–52.

6. Amarasingham R, Plantinga L, Diener-West M, et al. Clinical information technologies and inpatient outcomes: a multiple hospital study. Arch Intern Med. 2009;169(2):108–14.

7. Bridges to Excellence. Measuring what matters—electronically, automatically, (somewhat) painlessly. A report from the real-world field of innovation and implementation. Available at: http://www.rwjf.org/files/research/measuringwhatmatters2009.pdf. Accessed July 1, 2010.

8. deBrantes FS, D'Andrea G. Physicians respond to pay-for-performance incentives: larger incentives yield greater participation. Am J Manag Care. 2009;15(5):305–10.

9. deBrantes FS, D'Andrea G. Model predicts that HIT stimulus will have significant impact: two-thirds of physicians expected to participate. Available at: http://bridgestoexcellence.org/Documents/BTE-HITECH.pdf. Accessed October 3, 2009.

10. de Brantes FS, Rastogi A. Evidence-informed case rates: paying for safer, more reliable care. The Commonwealth Fund. June 2008. Available at: http://www.commonwealthfund.org/~/media/Files/Publications/Issue%20Brief/2008/Jun/Evidence%20Informed%20Case%20Rates%20%20Paying%20for%20Safer%20%20More%20Reliable%20Care/de_Brantes_issue_brief_SBA_final%20pdf.pdf. Accessed April 3, 2010.

11. Rosenthal MB, de Brantes FS, Sinaiko AD, et al. Bridges to excellence—recognizing high-quality care: analysis of physician quality and resource use. Am J Manag Care. 2008;14(10):670–7.

12. Jencks SF, Williams MV, Coleman EA. Rehospitalizations among patients in the Medicare fee-for-service program. N Engl J Med. 2009;360(14):1418–28.

13. The Institute for Healthcare Improvement. IHI map for improvement. Available at: http://www.ihi.org/IHI/about. Accessed September 15, 2009.

14. Agency for Healthcare Research and Quality. Available at: http://www.ahrq.gov. Accessed October 4, 2009.

15. Kohn LT, Corrigan JM, Donaldson MS, eds. *To Err Is Human: Building a Safer Health System.* Washington, DC: National Academies of Science; 2000.

16. Institute of Medicine. Available at: http://www.iom.edu. Accessed September 5, 2009.

17. Alliance for Patient Medication Safety. Available at: http://www.medicationsafety.org. Accessed October 4, 2009.

18. Pharmacy Quality Commitment. Available at: http://www.pqc.net. Accessed October 4, 2009.

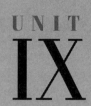

U N I T

IX

Pharmacy Informatics Ecosystem

UNIT COMPETENCIES

- Describe measures used to ensure the privacy, security, and confidentiality of health information.
- Discuss legal and ethical issues pertaining to health information.
- Discuss standards for interoperability related to medications, diagnoses, communication, and electronic data interchange.
- Discuss technologies used to automate the medication delivery process.
- Collaborate with other health care professionals to optimize informatics projects.
- Apply project and change-management principles and methods to informatics projects.

UNIT DESCRIPTION

This unit addresses topics that traverse multiple steps of the medication use process. These topics include the increasing role of patients as active contributors in their health care, the delivery of pharmacy services over distance, the security and privacy of patient health information as an increasingly important topic, methods for successfully managing health information technology projects, and the future of pharmacy informatics. Ultimately, every topic in this unit will impact readers regardless of their pharmacy practice environment.

Health 2.0 and Personal Health Records

Bill G. Felkey

OBJECTIVES

1. List at least five Health 2.0 tools for collaborating with patients.
2. Describe the key attributes of the Institute of Medicine's dimensions for quality improvement of health information systems.
3. Discuss the differences in information focus between patient, provider, and biomedical researcher communities.
4. Describe the available formats and attributes of the personal health record.
5. Describe the impact of personal health record adoption and Health 2.0 on the workflow and workload of pharmacy operations.

Previous chapters covered the systems that will help U.S. health care, in general, and the pharmacy profession, in particular, realize the vision of becoming a seamlessly connected digital field. Although it is imperative that all providers be able to collaborate effectively in a multidisciplinary team, the patient is often not chosen to be an integral part of the care team. The Institute of Medicine posits that the performance and quality changes necessary in health care information systems should utilize a set of dimensions that are captured in the acronym STEEEP—Safe Timely Effective Efficient Equitable Patient-centered. "Safe" assumes that all patients want their pharmacist to protect them from slips and mistakes that can cause them harm and to create a truly safe environment for their care. "Timely" promotes that information used for patient care needs to be not only accurate but needs to arrive at the point of care as close to real time as possible. "Effective" takes the position that evidence-based resources that use the best science possible will be available in the system. "Efficient" means the wasting of personnel time, money, and other resources will be eliminated or kept to a minimum.

The previous four dimensions focused on quality and cost considerations. Now the focus of the acronym switches to patients and patient populations, specifically access to the health care system and the philosophical and practical orientation of the system. "Equitable," therefore, promotes that the health care system will attempt to provide care, to the extent possible, to all patients. Finally, "patient-centered" advocates for patients to become fully involved in decisions regarding their health.[1]

The vision of health care becoming patient centered (or more personalized) is considered the driving force for **Health 2.0.** This new concept of health care uses a specific set of World Wide Web (Web) tools to provide better health education, promote collaboration between patients and providers, and help providers deliver desired health outcomes. Health 2.0 allows collaboration between patients and a network of nonprofessional caregivers as well as a full complement of providers who all have the most up-to-date information available when making decisions regarding the patient's care. Additionally, these data can be de-indentified for researchers to study to improve care processes for entire populations who are experiencing the same conditions. All of these attributes have a foundation of information access provided through electronic medical record components that include the patient-maintained personal health record (PHR).

Participatory Health Care and Information Age Medicine

Think for a moment about the ideal information system to support a pharmacy practice. Now try to imagine that the system's design leaves patients as uninvolved bystanders. Providers would have all the information they need to reduce uncertainty in making clinical decisions, but anything that happened outside of pharmacy operations would be disconnected and, therefore, unknown. Unfortunately, much of our health care system has historically operated in this manner. In this old system, the episode of care was the focus—at the expense of continuity of care. An analogy would be patients equating their health status with the operation of their automobiles. Many people drive their cars with little concern for how the cars work or how preventive maintenance keeps them working. When a problem occurs, the owners drop their cars off at a garage and pick them up at the end of the day, only to continue driving them hard until the next breakdown.

An article in the *British Medical Journal* described our previous approach to health care as being "industrial age medicine" in which the focus was on professional care that was segmented into primary, secondary, and tertiary layers with the use of specialist and more expensive care being encouraged. The new approach to health care is described as "information age health care" and encourages lower cost individual self-care, involvement of friends and family, and the use of self-help networks as the first-line approach. More discouraged, but still necessary, would be the role of professionals as first facilitators, then partners in the care process, and finally as authorities that fully take over the direction of patient care while still involving the patient in every decision.[2]

The label for this transformation of health care delivery is called "participatory care." In this approach, patients are not only involved in decision making about their care; they also are responsible for becoming highly active members of their own care team. The Web-oriented extension of this type of health care is called "Health 2.0." Health 2.0 is application of the tools provided by Web 2.0 for health care initiatives. **Web 2.0** refers to interactive and social media applications that comprise the second generation of the Internet, which developed after the 2001 collapse of the dot.com bubble. In the context of health, Web 2.0 is characterized by collaboration and interactivity among patients, caregivers, and providers; user-maintained content; and openness. Social networking is interaction among individuals using social media applications, which are Internet-based Web 2.0 software tools. Health 2.0 can be thought of as a subset of Medicine 2.0 (a Web 2.0 application for health and medicine that is used by physicians to carve out their responsibilities). Health 2.0 applies to an individual's use of Web 2.0 applications to manage his or her health.[3]

The year 2003 has been described as the time in which Internet use changed from the three "C's" of Internet functionality—content, communication, and commerce—to include a fourth "C," which stands for "community." In 2003, social networking began to gather strength, changing the way and the number of hours the Internet was utilized globally (versus the time spent using books, television, or other entertainment media).

For example, according to Alexa global traffic rankings (www.alexa.com), the top 10 most utilized Internet sites in 2005 included eBay, Amazon, Microsoft, AOL, and Go.com. In 2008, all of these sites had dropped out of the top 10 and were replaced by sites such as MySpace, Facebook, Wikipedia, YouTube, Blogger, and Live.com.[4] Although these sites were initially thought to be almost the exclusive territory of young people, interestingly, at the time this book was written, baby boomers were the fastest growing demographic on Facebook. In fact, much of the U.S. national pharmacy community is helping to organize professional networking and activities using this social networking site. In pharmacy school classrooms in an institution that requires each student to purchase a laptop computer, the old Microsoft game of solitaire is now replaced by Facebook screens whenever Doctor of Pharmacy students require a mental break from their studies.

Web 2.0 and Health 2.0

Pharmacists must learn a new vocabulary to effectively use and integrate Web 2.0 and Health 2.0 tools to develop social networking tools for the purpose of forming a trusted community component of their practice. These kinds of activities are always done in addition to traditional operations—not instead of them. Thus, a traditional Internet presence will still be maintained, but Health 2.0 tools will be utilized as an addition to normal patient interaction resources.

Answering the following questions should give pharmacists an idea of their literacy in this area:

- Do you find yourself reading blogs more than you do newspapers and magazines?
- Is Facebook your home page on your browser?
- Do you talk with your friends more on Skype than on your cell phone?
- Do you spend more time watching video on YouTube than watching network and cable programming on television?

TABLE 24–1

Web 2.0/Health 2.0 Application Tool Kit

Blogs	Music	Text/SMS broadcasting
Business networking	Office documents	Tools/widgets
Calls and VoIP	Photograph sharing	Travel
Chat	Really Simple Syndication (RSS)	Video
E-mail	Shopping	Virtual worlds
Games	Social bookmarking	Webinar programming
Micro-blogs	Social networking portals	Wikis

SMS = short message service; VoIP = voice over Internet protocol.
Source: Author.

- Do you plan on or are you currently getting your continuing education hours through an iPod?
- Has anyone sent you a tweet today?
- Are you keeping up with new literature by turning pages on journals or checking new listings on Connotea?

A resource called a "wiki"—a Web site that allows group participation in the creation and editing of Web pages—is the basis for some of the described Internet resources. Pharmacists can create or contribute to wikis, as well as monitor them for accuracy and alert users of any bias or conflicts of interest in the content of a wiki. (See Table 24–1 for other components of the Health 2.0 tool kit.)

Web 2.0 and Health 2.0 Resources Explained

Facebook is an example of a Web 2.0 social networking portal in that it tries to supply many of the resources listed in Table 24–1 for its members. Patientslikeme.com, another social networking portal, is an example of how Health 2.0 can provide a portal that allows people who are trying to cope with the same medical condition to communicate with each other. The same tools are used to build social as well as health Web sites. For example, one could use similar tool kit resources to plan a class reunion or to assist patients in navigating various treatment options for a medical condition. These sites not only connect people with similar interests or problems but, on health sites, allow everyone to share experiences and offer ways to cope with drug side effects, postoperative pain, and recovery of the ability to engage in normal daily activities.

Blogs, chats, and e-mails are all different methods for communicating. Typically, a blog is published on an Internet site in the same way a newspaper article would be created. Someone has something to say and posts those thoughts on the Internet. In a newspaper, readers can write letters to the editor, which would be published in a subsequent newspaper. In a blog, readers can comment in spaces provided directly below the published blog material. Blogs are very similar to discussion forums, but previously unknown bloggers can attract an audience of 1 million readers as word spreads on the Internet by a method called **"viral marketing"** in which people spread the word through their personal networks that a blog (or other Web 2.0 site) has interesting things to say. Web sites may also allow real-time instant messaging, cell texting, or "chats" to allow users to communicate in a conversational manner. E-mails on the other hand tend to be asynchronous and may typically be longer messages than those used in chat rooms.

"Social bookmarking" is also called **"social tagging"** in that people who have a common interest can denote Web resources that they deem to be valuable assets within their focus area. For example, delicious.com is a Web site that provides the user community's opinion of the best Internet locations on a given topic. Connotea (www.connotea.org) is a Web site that identifies published resources including, among other formats, peer-reviewed articles within a given focus area. Usually these articles are available in portable document format (PDF) for download and use in pharmacy practice. Sites such as Digg.com promote Web sites that contain breaking news or something that Internet searchers find interesting at that moment.

Wiki sites allow group participation in the publication of monographs that can be constantly updated. The most well-known is Wikipedia, which is frequently described as the encyclopedia of the people. Although contributions to any given monograph could be made by someone with a conflict of interest, moderators note when the potential for conflict could be present. Many scholars can understandably find the open nature of these community-contributed monographs to be problematic from an evidence-based standpoint. RxWiki is an example of pharmacist-contributed drug monographs. Some companies are using wikis to capture their employees' contributions for the purpose of knowledge management. If employees continually record their insights concerning clients and working processes of the business, then new hires can benefit from the employers' experiences by reading the wiki. Another advantage of this type of wiki is limiting the impact of having an experienced employee quit or retire from the business.

Having a trusted community utilize games to reach younger audiences is another tool employed on several sites (e.g., my online wellness [www.myonlinewellness.com] and Starlight Quest for the Code [www.starlight.com]) that address conditions such as diabetes and asthma. Learning self-management skills that include coping with sick days in diabetes or decreasing the incidence and severity of asthma attacks can be accomplished in a game format. In addition, using group-relevant photography, videos, music, and other multimedia formats can help build a sense of community in a social networking site. Another connection that can be made in a trusted community includes a shopping tool that allows community members to give feedback to the group on how well their purchase met their expectations. Travel considerations such as international equivalencies for drugs and immunization requirements can be communicated from a pharmacy site. Pharmacists can also choose to connect directly, in real time, to cater to the special needs of patients at remote locations globally.

Really simple syndication (RSS) offers news channels focused on specific topic areas that can be offered as "feeds" to a pharmacy Web page. For example, the American Diabetes Association sends out press releases and diabetes updates in this manner. This is just one way in which information on a trusted community Web site can be kept fresh while also giving people visiting the site a reason to return to it frequently.

Being able to send out short messages to groups is the sole focus of the Web site Twitter. A participant can either follow one or more members, or the participant may be followed by members who want to keep up with the insights of those they find interesting. This category of social networking site is called a "presence site" in that it lets others know what an individual is doing or thinking. There are many pharmacy applications for this kind of resource, including medication adherence uses, broadcasting new developments in research of interest to patients, producing warnings about drug recalls and other problems, and prompting health care management behaviors such as monitoring blood glucose levels on a regular basis. Communicating to a large audience by incorporating narrated

PowerPoint presentations can be accomplished through webinars that are either broadcast in real time or available as archives for viewing on demand.

Perhaps the largest concept of building a community is seen in those resources that actually create a virtual world online. For example, Second Life allows users to create a new entity (an avatar) that exists in a virtual world and interacts with other virtual beings. The University of North Carolina at Chapel Hill uses this resource to create a standardized patient that can be interviewed to allow students to take the virtual patient's medication history. The editors predict that it will not be very long before an enterprising pharmacist decides to open the first virtual pharmacy practice in this environment. Many other educational resources are being utilized by innovators in this environment.

The networking tools that can be used to reach a community of patients are being employed within businesses, corporations, and pharmacy practices. As stated previously, the use of wikis to enable knowledge management benefits can be one of many Web 2.0 tools that can be employed internally in a practice. Some businesses are using these resources to capture ideas and ways to improve operations. It is being reported, however, that using these resources can blur the lines of authority represented in a typical organizational personnel chart. In effect, the typical processes of scope of authority or chain of command are sometimes sacrificed so that a good idea from a front-end merchandise person concerning the prescription department will be freely communicated in the organization. Finally, several Web resources are considered professional networks that connect colleagues from different organizations. Two of these are LinkedIn and Plaxo.

Health 2.0 Macro Communities

Health 2.0 will ultimately serve the needs of three distinct communities. The first community will allow peer-to-peer communication between and among patients. Sites such as Revolution Health (www.revolutionhealth.com) have formed communities that address a particular disease or lifestyle issue, such as obesity. The second community comprises pharmacy and other health professionals who can interact on peer-to-peer patient sites such as Revolution Health and serve as expert bloggers. In turn, patients subsequently rate how well the advice worked for them.

Pharmacy professionals and medical professionals can also have peer-to-peer social networking sites for each discipline and sub-specialty. These sites allow consultation and discussion of relevant problems and issues. The third community type is that of biomedical researchers who analyze all data generated by the other two communities to determine best practices and apply what they learn to evidence-based decision support systems. The emerging bridge technology between patient and professional communities is becoming the PHR.

Role of Personal Health Records in Health 2.0

PHRs are, at the core, Health 2.0 applications. As described previously, a key characteristic of Web 2.0 is its focus on participation and collaboration. Similarly, the PHR provides the patient (or caregiver) the opportunity for greater participation in the collection, maintenance, and sharing of the patient's health-related information through a Web-based environment.[3] PHRs are anticipated to significantly impact the role of patients as active participants in their health care through collaboration with their providers.

The PHR is ideally housed in a Web-accessible, electronic format and is directly under the control of the patient while being universally available to any provider treating the patient. It should be designed as a life-long resource of health information needed by individuals to make health decisions. Individuals own and manage the information in their PHR, some of which comes directly from health care providers and includes data and commentary generated by the individual. The PHR should always be maintained in a secure and private environment, with the individual determining rights of access. The PHR is separate from and does not replace the legal record of any provider caring for the individual patient.[5]

The previous description of a PHR was adapted from the one used by the American Health Information Management Association (AHIMA). A work group conducted by the organization described current PHR formats that are based on paper, the personal computer (PC), or the Web, or a hybrid found on both PC desktops and Web sites. Some PHRs can also be displayed on and manipulated from portable devices such as smartphones.

Patients legally own the information in their medical records in most states. Unfortunately, patients are rarely made to feel as if they own that information. The ability to move information stored on inpatient and ambulatory medical records, results from laboratories, medication profiles from pharmacy systems, and images from imaging centers onto a PHR owned by the patient would go a long way toward getting patients involved in their own health care.

The most popular PHRs will allow patients to annotate the information that comes from their providers. In effect, this means a patient who is described as a poor historian can dispute this characterization by placing a comment beside the note. Or, if a provider writes an impression that the patient consumes alcohol to excess or is displaying hypochondriacal tendencies, the patient can then add annotations to the provider's notes. Notes usually cannot be entirely deleted in well-designed applications so that data can be preserved as a record. When an outright error is spotted by patients, they can seek a correction on both the PHR and native EMR that houses the error.

Increasingly, information systems and devices are being designed so that auto population occurs to PHRs as a byproduct of rendering care or using a self-monitoring device in the home. In a pharmacy, when a patient starts a new prescription, the relevant data would appear on the medication profile section of the PHR. Downloading the contents of a blood glucose meter log, electronically operated sphygmomanometer, or peak flow meter can occur through use of the synchronization cord to a computer or through a wireless connection such as Bluetooth. These connections help relieve the barrier of tedious data entry through a keyboard that would make it difficult for patients to keep their PHR up to date.

The best PHR is one that is secure, allows anyone reading it to see who entered each piece of information, permits easy exchange with other systems, and can be accessed at any time from any place. It is possible for information systems such as EMRs, laboratory data, pharmacy management systems, and PHRs to be interoperable only if standards for data communication are employed. Currently an agreed-upon document format called the Continuity of Care Record (CCR) and Extensible Markup Language (i.e., XML) are interoperability standards being used by the information technology industry. The CCR is a data communication standard accredited by the American National Standards Institute. Strong levels of encryption and strong passwords are being required by PHR applications to protect the privacy and confidentiality of stored patient information called for in the Health Insurance Portability and Accountability Act of 1996 (see Chapter 26 for discussion of the act).

In lieu of patients selecting their own PHR from sources such as Microsoft's HealthVault, Google Health, AHIMA's MyPHR, or dozens of other options, health systems have begun to offer branded patient portals that take the place of a patient-initiated PHR. This is being done, in many cases, to help increase patient affiliation and loyalty to the health system. The patient portal, which has all the functionality of a PHR, can also be used to promote existing services and develop new services of interest to patients. Health systems that have successfully implemented patient portals are finding significant savings in system personnel costs because a well-designed patient portal access can answer the kinds of questions patients typically ask over the telephone or in person.

One of the biggest challenges for health care providers who utilize PHRs and patient portals is the impact on their workflow and workload when patient-generated data and/or queries are performed through on-line channels. There are concurrent medical/legal issues concerning, for example, whether a pharmacist would be legally responsible for reading and acting on a patient's drug allergy reported in a PHR during the filling of a prescription for that patient. In this scenario, the patient might inform the pharmacist that he or she now has access to this record. Does this pharmacist have a duty to check this information even if it is not integrated into a pharmacy practice management system? The answer is that a jury may decide the answer to the question. Another consideration can concern the timeliness of a pharmacist's response to a patient's on-line query. If a pharmacist does not respond to a patient's question about a medication issue within 48 hours and the patient experiences a bad outcome during that time, would the pharmacist incur any liability? Again, this question may be addressed in a court of law someday.

Workload considerations should also be addressed. If all patients are given telephone, e-mail, chat room, fax, blog, and discussion forum access to a practice, in addition to face-to-face encounters with pharmacists, how will this added communication load be managed? Although systems can be designed to automatically refer patients to educational materials in response to identified key words in digital communication, and technicians can triage incoming communication on behalf of the pharmacist, the full impact of a collaborating, connected patient population is yet to be determined. One patient-centered medical home initiative found that adapting to increased patient communication was creating additional fatigue among providers.[6]

Conclusion

This chapter introduced the method in which social networking activities that are familiar to many can be focused on patient care and health-oriented purposes. These activities are designed to be conducted in addition to—not instead of—other traditional methods for patient care. A key document to promote participatory health care is the PHR. Pharmacists' advocacy for patients becoming actively involved in health care management and family caregiving should be a significant help in improving patient health outcomes.

LEARNING ACTIVITIES

1. Go to www.YouTube.com and search for the word *nebulizer* to see the potential patient education resources available from this source. Try to determine which resource would be appropriate/inappropriate to use with patients.
2. Go to the AHIMA myPHR site (www.myphr.com) and set up a PHR for yourself or someone in your immediate family.
3. Open up an account in Microsoft's HealthVault (www.healthvault.com) and compare its approach to the offering in #2.

References

1. The Institute for Health Policy Solutions. Health care quality measurement and monitoring features to consider. Supplement F to the report: challenges and alternatives for employer pay-or-play program design: an implementation and alternative scenario analysis of California's "Health Insurance Act of 2003" (SB 2). March 2005. Available at: http://www.ihps.org/pubs/2005_Apr_IHPS_SB2_FSup_Quality.pdf. Accessed August 26, 2009.
2. Smith R. Information technology and consumerism will transform health care worldwide. BMJ. 1997;314:1495.
3. Eysenbach G. Medicine 2.0: social networking, collaboration, participation, apomediation, and openness. J Med Internet Res. 2008;10(3):e22.
4. Alexa. Top Sites in the United States. [Web site traffic rankings.] Available at: http://www.alexa.com/topsites/countries/US. Accessed September 24, 2009.
5. AHIMA e-HIM Personal Health Record Work Group. The role of the personal health record in the EHR. JAHIMA. 2005;76;(7):64A–D.
6. Reid RJ, Fishman PA, Onchee Y, et al. Patient-centered medical home demonstration: a prospective, quasi experimental before and after evaluation. Am J Managed Care. 2009;15(9); e71–e87.

Telepharmacy: Changing the Practice of Pharmacy

Michael J. Brownlee and P. Neil Edillo

OBJECTIVES

1. Discuss the history of telepharmacy.
2. Explain key forces driving telepharmacy expansion.
3. Name the four potential areas for use of telepharmacy.
4. Discuss future direction for telepharmacy.

The history of telepharmacy is not a long one and its use is growing in pharmacy practice. The birth of telepharmacy came about through the necessity to provide medication-related services for patients with limited access to pharmacist resources. A recurring shortage of pharmacists has made it difficult to reach these patients and has continued to be a problem for the provision of pharmacy services. The increasing demand for pharmacy services by patients, lack of pharmacists to provide that service, and patient difficulties in physically accessing pharmacy services have created an opportunity for the growth of telepharmacy.

Telepharmacy has been broadly defined as the provision of pharmaceutical care through the use of telecommunications and information technologies to patients at a distance.[1] The definition has taken on many different meanings over the years as the types of telepharmacy have evolved with the growth of available supporting technology. In the first telepharmacy systems, a pharmacist had rudimentary connections with a patient and providers through telephones and grainy Web cams, and communications often where broken. The most common representations of telepharmacy solutions in the past were used in remote community dispensing of medications and counseling. The evolution of technology has allowed for growth of telepharmacy into many arenas, including hospital pharmacy and ambulatory care. The greatest improvements in technology have come in the form of improved camera resolution, faster computers, cutting edge monitors (e.g., LCD [liquid crystal display]), enhanced software, and most importantly—increased bandwidth and speed of the Internet. This ubiquitous availability of fast Internet connections, even in remote areas, has had a huge impact on the growth, expansion, and adoption of telepharmacy services.

Drivers of Telepharmacy

There are several reasons for the continued growth of telepharmacy systems in practice today. These reasons include medication safety, access to pharmacy services, financial issues, compliance with regulations, and addressing the shortage of pharmacists.

Medication Safety

From a medication safety standpoint, telepharmacy may be used in several ways. One is to use telepharmacy to prevent staff from coming in contact with a toxic substance (e.g., chemotherapy) in the IV room. Currently, a small number of sites in the country are using telepharmacy to protect their staff from the product they are checking.[2] Another way telepharmacy systems are used to enhance medication safety is the use of bar code technology to prepare medications. The system checks the bar code of the scanned product used in preparing an IV against the database to make sure it is the correct product. In addition, a photograph may be taken at all steps of preparation of the product so the pharmacist can verify that it was made correctly. In this scenario, the pharmacist is usually located in a room separate from the IV room. Finally, medication safety is enhanced when the pharmacist can talk directly to a patient who received limited pharmacist input previously and can provide counseling for the patient's medications. Usually, these patients live in rural communities where there is limited pharmacist access by patients.[3]

Financial Issues

Tightening reimbursement for pharmacies has caused consolidation, resulting in closing of some pharmacies in rural areas of the country. Patients in those areas are then forced to travel great distances to access a pharmacist as well as to potentially pick up their medications. Telepharmacy has been able to fill this void in which patients have minimal access to care. This has been demonstrated by several states, such as North Dakota, which have implemented state-wide strategies to provide telepharmacy services to those in need.[3] The financial impact of telepharmacy can also be beneficial because it reduces the need to hire additional staff or even build new facilities. There is an opportunity to use telepharmacy in unique settings, such as a freestanding kiosk, to provide contact between a pharmacist and a patient without requiring the building of a physical "pharmacy" space. Telepharmacy systems do not come without a cost, but in the long run, they can provide a financial benefit by minimizing the number of staff needed to provide the same types of service.

Compliance with Regulations and Shortage of Pharmacists

With the shortage of pharmacists and increasing demand for health care, some hospitals may be struggling to maintain pharmacist verification of orders 24 hours per day. This may be challenging for some smaller hospitals in rural areas or even larger hospitals with staffing issues. Telepharmacy may be used to connect a fully staffed hospital pharmacy with another hospital in need of help from afar to verify orders. Not only does this service help the nurses and patients of the receiving hospital, it also helps the hospital become compliant with regulations requiring the review of medication orders by a pharmacist.

The evolution and growth of telepharmacy are anticipated to be remarkable in the very near future. As described previously, multiple needs are unmet in the current health care market. With the continued aging of the baby boomers, there will be no shortage of medication management opportunities in the inpatient and outpatient arenas for pharmacy care. In addition, the aspects of health care reform that are focused on technology will increase pressure on pharmacy to improve access to care. Telepharmacy technology has transitioned from telephone calls to online video to streaming Web conferences on mobile devices. There is much to look forward to within the pharmacy profession and how pharmacists and pharmacy technicians can further connect with patients. The options are almost limitless—from online chatting, social networking, improved communication with other health care providers, financial verifications, language translations, and online quality assurance. Many models of telepharmacy are in the process of being created or have come to life in current practice. The next section will discuss some of the technology used in telepharmacy models that are currently in practice.

Telepharmacy Practice

To have a full appreciation of telepharmacy and its potential, readers must first understand the impact of pharmacy services on patient care. The basic medication use cycle outlines these services (Figure 25–1):

- A provider assesses a patient and determines that the patient is a proper candidate for medication.
- The provider then places an order for the required medication and the order subsequently travels to a pharmacist.
- If safe and appropriate for the patient, the medication is then dispensed by the pharmacist, and at that point, the medication may be administered to, or by, the patient.
- Once administered, the patient response is assessed by the provider, and the medication use cycle starts all over again.

At a glance, it might seem that the pharmacist is concerned only with the dispensing step of the medication use cycle. It is important to point out, however, that the pharmacist may directly impact each step of the cycle—not just dispensing. For example, a pharmacist might discuss with a physician a more effective form of a medication for a patient. In this instance, the pharmacist would affect the ordering phase of the medica-

FIGURE 25-1

Basic medication use cycle.

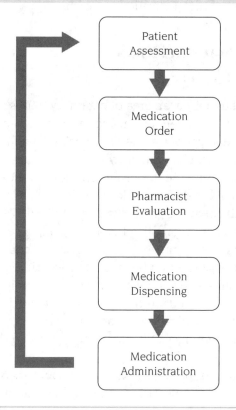

Source: Author.

tion use cycle because the physician now is more likely to order a different medication as a result of this collaboration. Another example is when a pharmacist counsels a patient to be aware of and to avoid potential drug-food interactions. Here, the pharmacist directly affects the administration phase of the medication use cycle by ensuring that the patient receives the full benefit of the medication.

Pharmacy services do not include just drug dispensing and distribution; they also include cognitive services supplied to both health care providers and patients. By extension, telepharmacy is not just remote dispensing or distribution of medications; it also involves the remote provision of cognitive services to other health care professionals and/or patients. This fundamental understanding will allow readers to look at different pharmacy settings and understand how telepharmacy currently plays a role in the various pieces of the medication use cycle.

Telepharmacy Settings

Mail Order Pharmacy

Mail order pharmacy is an area of pharmacy that is quickly gaining popularity.[4] The main benefits for using these pharmacies are convenience and privacy: Medications arrive at a specified mailing address in a short period of time (ideal for patients who have difficulty with transportation), and patients are not seen picking up their medication(s) at the local pharmacy. Mail order pharmacies can also save patients money by having a reduced copay for greater than a 30-day fill of their prescriptions. These pharmacies accomplish this by utilizing a central processing and fill model. In a central processing model, a prescription is faxed, mailed, or electronically prescribed to a central location staffed with pharmacists, technicians, and administrative staff. On receipt of the prescription, the pharmacist on hand remotely evaluates it and determines the appropriateness of the medication for the patient. Subsequently, in the central fill model, the pharmacist fills the prescription and ships the medication to the patient.

As you can see, patients receive pharmacy services without ever having to leave their home or physically touch the mail order pharmacy. They, or their provider, simply communicate to the mail order pharmacy that medications need to be filled and those medications will ship in the mail. Essentially, this whole pharmacy model functions only because of telepharmacy.

Community Pharmacy

Currently many functions qualify as "telepharmacy" in the community setting. Simply picking up the telephone and asking the physician to clarify an order because of concerns about a potential drug-drug interaction is considered telepharmacy; the pharmacist is remotely providing pharmacy service to the provider. Similarly, if a patient calls and describes feeling dizzy after taking a medication, the pharmacist can adequately assess if any of the patient's medications are the culprit and determine an appropriate course of action. This service, too, is considered telepharmacy because the pharmacist is remotely providing service to the patient.

In addition to these everyday activities, there are also innovative ways that telepharmacy is being used to assist in the provision of pharmacy services. Most people are aware that patients may request refills either over the phone or over the Internet by simply having access to their prescription number. When patients call the pharmacy, oftentimes an automated refill phone service (e.g., interactive voice response) can process the refill request by simply having the patient key in the prescription number. Alternatively, if the patient has ready access to the Internet, he or she can navigate to the community pharmacy Web site and request refill(s). Regardless of the mechanism, telepharmacy is used because the patient is communicating remotely to the pharmacy that a service is required.

As mentioned previously, another mechanism for using telepharmacy in the community setting is central processing. In the community setting, a pharmacist is still located in the pharmacy, but the prescription is sent via fax, electronic prescription, or mail to a central location. The pharmacy staff at the central location handle any and all issues pertaining to claims adjudication, contacting of physicians for clarification, and drug utilization review. Once deemed appropriate, this information travels back to the local pharmacist and allows dispensing of the medication. This process allows the pharmacist more time with the patient to understand any issues and counsel on appropriate medication use. The patient in this instance is indirectly impacted by telepharmacy.[5]

Taking this model one step further, a pharmacist might be available at a central location with only technicians manning the local pharmacy. This particular practice of telepharmacy in the community setting takes place at North Dakota State University as part of its overall telepharmacy project strategy.[3] In the setup for community telepharmacy, a central pharmacist can have videoconferences with the distant pharmacies and technicians for which the pharmacist is responsible. The distant technician is responsible for preparing the medication, whereas the centrally located pharmacist has complete oversight of the process. The pharmacist is able to manage the technicians and provide pharmacy services to patients by communicating in real time as if the pharmacist were physically present in the distant pharmacy.

Ambulatory Pharmacy

Typically, the term *ambulatory pharmacy services* brings many things to mind: a pharmacist providing anticoagulation services, a pharmacist checking chemotherapy in an infusion area, a clinic-based diabetes health educator, and the list goes on. The assumption is that a pharmacist is on-site to provide these types of pharmacy services. This assumption is usually correct; however, from a financial or practical perspective, sometimes an on-site pharmacist is not feasible and telepharmacy serves as a viable option.

Oregon Health & Science University (OHSU), located in Portland, Oregon, developed an innovative solution using an existing technology for a telepharmacy solution. In August 2008, OHSU joined with a physician-based oncology practice that had a set of five hematology/oncology clinics spread throughout the Portland metropolitan area. These clinics were staffed with compounding "technicians" to admix chemotherapy and other medications with no pharmacists on staff.

Because of limited resources, OHSU needed to implement a telepharmacy solution using an IV room manager software program. The software allows a pharmacy technician to compound a medication in the IV room, while taking pictures of the process according to a programmed protocol (Figure 25–2). The pictures and process are then analyzed by the pharmacist who is stationed outside the IV room. This prevents the pharmacist from having to enter in and out of the IV room, allowing for better compliance with USP <797> standards. Because the compounding information is electronically transferred to the pharmacist, conceptually there is no limitation on the distance that the pharmacist could be from the IV room and still verify these preparations.

With this telepharmacy practice, chemotherapy preparations could be verified by a pharmacist at a central location for all remote infusion clinics, with the most distant clinic being 30 miles away. OHSU currently has two centrally located pharmacists with technicians deployed at each clinic. In the prior physician-based practice model, no pharmacist checked any of the chemotherapy compounded for patient use. In the current model, all admixed medications are checked by the centrally located pharmacists by a process that is compliant with the Joint Commission and the Oregon Board of Pharmacy. Although the upfront cost of implementing this technology may seem expensive, it ends up being a cost-effective strategy in the long run relative to staffing each clinic with a pharmacist.

FIGURE 25–2

IV hood equipped with telepharmacy technology. The hood contains a camera to take photographs during the compounding process. Next to the hood is a touch screen monitor as well as a bar code scanner and a printer.

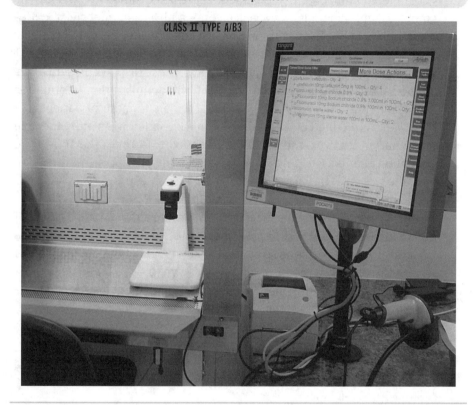

Source: Author.

Inpatient Pharmacy

Depending on the size of the hospital and the scope of pharmacy services, inpatient pharmacies may already deploy telepharmacy solutions in different ways. Pharmacies might utilize a central processing model in which a pharmacist will either receive a faxed order or an electronically transmitted order for a patient. Although it might seem that this is standard operating procedure, consider that the pharmacist may need to process orders for the entire facility or even across facilities where the pharmacist might not be anywhere near the patient or other health care professionals. In this scenario, a pharmacist is remotely providing pharmacy services to all facilities without potentially having to be on-site.

The intensive care unit (ICU) is an area that is experiencing increased use of telepharmacy as part of larger telemedicine initiatives. In one of the more common models (www.visicu.com), a physician intensivist, critical care nurse, and critical care pharmacist remotely monitor ICU patients. Specifically, the three providers sit together at a workstation area that is equipped with multiple computer displays. These displays present all the necessary patient information (medication administration information, vital statistics, telemetry, etc.) for the providers to monitor patients and intervene as dictated by the patients' clinical condition. As with other telepharmacy initiatives, this model is intended to address the shortage of qualified pharmacists (and intensivists and nurses) who are able to monitor the sickest of the sick. This model of care is occurring within hospitals, across hospitals, and even across state lines.

Automated dispensing machines (ADMs) are another form of telepharmacy in the inpatient setting (see Chapter 16). In this workflow, a pharmacist receives an order for a patient on a nursing unit. (The pharmacist may be on the unit or may be involved with central processing.) The pharmacist then verifies in the pharmacy information management system that the medication is appropriate for the patient. Once the medication is verified, a message is sent to the ADM that the medication is appropriate for a patient. The nurse then interacts with the ADM to remove the appropriate medication. In this instance, a pharmacist is able to dispense the correct medication to the nurse on the unit without having to be present physically on the unit.

Finally, the utilization of telepharmacy discussed in the ambulatory setting for checking chemotherapy may also be applied to the inpatient setting. A telepharmacy technology such as that used by OHSU for ambulatory chemotherapy may be used for chemotherapy and other doses prepared in the IV room. This will result in minimal contact with toxic substances, while also allowing staff to float to other areas of the health system and still be able to verify admixtures or other compounded products from a distance.

Telepharmacy Challenges

With telepharmacy still in its infancy, there will be challenges in overcoming perceptions about the quality of the care and the legality of pharmacists working away from their staff and patients. Progress is being made at the state level to work with boards of pharmacy to write rules and regulations that support the use of telepharmacy applications and technology. It will be critical for those developing and using such technology to work closely with the boards of pharmacy to ensure that pharmacy services are maintained through the process. Telepharmacy approaches that remove the pharmacist from the process completely may compromise patient safety by preventing adequate monitoring and counseling for the patients' medications. These types of systems should be implemented under strict supervision of a provider in a clinic. It would be dangerous for such systems to start appearing at local shopping malls. These systems may accurately dispense a medication, but they cannot perform drug utilization reviews, answer a patient's questions about side effects, and provide general care to a patient.

Telepharmacy provides pharmacists and their staff the ability to collaborate with health care professionals and take care of patients from a distance. Emerging technologies, proactive boards of pharmacy, economic pressures, and a growing number of patients will continue to demand telepharmacy services for all areas of the country. The profession of pharmacy should embrace the use of technology when it provides a means to deliver safe and effective care to patients.

Conclusion

The concept of telepharmacy is still in a relative state of infancy. The explosion of technology since the late 1990s has allowed software and hardware vendors to work with pharmacies to fill the unmet need of medication management for patients without access to pharmacy resources. Telepharmacy can serve our patients in many ways such as improving medication safety, providing access to medications and clinical counseling, and addressing distribution challenges. It is exciting to think about where telepharmacy will be in the very near future and how pharmacists can be involved in the care of patients who have had limited access to medication management in the past. Pharmacy patients will continue to be more "connected" through technology, and pharmacists have a unique opportunity and responsibility to leverage their expertise to work not only with patients but with other health care providers. It will not be long before patients walk into pharmacies holding a storage device (e.g., a thumb drive) that contains their personal health record (PHR) or provide their log-in information to access their PHR online. The profession of pharmacy needs to be proactive about its approach to being involved in patients' care when it comes to technology. Soon pharmacists will be able to download their telepharmacy application from the application catalog of their smartphone provider and get connected in no time. The use of mobile devices and blazing wireless Internet speeds will make access to a pharmacist a reality for patients in remote locations who want to connect with their pharmacist.

LEARNING ACTIVITIES

1. Review Figure 25–1. On the basis of the concepts and descriptions presented in this chapter, identify three potential telepharmacy activities that could occur at each step in the medication use cycle. What challenges exist to the use of telepharmacy at each step?
2. In the pharmacy where you work/intern, what telepharmacy services are being provided? Discuss these services with one of the pharmacists. Does the pharmacist consider these services to be critical to the delivery of patient care? What alternative options would exist if the telepharmacy services were no longer available?
3. Contact your state board of pharmacy and determine the current regulations regarding telepharmacy. What constitutes the "practice of pharmacy"? Does the combination of the definition of pharmacy practice and the current telepharmacy regulations limit pharmacists' ability to provide care over the phone? What provisions exist for delivering pharmacy services across state lines?

References

1. National Association of Boards of Pharmacy. Available at: http://www.nabp.net. [Click on "Accreditation Programs," then "VIPPS," and then "Definitions."] Accessed September 10, 2009.
2. O'Neal BC, Worden JC, Couldry RJ. Telepharmacy and bar-code technology. *Am J Health Syst Pharm*. 2009;66(13):1211–6.
3. NDSU. What Is Telepharmacy. Available at: http://www.ndsu.edu/telepharmacy. Accessed September 11, 2009.
4. J.D. Power and Associates. 2009 national pharmacy study. Available at: http://www.jdpower.com/healthcare/articles/2009-National-Pharmacy-Study. Accessed September 29, 2009.
5. AmerisourceBergen. AmeriSource completes development & testing of autonomics central processing program. Available at: http://www.amerisourcebergen.com/investor/phoenix.zhtml?c=61181&p=irol-newsArticle&ID=197979&highlight=. Accessed September 25, 2009.

Security and Privacy Considerations for Pharmacy Informatics

Bradford N. Barker

OBJECTIVES

1. Understand the terms associated with the privacy and security rules of the Health Insurance Portability and Accountability Act (HIPAA).
2. Describe the basic requirements of HIPAA that health care personnel must fulfill.
3. Describe the importance of HIPAA.
4. Describe common mistakes related to HIPAA that health care workers make.
5. Apply knowledge to real-life scenarios in determining how to follow HIPAA guidelines.

The makers of the Constitution conferred the most comprehensive of rights and the right most valued by all civilized men—the right to be let alone.[1] This statement by Supreme Court Justice Louis D.

Brandeis in 1928 reflects the current predominant view in America—that our culture was founded on principles of freedom and individual rights. However, the right to privacy is not explicitly stated in the Constitution or the Bill of Rights. Privacy was not developed as a legal concern until 1890, when Louis Brandeis and Samuel Warren published their article "The Right to Privacy" in the *Harvard Law Review*.[2] Using the Fourth Amendment as the basis of a right to privacy, Brandeis later argued in the Supreme Court case Olmstead *v* United States[1] that wiretaps executed without a warrant should be illegal. In the late 1950s, the Supreme Court's majority opinions regarding privacy started to change and some amendments to the Constitution were interpreted as providing privacy protection. In the 1960s and 1970s, the U.S. Supreme Court defined the concept of privacy to include personal decisions concerning reproduction, sex, and marriage.

Privacy and security go hand in hand. The right to privacy is recognized today in all U.S. states and by the federal government, although the level of privacy protection varies from state to state. Generally, federal laws provide a minimum legal standard and stricter state law takes priority.

Although most people agree that privacy is to be respected, their definitions of privacy vary and few see eye to eye on what measures are reasonable for maintaining a person's private information. International courts interpret laws relating to privacy and confidentiality of medical records and information in several ways. The Health Insurance Portability and Accountability Act (HIPAA) of 1996 attempts to provide a standard for both the courts and the health care industry's interpretation of privacy.[3]

Privacy

In the realm of informatics, privacy has to do with collecting, storing, and disseminating information. For both health care professionals and patients, privacy means being free from unauthorized intrusion and protecting personally identifiable information, including name, birth date, Social Security number, and financial data. Thus, privacy in health care organizations involves policies that determine what information is gathered and stored, how the information is used, and how patients are informed and involved in this process.

Organizations that fail to address privacy issues can suffer substantial financial loss and significantly damage the trust of their patients. For example, if personal information is stolen, such as records indicating that a patient has a sexually transmitted disease or terminal cancer, it is a problem of both privacy and inadequate security, not to mention a situation that would make the patient angry.

Security

Before the age of electronic information, most health care information security needs were limited to corporate accounting and medical records—needs that could be met by a shredder. Now an organization's information usually permeates its infrastructure, potentially including business partners' and employees' home computers. As access to electronic information expands, all information technology components are potential security risks. Examples of potential risks include:

- Discarded hospital computers that are given to schools and have had their hard disks reformatted but not wiped clean of information.
- Buildings formerly rented by a hospital that still contain direct, unsecured connections to the hospital's intranet.
- Unsecured access to a corporate network through wireless access points and a personal router with an open wireless connection.
- A laptop computer that is accidentally left on a plane and contains 5 years' worth of an entire hospital's patient data and laboratory reports.
- A 12-year-old using an Internet workstation in a school library to hack into a hospital's medical records.

Most health care organizations have thousands of potential risk points like these, and the risks will become greater as the means for capturing and transporting data become cheaper and more prevalent. The growing use of cell phones containing digital cameras and video recorders demonstrates the speedy onset of new security issues. Anyone can quickly take a picture of a computer screen, for example. As these devices pervade our lives, how will hospitals handle the need to protect patients' identities? Will tinted windows or a lack of external windows become the norm? Will visitors be allowed in patient wards at all?

Data Access

Traditionally, the method for dealing with data security has been compartmentalization, which used to be accomplished physically. Locked filing cabinets and keyed or number-punch door locks were sufficient to secure most areas, keeping out everyone except authorized employees. Now, electronic tools (e.g., log-in identifications or passwords) are used to restrict who can view material.

In health care systems, physical security issues can be a major challenge. For example, nurses can pull up a patient's electronic chart at the nursing station, get the information they need, and walk away, leaving the patient's information on the screen. Although screen savers with password protection (which come on after a predetermined time of no activity, requiring the user to type in a password to get back to the data) are security aids, they can be annoying and detract from patient care. Some health systems restrict access to data by giving authorized users electronic name badges that have a short-range radio frequency or infrared identification signal. When no one with the correct security rights is in range, the computer screen goes blank.

To help protect data and keep different data elements separate, most organizations have an intranet that is connected to an external network, usually through the Internet. The intranet allows data to be transferred with minimal risk because its connection to the Internet is protected by one or more layers of firewalls. **Firewalls** usually consist of a set of security-related programs that protect a network from unauthorized users. These programs can either run on individual computers (primarily on home computers) or are installed on a computer linked to a network, usually for a business, where the firewall acts as a single gatekeeper for all computers on the network. Firewalls can determine whether to forward messages between the personal computer (PC) or internal network and the Internet. A firewall is usually installed in the electronic "no man's land" between networks so that no incoming request can reach the organization's protected network resources directly. Firewalls also screen messages to make sure they come from previously identified computers. Mobile users can get remote access to private networks that have firewalls by using secure log-on procedures and authentication certificates (this is called **virtual private networking,** or VPN).

TABLE 26–1
Common Computer Crimes

- Unauthorized network access, such as using wireless computers to find and access wireless networks without the owner's permission or knowledge.
- Unauthorized computer use, such as infecting a computer with a virus that allows it to be controlled by others to retransmit spam e-mail or store files remotely.
- Theft or inappropriate use of data.
- Theft of computer equipment or programs.
- Malicious damage or sabotage, including causing destruction via computer viruses or worms.

Source: Author.

Computer Crimes

Computer crimes are increasing exponentially; examples are listed in Table 26–1. Computer crimes occur in several different ways: by employees misusing privileged information; by hackers breaking in through an institution's network or Web site; or by hackers masquerading as trusted individuals, also known as identity theft. The methods range from passively viewing protected data to modifying data. The more sophisticated crimes involve installing **malware,** malicious software (e.g., viruses, spyware, worms) that is designed to infiltrate or damage a computer system without the owner's informed consent.[4]

Viruses are software programs that are capable of reproducing and infecting computer files and programs: executables, documents, or the boot sectors on floppy and hard disks.[5] A form of electronic vandalism, viruses do not target only desktop or laptop computers—they have now been found on handheld computers, cell phones, automated teller machines, and high-end cars.

Spyware secretly tracks computer users' activities, key strokes, log-in names, passwords, and Internet usage. **Worms** automatically copy themselves and distribute the copies to other computer systems via e-mail attachments or direct connections. Worms do not necessarily infect other executables; instead, they proactively spread themselves over a network (possibly by mass e-mailing). A specialized type of worm or virus is a **Trojan horse,** which performs malicious acts while seemingly running as an innocent program. Worms and viruses are now globally distributed via the Internet. A virus or worm runs on a PC like any other program but usually masks its use of the operating system's resources so that the operating system is unaware of the presence of malware.[6]

Programs to protect against viruses, such as Norton Antivirus, Symantec Security, and McAfee VirusScan, are constantly updated by the manufacturer as new virus threats emerge. Whether a virus on your computer can be detected depends on the virus's speed in spreading over the Internet (formerly measured in months, now in days or even hours) versus the ability of these companies to recognize the threat and update their software. Most virus protection programs now have software built into the virus checker that allows the program to automatically download updates.

More subtle viruses are starting to be introduced. Like the common cold virus, these viruses "rewrite" themselves every time they propagate, making each strain harder to detect. Viruses can be automatically programmed to tell a computer to access a targeted Web site continuously, which a computer does in a way that masks this interaction from the user. When hundreds or thousands of computers are infected with such a virus, they can disable even a very large Web site. Known as a **"denial of service"** or DOS attack, this is now one of the most prevalent uses of viruses. Incorporating the code for a DOS attack into a worm or virus is relatively easy. During the time the Web site is being bombarded by requests from the infected computers, the system is unavailable, which could result in lost revenue or inability to access a patient's records.

Phishing is a form of identity theft in which a scammer uses an authentic-looking e-mail to trick recipients into giving out sensitive personal information, such as a credit card, bank account, or Social Security number. Recipients may receive a note from a bank asking them to go to its site (link provided, of course) to reenter personal information. Usually, this Internet address differs from that of the authentic site by only one character. In initial phishing attempts, the facts requested might have tipped off the recipient (a bank would not really need a mother's maiden name), or there are misspellings in the phony e-mail, but these scammers have gotten much savvier.

Pharming is much more dangerous than phishing in that no action has to be performed to hand over personal information to identity thieves. Rather than sending e-mail requests for information, pharmers attack the servers on the Internet that direct network traffic (i.e., DNS [Domain Name System] servers) and instruct the servers to redirect the computer user's request for a Web site to a site set up by the pharmer. As far as the browser is concerned, it is connected to the right site because the bogus site has the same look and feel of the requested site.

Security Administration

Security systems are only as good as their ability to adapt to a changing environment. The best security system in the world is nonfunctional if it allows an employee who was fired yesterday to access the company's information today. Yet many health care systems do not link the databases between their personnel files and the security systems. For example, a corporation very likely will change the employment status of a terminated employee in the personnel database (the database that processes payroll checks). However, the person's name may not be deleted from the security database (the database that determines which doors can be automatically opened by keycard or number pad) or the databases that determine whether a person can log in to a particular system. In the latter instance, the person's name may be deleted from the main computer system but not from a specialized, non-connected system such as the blood bank or pharmacy system. Table 26–2 lists questions that can be part of an audit to help improve security in any health care environment.

The results of the questions listed in the table, especially for computer systems that have an automated connection to the personnel computer (and therefore are rarely checked manually), can be highly informative.

In addition, protection against viruses and other potential threats is only as good as the latest software update of the organization's firewall and servers, as well as the individual PC's antivirus software. These updates include software installed in the network components (known as **firmware**), as well as software installed on the PCs. Many viruses exploit security holes in software programs that have not been "patched" by users, even though the software manufacturers have made a patch available.

TABLE 26–2

Computer Security Questions to Consider

- How long does it take new employees to gain access to the network and the applications needed to do their jobs?

- When employees are transferred or promoted, how long does it take to provide them access to the applications they need? Are they still allowed access to applications that are not used in their new position?

- How often are manual audits performed to ensure that the people who have access to applications should have that access?

Source: Author.

Other Security Risks

Any information technology concern that could lead to data being transferred to a person who has no legitimate reason to see the data is a security concern. Sometimes, this can be as simple as ensuring that none of the terminals at the nursing stations are in a position to be viewed by unauthorized personnel, such as visitors or patients. Another recognized concern is the need to secure wireless local area networks throughout a hospital. A less recognized threat (and a more complex and problematic issue) is whether Universal Serial Bus (USB) flash drives should be allowed to store and transport patient information. Compact USB flash memory drives are small enough—about the size of a pack of gum—to slip easily into a pocket, on a lanyard around a neck, or on a keychain. They are relatively inexpensive and readily available, will work on most computers today, and are able to store and transport large amounts of computer data.

Advance planning is critical to ensure that procedures or technologies with security concerns do not become security breaches. With forethought and planning, health care providers can have access to the information they need to care for patients, and unauthorized users can be barred. Waiting until there is a fire, flood, power outage, or computer system failure is not the best time to inquire about how to safeguard your data and make your system secure.

Any computer operation that involves transmitting data off-site should be reviewed for possible security concerns, including how these data will be restored during a crisis. Whatever security measures are used should not delay data restoration because such delays can disrupt computer operations, which can have far-reaching consequences for the organization, including long waiting periods for the data to be available again and exorbitant system-wide costs. Table 26–3 lists common security mistakes, and Table 26–4 contains helpful, special security precautions.

HIPAA: Health Insurance Portability and Accountability Act

The Health Insurance Portability and Accountability Act (HIPAA) of 1996 was originated to protect health insurance coverage for workers and their families when they change or lose their jobs. When the act was proposed, there

> ### TABLE 26-3
> Common Security Mistakes for PHI

- Use or disclosure of patient information without prior, written patient authorization for a purpose other than treatment, payment, or operations.
- Failure to log off or secure computer screens when the computer is not in use or unattended.
- Failure to close computer files when not in use.
- Performance of inappropriate and unintentional actions and disclosures of PHI through e-mail, Internet, and fax transmissions, such as sending a fax without verifying the fax number beforehand.
- Posting of passwords on the computer in a file or e-mail.
- Sharing of passwords.

PHI = protected health information.
Source: Author.

was little federal regulation that related to secure and private communication between health care providers and third-party payers. HIPAA's scope grew as it passed through committees in the U.S. House of Representatives and the U.S. Senate—ultimately affecting other programs, including the Internal Revenue Code, the Social Security Act of 1999, and the Public Health Service Act of 1994. To decrease the administrative cost associated with health care, HIPAA standardized transactions between third-party payers and health care facilities, while providing strict policies for the privacy and security of patient information.

> ### TABLE 26-4
> Special Security Precautions for Computers

- Do not disclose passwords.
- Verify recipient of faxes.
- Do not view electronic PHI in public areas.
- Do not send electronic PHI via the Internet unless the data are encrypted.
- Do not view electronic PHI inappropriate to your job.
- Do not e-mail electronic PHI to anyone, including internal staff or external requesters of data.

PHI = protected health information.
Source: Author.

HIPAA called upon the U.S. Department of Health and Human Services (DHHS) to publish new rules to[3]:

- Standardize electronic patient health, administrative, and financial data.
- Establish unique health identifiers for individuals, employers, health plans, and health care providers.
- Set security standards to protect the confidentiality and the integrity of "individually identifiable health information"—past, present, and future.

HIPAA is a very diverse law and affects not only health care organizations—including all health care providers, health plans, public health authorities, health care clearinghouses, and self-insured employers—but also life insurers, information systems vendors, various service organizations, and universities. The act covers topics such as continuance of health care coverage for existing conditions from one employer to the next, as well as protection of patient medical information. The act also defines privacy as an individual's right to control access and disclosure of his or her protected, individually identifiable health information. Privacy and security regulations have been put in place to protect the patient's confidentiality and privacy.

HIPAA Privacy Rule[7]

HIPAA contains several components, but the Privacy Rule will affect most health care associates at one time or another. Health care organizations that are in any way funded by the U.S. government have committed themselves to ensure that patients receive the best possible care, including protection of the patient's rights (including privacy).

As health care providers, pharmacists want patients to be confident that their information will be protected so that the patients will be comfortable disclosing complete and accurate information such as medication history, condition, and symptoms. Patient care could be compromised if the patient does not fully disclose the necessary information because of mistrust.

Overview of Privacy Rule

HIPAA is a federal privacy law that, combined with state privacy laws, establishes how health care workers should handle medical information.

The law requires health care organizations to notify patients of their rights and provides them a process in which to exercise those rights. The law defines patient identifiable medical and billing information or "protected health information" (PHI), outlines how health care organizations can properly use and disclose PHI, and defines the requirements of a health care organization to protect PHI from misuse or inappropriate disclosure.

Notice of Privacy Practices

Patients will receive the Notice of Privacy Practices for Protected Health Information ("notice") upon receiving services at a health care organization. The notice explains that the patient has a right to know how his or her PHI can be used or disclosed, and how the facility will use and disclose PHI, including providing treatment, obtaining payment for health care services provided, operating or administering the facility, and complying with legal requirements.

The notice will inform patients about additional rights concerning their PHI. For example, patients can view and obtain a copy of their medical records, request to have their medical records amended, specify a list of persons outside the facility to whom their PHI has been disclosed, and file a complaint with any health care facility or DHHS if they believe their PHI was mishandled or their privacy rights were violated. It is important to note that patients can obtain copies of their records but cannot take the originals home.

Right to Request Alternative Communications

Each patient has a right to request that the health care provider send communications to the patient in a way that differs from standard procedure or to a location other than the address on file. Most health care organizations will accommodate reasonable requests. Patients will be asked to sign an acknowledgment stating that they have been shown and offered a copy of the notice.

Protected Health Information

Protected health information includes any information that can identify the patient, including information related to past, present, and future physical or mental conditions, and to any health service or treatment. This information can be in any form: written (not necessarily on paper), oral, electronically transmitted such as a fax or e-mail, or stored in a database.

Examples of PHI include patient name, photograph, address, Social Security number, birth date, telephone or fax number, e-mail address, or any part of a medical record that would make the patient identifiable (occupation, country of origin, etc.). A patient number (assigned by the health care organization) alone is not PHI and *can* be used.

PHI can be transmitted and used for **treatment, payment** (billing and collecting for treatment), or **operations** (TPO) processes. TPO includes general health care operational use, such as quality improvement, infection control, credentialing, peer review, case management, clinical training, customer service, and some fund-raising activities. What constitutes treatment with regard to use of PHI can be defined as providing, coordinating, or managing a patient's health care. Treatment includes consultations between health care providers about a specific patient and referral of a patient from one physician or facility to another. In these cases, using PHI data is permitted under the Privacy Rule without the patient's authorization.

As a general rule, organizations should review the proposed use of PHI data with the staff person responsible for complying with federal and state law. It also may be necessary to obtain the patient's prior written permission.

Incidental Disclosures

The Privacy Rule is not intended to prohibit providers from talking to each other or to their patients in a treatment setting. Some incidental disclosures are permitted. A disclosure may not be considered incidental if it was preventable. All health care providers should use reasonable safeguards to limit incidental disclosures, which include speaking in a low voice, turning away from others when discussing a patient, closing a paper or electronic chart or schedule, or turning a computer screen so that unauthorized persons cannot see the screen.

Disclosures Permitted by Law for Public Health Activities

Health care facilities are allowed, but not required, to report certain information to governmental agencies—without obtaining patients' authorization—for 12 national priority purposes:

1. Required by law (but not by the Privacy Rule)
2. Public health activities
3. Victims of abuse, neglect, or domestic violence
4. Health oversight activities
5. Judicial and administrative proceedings

6. Law enforcement purposes
7. Decedents
8. Cadaveric organ, eye, or tissue donation
9. Research
10. Serious threat to health or safety
11. Essential government functions
12. Workers' compensation

However, these types of disclosures must be documented and tracked.

Patient Authorization

While under the care of a health care organization, patients should be given the opportunity to agree or object to uses/disclosures of their PHI, such as listing of the patient's name, room, general condition, and religious affiliation in the inpatient directory; notification of family members and persons assisting in the patient's care; or disclosures for disaster relief purposes. If a patient objects to disclosure of his or her PHI, any person inquiring about the patient must be told that the organization has no record of that patient.

The "need to know" rule pertains to disclosing PHI only to individuals who are involved in the direct care of the patient. The "minimum necessary" rule pertains to disclosing only the minimum amount of PHI needed to accomplish a task. Table 26–5 lists tactics to help avoid improper

---

TABLE 26–5

Steps to Help Prevent Improper Disclosures of Medical Information

- Avoid discussing patient medical information with friends or family, or in public places.
- Be careful to e-mail or fax information to the proper address or number.
- Avoid leaving information on fax machines and printers for long periods of time.
- Be sure to close computer files that contain PHI before leaving the computer if the file can be seen or accessed by unauthorized people.
- Avoid leaving clipboards with medical information and medical records in places where they could be looked at, altered, or stolen.
- Follow the health care institution's policies for retaining and discarding PHI.
- Always dispose of PHI data in designated containers.

PHI = protected health information.
Source: Author.

disclosures of medical information. Federal and state governments have fined both health care workers and facilities for improper disclosures. Both civil fines and criminal penalties have been involved in some cases, along with loss of professional licensure.

Communication Security

Many communication tools are used by health care professionals in today's health care environment. These tools help clinicians communicate with each other but open up the possibility for patients or visitors to overhear PHI. The following tips offer suggestions to help abide by HIPAA guidelines when discussing PHI on a telephone:

- If the device can be overheard, always let a caller know when the speakerphone mode is in use.
- Keep the volume at a level that allows you to hear the caller but does not allow the caller to be overheard.
- Put the device in "do not disturb" mode when entering a meeting.
- Before transferring an outside call to a communication device, check that the receiving user wishes to accept the call.
- Do not leave confidential information in a message.
- Do not initiate a confidential conversation before asking the person receiving the call if he or she is in a private area to converse.

HIPAA Security Rule[8]

The Security Rule covers **electronic protected health information** (ePHI), that is, PHI stored in an electronic form. ePHI includes any transmission media used to exchange stored PHI, such as the Internet, intranets, or any network. A health care organization is required by the Security Rule to ensure the confidentiality, integrity, and availability of all ePHI that the organization creates, receives, maintains, or transmits. The organization also must protect against any reasonably anticipated threats or hazards to the security or integrity of ePHI, including disclosures permitted for the 12 national priority purposes. The organization is responsible for its workforce's compliance with the Security Rule.

In general, patients should not access their medical records on the computer. Although they have the right to see their records, the health care organization must ensure that the records are accessed in a manner that conforms to state and federal law. Patients can view their records in the medical records department, or they can receive test results from their physician. Friends, relatives, or co-workers who visit a patient in the hospital should not access the patient's records. This is most likely to occur if the patient's paper chart is inadvertently left in the room or close by. The patient should decide if the information is to be shared. This area will continue to evolve as national efforts to increase patients' involvement in their health care lead to more options for electronic management of PHI.

Faxes

Faxes are vulnerable to unauthorized access. Because faxes were one of the first electronic transmission methods, many states have very strict laws that pertain specifically to transmitting PHI data by fax. As a general rule, personnel should always check the health care organization's policy for using a fax to transmit PHI data (some prohibit this practice). If a policy is not specified, a good practice is to always verify the fax number by calling beforehand, confirm receipt of the fax by an authorized person, use a cover page with a printed disclaimer, and follow the minimum necessary rule.

E-mail

Most organizations will have Internet and e-mail policies that outline appropriate use of the e-mail system. In general, ePHI should never be transmitted by e-mail, either internally or externally. E-mail transmissions are vulnerable to interception or receipt by unauthorized persons. In addition, the information is stored and can be reviewed later. There is currently no universally accessible and accepted secure e-mail technology in the health care industry. Most health care organizations audit e-mails for inappropriate ePHI disclosures; therefore, employees should not expect e-mails they sent, received, and stored at work to be private.

Security Incident

A **security incident** is defined as unauthorized access, use, disclosure, modification, or destruction of ePHI and includes interference with the health information system, improper network activity, and misuse of PHI data. A security incident does not have to be related to a malicious action. A service disruption such as a natural disaster is considered a security incident if data are accidentally modified or destroyed. Security incidents include the presence of computer viruses or worms, theft of ePHI by hacking, or any unauthorized use of the health care organization's system for processing, transmitting, or storing data. In all cases, a security incident should be reported to the person responsible for ensuring compliance.

In general, a health care professional should limit physical, oral, and electronic access to PHI data. Measures to limit physical access to PHI include:

- Do not leave files open and unattended, and be sure to lock cabinets and drawers.
- Turn computer screens so that unauthorized persons cannot view the screen.
- Do not leave copies/originals of PHI in a copy machine.
- Do not leave printouts in unattended fax machines.
- Shred and dispose of confidential information in the proper container (shredder bins).

To limit oral communication of PHI, health care professionals should:

- Discuss PHI only when it cannot be overheard.
- Discuss PHI only with individuals involved with the patient's treatment.
- Disclose only the minimum amount of information necessary.

To limit electronic access to PHI, health care professionals should:

- Log off computers that are not in use.
- Keep all passwords private.
- Refrain from viewing ePHI in public places.
- Refrain from e-mailing ePHI to anyone.

Anyone who overhears or comes across PHI that is not related to that individual's job should not use or share the information and should report any possible privacy policy violations to the appropriate person (supervisor, privacy officer, or corporate compliance officer).

Enforcement and Consequences

In August 2009, the DHSS Office for Civil Rights took over enforcement of the Security Rule.[9] There are many reasons why an individual caregiver should not violate these laws besides avoiding disciplinary action by the health care organization, which could range from counseling to a warning to termination. Patient care can become compromised if patients learn of the violations and consequently keep information from their caregivers (e.g., medication history, condition, and symptoms). In addition, violations could subject an individual to civil and criminal penalties, including fines and imprisonment.

State Laws

With regard to HIPAA, each state's medical privacy laws must be analyzed by affected organizations to determine what steps are important to ensure health information privacy. The effect of the law for each situation depends on many factors and varies widely by state, so it is best to engage legal counsel with experience in this area to assess and help minimize legal liability on the basis of an organization's particular requirements. The information in this chapter is in no way a substitute for legal advice.

Physician-Client Privilege

At one time, a physician (and by relation, other health care professionals) could assume that any health care-related information communicated between the patient and the physician could be treated as confidential, even in a court of law. However, the legal statute for this privilege is not federal and varies widely between states. Many states use a system accepted by the Canadian Supreme Court, called the Wigmore test, to determine whether physician-patient confidentiality exists. Communication is privileged under the following circumstances[10]:

- The communications must originate in confidence with the understanding that they will not be disclosed.
- This element of confidentiality must be essential to the full and satisfactory maintenance of the relationship between the parties.
- The relationship must be one that, in the opinion of the community, ought to be assiduously fostered.
- The injury that would result from disclosure of the communication must be greater than the benefit that would be gained by correct disposal of litigation.

One interesting legal interpretation of the physician-client privilege has evolved from decisions in some court cases. According to these decisions, the physician-client privilege can be waived if the physician asks a patient to sign a "limited confidentiality consent statement," which includes a clause recognizing that ". . . as a result of legal action, the physician may be required to divulge information obtained in the course of this research to a court or other legal body."

Ethical Issues

Why should health care professionals care about ethics in information services? If these individuals do what is generally considered right with regard to patient privacy, their conduct will be explainable to their peers and defensible in a court of law. Most importantly, complying with professional ethics will allow them to sleep well at night, knowing they have done the best they could in a given situation.

It is essential to make the distinction that health care professionals cannot subscribe to one set of ethics at their facility and another outside their profession: An individual's ethics define who they are. Ethics is the science that points out standards and ideals of life in harmony with natural law. It helps health care professionals to answer the question "what ought I do?"

Ethics is arguably the most important component of a profession, especially one that deals with people's lives, as health care professions do. What is unethical is not necessarily illegal. Thus, an individual or organization faced with an ethical decision, such as what to tell the family about a patient's condition or whether to share patient-related information with a colleague who can help the patient, is not necessarily breaking the law. Adopting health care information technology without considering patient risk is an unethical decision, but it is not (at the time of this writing) illegal. Each profession's code of ethics serves as an important guide. Codes are inspirational—aiding young members of a profession and inspiring its elders—and they help to maintain a high moral tone among those in active practice. Codes of ethics should delineate principles underlying a profession's duties and the practitioners' responsibilities and rights. These principles apply to relationships with administrators, medical and nursing staffs, pharmacy committees, rank-and-file personnel, students, visitors, the health care facility, the general public, the community, and others such as paramedics, the medical record librarian, the social worker, the dietitian, and others in the health care field.

Conclusion

A career in pharmacy practice will be impacted by the topics discussed in this chapter. In fact, the topics in this chapter will continually change—through additions, modifications, and deletions—over the years of a practice. The topics in this chapter can be quite daunting and potentially can cause uneasiness among pharmacists as they try to do what is best for their patients in an ever-changing legal and regulatory environment. The first step is to follow state pharmacy practice laws; however, appropriate federal laws (e.g., HIPAA) should also be heeded. Professional pharmacy associations, state boards of pharmacy, and the federal government are all sources to help determine the implications of laws that impact pharmacy practice.

Additionally, with regard to use of information technology in practice, pharmacists should exercise caution to ensure that they do not expose their practice to unwanted electronic risks: intruders, malware, and so forth. Finally, while maintaining a practice that is compliant with appropriate federal and state laws, pharmacists should adhere to ethical principles that always place the patient in the center of their efforts.

LEARNING ACTIVITY

1. Vocera is an example of a helpful communication tool used in many health care organizations today. However, Vocera poses a significant challenge to preventing disclosure of PHI data because the caller does not know the location of the badge user (nurse) at the time of the call, and the nurse is usually at the patient's bedside. In addition, Vocera devices are generally used without an earpiece. How would you recommend simultaneously using Vocera and protecting PHI data? (See www.vocera.com.)

2. Go to the Web sites www.legalarchiver.org and www.gpoaccess.gov/cfr, respectively, to review HIPAA and the Privacy and Security Rules. Note the numerous amendments to the act. Also, search for non-government references such as Reference 9 to determine the effects of the act and the Privacy and Security Rules on health care organizations, life insurance companies, information systems vendors, other businesses, and health care costs.

References

1. *Olmstead v United States*, 277 U.S. 438, U.S. Supreme Court (1928).
2. Brandeis L, Warren S. The right to privacy. *Harvard Law Rev.* 1890:4(5):193–220.
3. Health Insurance Portability and Accountability Act of 1996. The 104th Congress. Public Law 104-191. Available at: www.legalarchiver.org. Accessed May 5, 2010.
4. Wikipedia. Malware. Available at: http://en.wikipedia.org/wiki/Malware. Accessed March 4, 2010.
5. WordNet Search. Available at: http://wordnetweb.princeton.edu/perl/webwn?s=computer %20virus. Accessed September 28, 2009.
6. Cisco. What is the difference: viruses, worms, Trojans, and bots? Available at: http://www.cisco.com/web/about/security/intelligence/virus-worm-diffs.html. Accessed September 28, 2009.
7. 45 CFR Part 164 Subparts A and E.
8. 45 CFR Part 164 Subparts A, C, and D.
9. Beluris TAM, Durie BA, Gosney A. Heightened enforcement of privacy and security laws creates new liability and compliance challenges for providers and business associates. BNA's *Health Law Report.* 2009:18(37). Available at: http://www.mwe.com/info/pubs/BNA_092409.pdf. Accessed May 5, 2010.
10. Lowman J, Palys T. Going the distance: lessons for researchers from jurisprudence on privilege. May 7, 1999. Available at: http://www.sfu.ca/~palys/Distance.pdf. Accessed September 28, 2009.

Pharmacists' Role in Managing Medication Use Projects

Christopher R. Fortier and Sandi H. Mitchell

OBJECTIVES

1. Understand the importance of pharmacists leading implementation projects for medication use technologies.
2. Describe the various types of pharmacy informatics staffing structures.
3. Describe each phase of the project life cycle, including project initiation, planning, execution, and closure.
4. Discuss the project management skills that pharmacists need to be successful in project leadership and implementation.
5. Define the various project management pitfalls for project leaders to avoid.

Implementation of medication use technology projects in health care settings across the country is gaining momentum. These projects typically comprise various systems such as computerized provider order entry (CPOE), electronic prescribing (e-prescribing), and bar code medication administration (BCMA). In a recent survey, the percentage of health information technologies implemented across the country was less than 50%: electronic medication administration record (eMAR) (13.7%), CPOE (12%), BCMA (24.1%), smart pumps (44%), e-prescribing (20.7%), IV robotics (10.1%), and carousels (12.7%).[1] Technology and automation are major components of the pharmacy practice model of the future and will play an integral role for everyone involved in pharmacy practice—community pharmacists, clinical specialists, operational pharmacists, and directors of pharmacy. It is essential for pharmacy students, residents, and practitioners to have a solid understanding of and the associated skills for project management, change management, problem solving, and program leadership.

Currently, colleges of pharmacy and residency programs are developing pharmacy informatics curricula that include project management. Project management principles are essential components to the success of any project implementation, no matter the project size. Having the necessary skills to lead and participate in pharmacy informatics projects will benefit student or practicing pharmacists throughout their educational or professional careers. The pharmacy profession must lead the oversight for all medication use technologies. This role will require project management skills to design, develop, implement, and manage these systems to ensure that these technologies provide optimal medication and patient safety. However, no matter which technology is being evaluated, pharmacists will need to collaborate with various other disciplines, including information technology (IT), and with clinicians (physicians, nurses, and respiratory therapists) to achieve optimal outcomes. The implementation of these technologies will hopefully create more efficiency, streamline workflow, and provide patient and drug information 24 hours a day.

This chapter will provide a formalized understanding of project management, the required skills, lessons learned, and potential pitfalls. This information will help pharmacists to be successful in leading and managing all medication use technologies from the request for proposal (RFP) phase to full system optimization. First, pharmacy informatics staffing models, allotted resources, and ensuring that pharmacy is at the table when decisions are being made will be discussed. Then, each phase of the project life cycle will be broken out into sections and discussed in detail. Within each phase, specific strategies and tools to use when leading and organizing a project will be discussed. Finally, the essential management skills and the top project management pitfalls will be outlined.

Positioning the Pharmacy to Lead

Before project planning begins, the pharmacist must first assess the current pharmacy position concerning the proposed informatics project. Unfortunately, when new technologies are being discussed and possibly even being evaluated, pharmacy may not have a seat at the table. Being a part of the initial discussion and having the ability to consistently participate in the RFP process and the on-site testing period are critical in selecting the right product. No matter which pharmacy informatics structure an organization has, pharmacy teams must strategize to ensure that they are represented and can provide feedback on the technologies being evaluated. A collaborative relationship with IT and other key leaders within the organization is critical to putting pharmacists in a leadership role.

Pharmacy must communicate and, in some cases, justify to key organizational leaders that pharmacists must be a major participant in the multidisciplinary medication use electronic initiatives. Organizational leaders need education on how the medication use process connects pharmacy to the rest of the health care setting.[2] Pharmacy must emphasize the complexity, risk, and medication error prevention strategies, and ensure that implementation of new technologies leads to safe and more effective medication use. Finally, pharmacy needs to capitalize on pharmacists' well-rounded skills in computer systems, the medication use process, project management, medication safety, clinical management of medications, drug distribution, drug administration, workflow, and staff education. Organizational leaders must assess the risks of not having a pharmacist team integrally involved in the process.

Variability of Pharmacy Informatics Staffing Models

In addition to the variable adoption rates of medication use technologies within health care, pharmacy informatics reporting and staffing structures are also widely variable. Community pharmacy and organizations such as

Veterans Affairs have more of a centralized informatics model with collaboration between pharmacy and IT staff. Hospitals and health systems have mixed informatics models; consequently, the best practice recommendations have not been developed around a defined infrastructure. The position of pharmacists in informatics models across the country varies: Pharmacists and/or pharmacy technicians may work within a pharmacy informatics division, or pharmacists may report to IT staff, the chief information officer, or the chief medical information officer. Pharmacists are excluded in other models in which IT analysts work in IT and lead pharmacy informatics projects outside of the pharmacy department.

The advantages in having informatics pharmacists reporting to pharmacy consist of ensuring a full-time focus on medication use technologies, having participants with a well-rounded background in computers and medication use, and owning the pharmacy information management system, which is the central interface to all medication use technologies. Additionally, pharmacy controls the formulary process, approves medication use policies/guidelines, and understands the workflow for ordering and dispensing of pharmaceuticals. Staffing resources allotted to a pharmacy informatics division differ by size of institution or pharmacy organization. One survey found that, on average, hospitals have 1.9 full-time equivalent (FTE) pharmacy informatics technology personnel, with a range of 0.9 to 4.9 FTEs, depending on hospital size.[1] The survey also reported that the FTEs consisted of a mixture of position types including pharmacy managers, pharmacists, pharmacy technicians, and/or IT analysts. Again, best practice recommendations for informatics staffing within hospitals have not been developed, but research is being conducted to determine suggested staffing levels based on specific technology implementations.

Project Management

Project management is a process that consists of a variety of tools to help the project leader and team to organize, document, track, and report on project tasks and progress. During implementation of medication use technologies and automation, project management begins with system identification and vendor selection, as well as application, design, development, implementation, and system maintenance. Project management contains a defined project scope that includes a roadmap for deliverables to achieve the expected outcome of the project. For a technology project to be successful, several components must be in place and be communicated to all project participants. First, there is an empowered process owner to lead the project, a defined reporting structure, accountability, and decision making. The process (project) leader is responsible for (1) expected system benefits and integrity of the process design; (2) planning, implementing, orientation, and training to provide awareness and acceptance of the process; and (3) measurement and reporting of compliance across organizational departments.[2]

Additionally, participation must be collaborative across all disciplines throughout the implementation process, and the participants need to include those who will be affected by the project, such as the nurse or staff pharmacist. Effective project leaders will have a formal process for communication, know how to motivate stakeholders to complete the work, facilitate issue resolution, and resolve the risks that develop throughout the project. A formal project management outline can be broken down into what is called a project life cycle that includes project initiation, planning (analysis, design), execution/control (build, test, train, activate), and closure.

Project Initiation

The project initiation phase sets the direction for the rest of the planning, execution, and closure of the project. At this point, the project team and its leader have not been identified because the initiation begins first with the commitment of the organization to support the project. In some cases, pharmacists or others may need to demonstrate to administration the need for project resources and the feasibility to support and provide these resources. A business plan and/or return on investment (ROI) document may be developed to further justify and outline the project goals and purpose for those administrators.

Once authorization to move forward is obtained, a project leader will need to be identified and a project team created. It has been postulated that implementation of technology and automation is driven 90% by people and 10% by technology, so it is critical to have the right people involved from the beginning.[3] This group will need to identify what resources it will take to complete the project and who will develop the plan, design, and analysis that will guide the process. Additionally, depending on the size and complexity of implementation, some projects may require the establishment of subcommittees to accomplish more detailed work on a certain aspect of the project. For instance, a subcommittee on handheld devices may be needed to determine which products will work best for nursing and with a hospital's wireless infrastructure for the larger BCMA project.

The first major initiation task for the stakeholders will be to create key documents around the vision and proposed outcomes for the project. The project scope, mission statement, and charter should include:

- Project scope: Many projects run into problems because they are not well defined. The purpose of the scope is to connect the project team, project leader, and staff by using the scope as an agreement. Defining the scope requires determining the overall goals, the background, the "geography" of the clinical areas included, the opportunities for improvements, other related projects in process, and changes that will result from implementation of the project.
- Project mission statement: The statement should provide a clear and concise description of the need that exists to justify a project and what the project hopes to achieve.
- Project charter: The charter should identify the project vision and objectives, scope, critical deliverables, organizational structure, stakeholders, key roles, and risk points. It should also include the names of the stakeholders involved. It may also include how the project could have an impact on other technologies.

Finally, most informatics projects will require purchase of a technology or automation product from a vendor. Evaluating vendors for a needed product will require a process to properly evaluate, test, and use the product. A common structure for vendor assessment will be to first conduct a review of the current marketplace to identify which vendors provide the technologies of interest. The review is accomplished by asking vendors to respond to a formal request for information (RFI). Once the team has determined which vendors are the best candidates to provide the product, the next step is to develop a formal RFP that outlines exactly the contract terms, pricing, vendor support, software, and other system features and functionality. A short list of vendors to be invited for an onsite demonstration visit is created. Visits to other vendors' sites and an onsite vendor showcase for staff to test and score the technology on a formal survey will need to be conducted.

Project Planning

This phase of the project life cycle involves the development of a path to accomplish the goals set forth during the initiation phase. Project planning requires great organization and the utilization of tools to track progress, identify and resolve risks, and provide a strong method of communication. Along with the project team, the leader must first begin to outline the sequence of project activities, estimate the duration for those activities to be completed, and more specifically define the resources (personnel and technology) required. During development of the outline, the project scope document can serve as a baseline for the plan and resources. A Gantt chart (Figure 27–1) is a useful tool to outline project tasks. Gantt charts include multiple columns that are designed specifically for each project. A standard chart will include a task description, start date, finish date, resources, percentage of completion, status, and milestones. As challenges develop, the project team has the option to modify the project plan. When these challenges or new ideas arise, they are reviewed by the project team, and

FIGURE 27–1

Sample Gantt chart for a pharmacy informatics project.

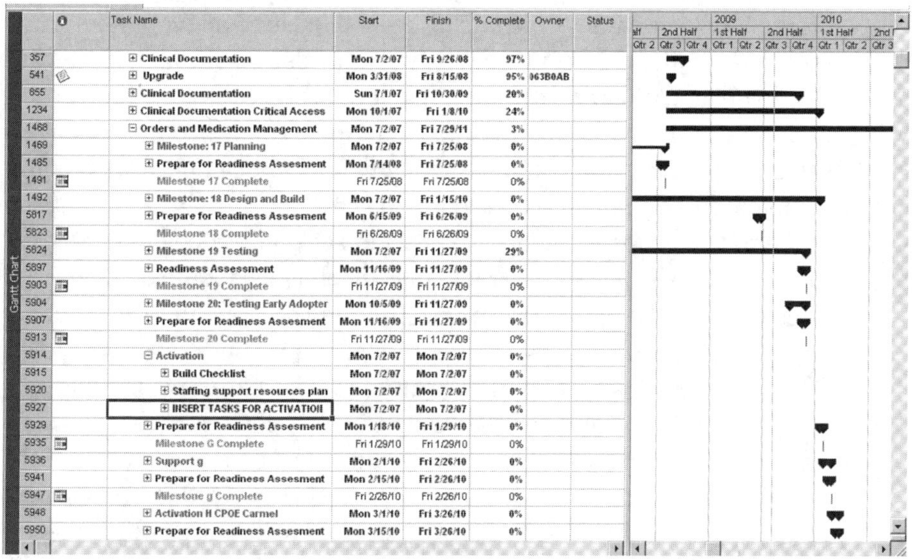

	Task Name	Start	Finish	% Complete	Owner	Status
357	Clinical Documentation	Mon 7/2/07	Fri 9/26/08	97%		
541	Upgrade	Mon 3/31/08	Fri 8/15/08	95%	063B0AB	
855	Clinical Documentation	Sun 7/1/07	Fri 10/30/09	20%		
1234	Clinical Documentation Critical Access	Mon 10/1/07	Fri 1/8/10	24%		
1468	Orders and Medication Management	Mon 7/2/07	Fri 7/29/11	3%		
1469	Milestone: 17 Planning	Mon 7/2/07	Fri 7/25/08	0%		
1485	Prepare for Readiness Assesment	Mon 7/14/08	Fri 7/25/08	0%		
1491	Milestone 17 Complete	Fri 7/25/08	Fri 7/25/08	0%		
1492	Milestone: 18 Design and Build	Mon 7/2/07	Fri 1/15/10	0%		
5817	Prepare for Readiness Assesment	Mon 6/15/09	Fri 6/26/09	0%		
5823	Milestone 18 Complete	Fri 6/26/09	Fri 6/26/09	0%		
5824	Milestone 19 Testing	Mon 7/2/07	Fri 11/27/09	29%		
5897	Readiness Assessment	Mon 11/16/09	Fri 11/27/09	0%		
5903	Milestone 19 Complete	Fri 11/27/09	Fri 11/27/09	0%		
5904	Milestone 20: Testing Early Adopter	Mon 10/5/09	Fri 11/27/09	0%		
5907	Prepare for Readiness Assesment	Mon 11/16/09	Fri 11/27/09	0%		
5913	Milestone 20 Complete	Fri 11/27/09	Fri 11/27/09	0%		
5914	Activation	Mon 7/2/07	Mon 7/2/07	0%		
5915	Build Checklist	Mon 7/2/07	Mon 7/2/07	0%		
5920	Staffing support resources plan	Mon 7/2/07	Mon 7/2/07	0%		
5927	INSERT TASKS FOR ACTIVATION	Mon 7/2/07	Mon 7/2/07	0%		
5929	Prepare for Readiness Assesment	Mon 1/18/10	Fri 1/29/10	0%		
5935	Milestone G Complete	Fri 1/29/10	Fri 1/29/10	0%		
5936	Support g	Mon 2/1/10	Fri 2/26/10	0%		
5941	Prepare for Readiness Assesment	Mon 2/15/10	Fri 2/26/10	0%		
5947	Milestone g Complete	Fri 2/26/10	Fri 2/26/10	0%		
5948	Activation H CPOE Carmel	Mon 3/1/10	Fri 3/26/10	0%		
5950	Prepare for Readiness Assesment	Mon 3/15/10	Fri 3/26/10	0%		

Source: Author.

the impact of these additions to the plan can be clearly delineated before they are added into the project plan. For example, if a task is taking more time, additional people can be assigned or the functionality level can be decreased.

Information technology projects usually have their own language and acronyms. All project matters need to use the same language and definitions of terms, so a project glossary is a useful document. These terms need to be included in the project communication plan that is developed during this phase. A communication plan delineates how the project information will be communicated throughout the organization and for the duration of the project. A clear communication plan is a basic component for project management and builds trust among all levels of participants. A lack of communication will have significant effects on the project, including delays and team dissatisfaction, and can inhibit staff buy-in for the new technology.

Communication plans include a variety of methods to keep the project team, organizational leadership, and end users informed of the project status. Methods that best deliver this information to the team as effectively and efficiently as possible will be most beneficial. These methods include regularly scheduled meetings with an organized agenda and follow-up minutes; the meeting minutes can refer back to a later time or provide an update for individuals who were not able to make the meeting. E-mail, blogs, Web casts, videoconferencing, and other electronic communication tools to keep the project moving forward can also be used.

A subset of the project planning phase is analysis of the project's or organization's readiness for implementation and forthcoming changes. Conducting an analysis during the planning phase can provide the project team with information on preexisting challenges. Using a current and future state functional validation process is a recommended method to perform this formal analysis. **Current state functional validation** begins with interviewing end users who will be most affected by project implementation. The interview process should include predetermined questions about roles, automated systems, technologies, staff knowledge base, and possible pain points (problems). Interview data can be entered into electronic workflow systems, such as Microsoft Visio, to provide a visual representation of the workflow and the current pain points. Figure 27–2 uses "swim lanes" (rows) to indicate user roles. The shapes of boxes (in this case) used within the row will explain the type of process (tasks) involved, and the arrows connect the tasks to accomplish the process.

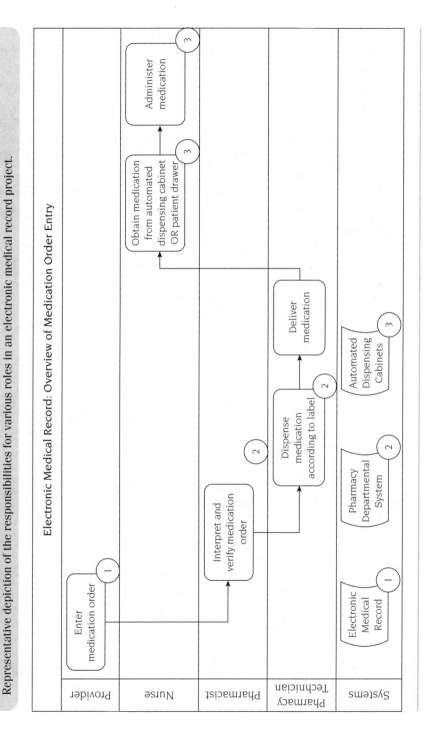

FIGURE 27-2

Representative depiction of the responsibilities for various roles in an electronic medical record project.

Electronic Medical Record: Overview of Medication Order Entry

Once the current validation is completed, the stakeholders must work together to review the information to build a consensus on the final plan for project design. Following completion of the design sessions, the team will then need to conduct an evaluation of the **future state functional validation.** The same template used in the current state validation can be used to identify and resolve the identified current state pain points, plan for integrated testing, and project the future staffing roles and technology functionality.

In addition to these specific strategies to plan, communicate, analyze, and design the current and future workflow, development of a financial assessment may be required. Administration could ask for a project budget containing estimated costs and a spending plan. The budget needs to include the vendor and organization-specific costs listed in Table 27–1. Again, the project team should be involved in identifying and estimating the project budget.

Before the project execution phase begins, the project team should ensure they are aware of the potential project management pitfalls (Table 27–2). A solid plan for each of the potential dangers should be in place.

Project Execution/Control

Execution consists of following the plan actions set forth in the previous phases to achieve the predicted results. Project execution requires incor-

TABLE 27–1

Cost Considerations for Project Implementation

Vendor Costs	Infrastructure Costs	Organizational Costs
Software	Network	Printers
Installation	Wireless infrastructure	Extra staffing/overtime
Maintenance/upgrades	Workstations/computers	Activation support
Server	Devices/hardware	Training resources
Customer support	Additional FTEs	
Activation support		
Customer support	Additional FTEs	

FTE = full-time equivalent.
Source: Author.

TABLE 27-2

Top Pitfalls in Project Management

- Change in scope of project.
- Failure to involve the right people.
- Insufficient communication within project team and with future users.
- Failure to develop a sound project plan and timeline.
- Failure to use standardized tools.
- Lack of early staff involvement or buy-in.
- Failure to map out workflow process changes prior to go-live.
- Failure to continue adequate training and education programs throughout activation.
- Failure to resolve issues or tracking decisions.
- Failure to provide continuous project improvement.
- Lack of champions.

Source: Author.

porating the method of control to steer the project, track results, and overcome challenges that arise. Control is the assessment of the health of the project, as well as collection and reporting/updating of project status information to the sponsors and stakeholders. The project leader will continue to push information through the project communication plan and update project tasks and deliverables. The project leader will also assess team performance to determine areas that need improvement. Control requires monitoring and resolution of the project risks. When issues arise, documenting the risk in an easy-to-understand format is useful to effectively present the information to a review committee. Figure 27–3 categorizes the project risks and reports on patient safety, probability of each type of risk, and the impact of the risk. The chart allows documentation of a mitigation strategy that details the steps that can be used to lessen the probability and impact of risk.

The execution phase can be broken into two phases: activation preparation and actual project activation.

Activation Preparation Phase
Prior to activation of the technology and after the planning phase, the project team will possibly need to build and test the technology that is

FIGURE 27-3

Sample project risk assessment model.

RISK Associated with Current Strategy to Maintain Project Timeline	Patient Safety Risk?	Risk Category	PROBABILITY OF RISK (Low, Medium, High)	IMPACT OF RISK (Low, Medium, High)	MITIGATION STRATEGY
Leadership mandate for additional order sets for activation	Yes	Build	High	Medium	Identify additional available resources, or switch the priorities of builders toward order sets
Clinical decision support (CDS) functionality does not have a governance committee to prioritize the functionality requests	Yes	Order entry	High	Medium	Pharmacy advocate for several slots on CDS committees
Testing requires departmental resources	Yes	Testing	High	High	Site leadership needs to champion all departments to provide front line staff to do the user acceptance training

Source: Author.

being implemented. Both of these processes can take time, but they ensure that minimal risks and issues exist when the technology is activated. Normally, a certain subset of the project team will be involved in this function, and the project leader will need to guide this effort according to the same process used for the actual activation. Using the tracking document, the project leader continues to communicate the status to the team and works to resolve issues that arise during this build and test period.

Additionally, in the activation preparation phase, the team will need to develop a training and education plan for end users. Training and education for the implementation of new technologies have the greatest impact on project success, but unfortunately these materials often are not well planned or all encompassing. The project leader needs to create a training subcommittee who can focus solely on this task to ensure that end users have comprehensive education, which in turn will ensure user knowledge and confidence and patient safety. The subcommittee should consist of various levels of users to develop the training structure. This group should work to develop a training agenda, content, training materials, and technology competencies. Training could begin with didactic classroom training on the background of the technology and likely changes to the workflow process. This is also an opportunity to educate staff on policy changes and to justify the benefit of and reasons for the new technology. Following classroom training sessions, end users should be provided with real-life and real-time training within the environment that the technology is going to be used. During the activation preparation phase, smaller pieces of the technology, such as scanners for BCMA, could be incorporated to make staff comfortable with the technologies instead of incorporating all of the changes at once. The logistics of mandatory training could be difficult; therefore, the subcommittee needs to work with other divisional leaders to incorporate this education into a staff training schedule. Once the schedule is finished, all staff should complete the established technology training activities.

Activation Phase

At this point, the majority of the work and planning is done, and once activation is scheduled, the process will move itself forward. However, the team must consider some critical path steps to support and receive feedback during the activation phase. First, staff should be consulted to set an implementation date and the expectations for the go-live period. The project team needs to be visible during the activation to help support the end users. A method for staff to bring up questions or issues is needed; the project leader could hold daily or regular meetings with the staff and project team to track the project status, identify risks, and troubleshoot. A daily shift meeting led by the project team can capture issues and identify resolutions and interim workarounds until those resolutions can be implemented. Upon completion of the go-live and as the project moves into the maintenance phase, the leader should collect feedback through staff surveys, e-mail, or focus meetings to determine how the training and go-live processes could be improved. This information can be used for the next project rollout.

Project Closure

As the project is coming to an end, an effective strategy is to continuously provide project status updates not only to the project team but also to staff and organizational leadership. This is the time to promote the successes achieved at each step of the project, outline the new process, discuss how it will improve performance, and work to reeducate staff on key points to ensure optimal system use. The project leader should publicly recognize staff and supporters for their work and celebrate the project accomplishments.

Even though it may seem that the project may never come to an end, certain methods need to be used during finalizing of the project. Following full implementation, the project will come to its closure phase but continue into the maintenance and optimization phases. These two phases will still require aspects of the project plan and execution, including involvement of some of the stakeholders. During closure, the project leader and team will consider a cut-over plan and a transition to either some type of support function or implementation of the next project. Before this can happen, stakeholders must complete the documentation, training, and knowledge transfer for the project, all while working to close out the final tasks and pending issues. When those pieces are complete and full closure has occurred, it will be important for the team to conduct a final project evaluation and review. The first steps are to agree on the criteria included in the evaluation, survey as many participants as possible, and develop an executive summary of what went well (and what did not) and what should be considered for the next technology implementation.

Conclusion

This chapter introduced a basic structure of the life cycle of a technology project, although the process relates to any and all projects. Use of the formal strategies and methods outlined will equip the pharmacist with the tools and processes to lead and participate in a technology project implementation. However, project management is much more than just understanding the project structure. Potential future project leaders will need to develop and refine certain project management skills throughout their career. They should look for opportunities to obtain experience, read the literature, and seek advice from mentors that focus on the essential project management skills:

1. Communication (listening, persuading)
2. Organization (planning, goal setting, analyzing)
3. Team building (empathy, motivation)
4. Leadership (setting an example, vision, delegation, attitude)
5. Coping (flexibility, creativity, persistence)
6. Technology knowledge base

LEARNING ACTIVITIES

1. Build a strategic plan for implementation of an e-prescribing software and workflow that includes project scope, charter, and project team.
2. Develop a tool to evaluate and select a BCMA system.
3. Design a database tool to collect, track, share, and report on an implementation process for medication management technology.
4. Evaluate the strengths and weaknesses of two medication use systems that are in direct competition for implementation. Use formal survey tools to quantify the input. Justify the selection of one technology over the other using the literature, system advantages, and the current technology status of the organization.

5. Review the risk factor document on bar code scanning (Figure 27–3) and discuss the value of each column.
6. Capture a current functional state workflow of the technology using the case study below. Using a document similar to Figure 27–2 (Microsoft Visio), identify each of the roles in the swim lanes; then, using boxes or icons of various shapes, outline the different steps or tasks that are required to complete a technology process.

Case Study

- A community hospital has 300 beds and an EMR.
- Providers enter medication orders into the EMR.
- Pharmacists verify medication orders.
- Pharmacy technicians dispense medications according to the labels.
- Nurses document medication administration in the EMR.

References

1. Pedersen CA, Gumpper KF. ASHP national survey on informatics: assessment of the adoption and use of pharmacy informatics in U.S. hospitals—2007. *Am J Health Syst Pharm.* 2008; 65(23): 2244–64.
2. Siska MH, Meyer GE. Pharmacy informatics: aligning for success. *Am J Health Syst Pharm.* 2008; 65(15):1410–1.
3. Tribble DA, Poikonen J, Blair J, et al. Whither pharmacy informatics. *Am J Health Syst Pharm.* 2009; 66(9):813–5

Coming Challenges and the Future of Pharmacy Informatics

Bill G. Felkey

OBJECTIVES

1. Describe challenges and approaches to predicting future trends in informatics.
2. Describe drivers of change in informatics.
3. Describe organizational challenges to the adoption of new technologies.
4. Describe informatics innovations that are related to wireless connectivity.
5. Describe radio frequency identification as an innovative health care technology.
6. Describe future changes in informatics.
7. Develop strategies to keep up with future changes in informatics and pharmacy practice.

Expect Whitewater Change

The quote "It's difficult to make predictions, especially about the future" has been attributed to Yogi Berra. With health care technology, however, there tends to be a steady stream of innovations to learn about and evaluate. Then, there is the problem of getting people to adopt the new technology and incorporate it into their lifestyle and practice setting. Another issue is that people tend to use only a small percentage of the capability of a new technology such as a computer, smartphone, or personal digital assistant. So many wonderful technologies and technological capabilities are available right now. Because of this abundance, people seldom feel the need to look very far into the future to be amazed at what is coming next. There are, however, those who speak and write about "disruptive technologies." Technology can be disruptive to a pharmacy practice in that it has the capability to fundamentally change the way in which a pharmacist operates.

People who label themselves as futurists typically get into trouble when they make predictions rather than attaching probabilities to possible outcomes. The tendency is also to extrapolate current trends or to attempt to paint a picture of only one future scenario. Sometimes futurists make additional errors in their predictions by overestimating the impact of recent short-term changes. Things that seem big in current events frequently turn out to be fads or a "flash in the pan" phenomenon. It does seem, however, that change is truly the only constant. If larger blocks of time are considered, such as time periods of a decade, the way things were done 10 years ago is seldom the way they are done now.

The focus then should not be to predict the future but to prepare for it and shape it according to a predetermined set of goals. To do this, pharmacists need to look at the drivers of change that could create different scenarios of the future. These scenarios will usually look like wildly optimistic, moderate, or "doom and gloom" versions of the future. Pharmacists who reflect on these possibilities will usually try to determine how to prepare now for the challenges that each version represents.

Driving Forces of Change

Driving forces that should continue to shape health care for a very long time include the recent large government involvement in the industry, aging baby boomers and their ability to use technology to connect to people and information, work on the human genome, progress in biotechnology pharmaceuticals, and consumer electronic versions of expensive medical devices.

Information system-related drivers include (1) the Internet and its role in connecting the planet in an information age, (2) increasing accountability for patients regarding their lifestyle choices that ultimately impact health insurance copays, (3) larger buyers controlling a greater percentage of market purchases, and (4) the continual push toward cost containment as the health care sector consumes a greater percentage of the gross domestic product. If we consider only the information technology aspects of the three potential scenarios, then the wildly optimistic scenario would result in excellent outcomes from information system investments that are responsible for delivering most, if not all, of the vendors' claims about their product offerings. Health care providers in a wildly optimistic scenario would embrace these technologies, and patients would fully participate in both disease management and wellness opportunities by actually focusing on accountability and self-care management.

In the moderate scenario, one could imagine that information technology will be implemented in a standardized fashion, but the technology is not fully embraced because it seems to be more focused on saving money than providing care in meeting the needs of people professionally and personally. Some providers and patients would be enthusiastic, but many would respond with apathy to new opportunities. The cost of health care in this scenario would probably continue to rise and consume more of this country's gross domestic product.

In the pessimistic scenario, information systems would not provide a return on the investment, and health care providers would find that being more connected to patients is the chief cause of provider burnout. Patients would continue to live unhealthy lifestyles. Obesity-related diabetes would move from the current 50% level in some states to a 60% level. Applicants to pharmacy schools would decrease as practitioners warn young people to steer clear of health care occupations.

Organizations such as the HealthTech Center currently look at least 2 to 5 years into the future in an attempt to prepare members of their organization for these disruptive technologies.[1] In the same way that medications flow to the market in a pipeline, technologies in various stages of research and development can be tracked as patents are filed and research reports are published. In our experience, health care providers cherish the notion that technology can be pre-certified and preselected for their use. Organizations can choose to prepare for coming disruptive technologies just as they would for a potential future scenario.

Most health systems and ambulatory providers do not want to make a mistake by selecting and purchasing technologies that do not produce a return on investment. A real leadership challenge exists to prepare an organization for both the positive and negative impact of technological innovation. Determining whether a new technology is consistent with the mission and values of a health care organization should be approached both strategically and tactically.

The HealthTech Center promotes that organizations select strategies for dealing with new technologies before they engage in selecting the technologies they will employ.[1] Monitoring technology trends and trying to identify the strategic and tactical implications of these trends may make it possible to prepare for disruptive technologies. It is important to remember that capital investment, workforce considerations, facility considerations, and clinical program impact will need to be considered for any future technology.

The editors of this book constantly engage in environmental scanning to determine the potential of emerging technologies to have a positive impact on everyday practice. We have found that many organizations avoid innovator or early adopter roles with regard to technology. While some step out as leaders, others reactively acquire technology only because of perceived threats from competitors in their market. We know that careful consideration is the only hedge for the inherent capital risks involved in selecting and purchasing new technologies.

One very positive aspect of health care organizations adopting new technology is that Americans are particularly interested in learning about new developments in health care technology as they emerge. It should be very easy to have local media promote, in both print and electronic formats, the new acquisitions adopted in a pharmacy practice. Specifically, we recommend that you promote the scientific advances made possible by the technology acquired from the perspective of patients. Explain how changes in the therapeutic outcomes of patients and their overall positive health care experience can be enhanced by these technologies.

Organizational challenges will follow the adoption of new technologies. The need for continuing education and intensive on-site training will increase. Support and servicing of health care devices that connect patients to their health care system will require implementation of a new infrastructure in health care. Technicians will be required to repair and adjust technologies to keep these devices operational. Some of these adjustments will take place in the home of patients, whereas others will occur remotely via telecommunication channels.

From an organizational perspective, we believe that creating a culture of change is necessary in every pharmacy practice setting. When change is a constant in an organization, it gathers a certain momentum over time. From a leadership perspective, it is almost always easier to redirect a moving organization. It is, however, very difficult to start a stagnant, "stuck," or frozen organization moving. For this reason, we believe that there are many opportunities for pilot testing and infusion of new technologies into the organization while we wait for the "perfect" technological solution to emerge.

Wonderful Wireless Connectivity Changes

How does the expression go? There is something in the air. We see a future in which lots of data in the air are directed toward the improvement of patients' health outcomes. Everyone was very enthusiastic when the first wireless networks came online in the 1990s. People were actually drinking coffee in a local restaurant and concurrently surfing the Internet, and we were all amazed. Health systems, clinics, and homes put access points in their buildings, and connectivity at reasonable speeds was a reality. In the 1890s, Marconi paved the way with his "magic box" radio. Little did we know that another revolution in wireless communication would take place in the early 2000s.

Early cellular telephones created problems because scanners could listen to the traffic on the cellular tower, making privacy impossible. As digital communication became routine, we started living with speeds that were a fraction of the speed of a dial-up modem (14 Kbps). The Federal Communications Commission has opened up the frequency for a WiFi variant called WiMax, which should allow broadband Internet services (cable modem and digital subscriber line [DSL]) to broadcast out to approximately a 30-mile distance. Cellular companies now provide DSL-like speeds in networks that saturate more than 95% of the country with wide-area network broadband data coverage. Health care applications for smartphones are being launched on almost a daily basis. Wireless connectivity is beginning to include automobiles, public transportation, and even kitchen appliances. From a connectivity standpoint, an end-to-end global connection is almost possible. Satellite phones can call from even the remotest mountaintop, even when the cell phone towers are hundreds of miles away. Samsung has announced a phone that will receive 40 satellite television channels. Now we never have to miss the broadcast of our favorite team's game or that reality program we love to watch.

Wireless-friendly cities and even rural towns are making it possible for people to connect wirelessly (and sometimes freely) throughout the community. The repertoire of wireless options includes 802.11X (or WiFi), Bluetooth, GPS (global positioning system), SMS (short message system), 3/4G, VoIP (voice over Internet protocol), and even more ways to connect around the world. This year, airlines have begun to offer WiFi networks on their flights. The GPS personal locator Wherify is a digital watch that requires cellular activation and costs approximately $100. It can be placed on a small child or a loved one with Alzheimer's disease and allows caregivers to instantly locate their charges on demand. A small rivet in the band prevents the watch from being easily removed.

SMS is being used to enable alerts and prompts for wireless synchronization of people and information. Text messages are being sent at a rate of more than 6 billion per day, which is approximately the number of people on the planet. The paradigm that we are starting to recommend now has been coined by a company called Cogon Systems and is labeled "always available, strategically connected." The company takes important information from health care organization databases and transfers it to health care providers whenever significant information becomes available. Although this model is feasible only in target markets in which a pervasive wireless network is available, it is the best model for the use of current technology in health care. In this model, data are "pushed" every 30 minutes or when required by programmable alerts (for abnormal laboratory ranges, etc.). Data can also be seamlessly transferred to a system by means of the traditional sync function any time a provider requires the information. This system represents a compromise from the perspective of both data availability and battery life and is generally a good mix of both.

Some health systems are reporting savings of several hundreds of thousands of dollars from the use of VOIP technology. This technology allows use of the Internet for voice communication. Telephones or radio frequency devices use the infrastructure of the Internet for telecommunication. Charges to corporate clients for telephone communication have risen to the point at which even the installation costs of VOIP have become reasonable.

Some report that the quality of the communication is somewhat diminished but is acceptable.

Wireless communities and institutions open up the possibility that the Vocera company has seized. Vocera offers a small badge with an activation button that allows users to communicate with other personnel within a network in a hands-free fashion. Users are able to say the name of the party with whom they wish to communicate or the role of the individual they are seeking in the wireless network. The device then locates and informs that individual of an impending call. The individual can then accept the call by voice and communicate with the person initiating the contact. Health systems who have employed the technology have reported faster response times and cost savings.

First responders include police, firefighters, emergency medical technicians, and so on. A new type of memory chip has just been introduced for cellular telephones. We can see a scenario in which the cellular telephone of the injured person would be a potential storage site for an individual electronic medical record. Most cellular telephones have single-key dialing for 911 (the 9 key of the telephone). It is possible that the medical record of an injured person could be transmitted to first responders by pressing an additional key. Alternatively, once the identity of the patient is known, electronic medical records can be accessed and transmitted to the trauma team caring for the patient.

Remote monitoring of patients is already taking place in the virtual intensive care unit. A medical specialist, called an intensivist, can virtually monitor as many as 90 patients in five hospitals. Telemetry monitoring algorithms would bring patients to the attention of the virtual care center on a priority basis. If a vital sign was significantly out of normal range, the patient's profile would be brought to the display array, which is made up of nine screens. In addition to live monitoring of data concerning the patients' health status, the physician would be able to zoom in to examine the patient by telemedicine video, and additional voice and video connections would be utilized to coordinate care on-site.

Robotics and Artificial Intelligence

Robotics is currently used in several health care arenas. Surgical robots, pharmacy dispensing robots, patient-mover robots, and other types of robots are fairly commonplace. Robots that dispense after-hours refills operate from within a kiosk placed outside a prescription department in a community pharmacy when the department is closed but the front end of the pharmacy is still operating. HelpMate robots serve as couriers in some health systems. They navigate busy hospital hallways and operate elevators to move STAT medicine and dietary trays throughout the facility.

The use of artificial intelligence in health care has also been around for years. Helping to make decisions concerning end-of-life support is the substance of software such as APACHE. There are several diagnostic software programs, ranging from pathology interpretations of the KEEL application to automated electrocardiogram consults that render a diagnosis. Progress has been slow, but the emphasis on the practice of evidence-based medicine promises to build the need for matching variables from the literature to individual patient cases.[2]

Gadgets and Gizmos

Oh my! Where to start? A Swiss army knife/USB memory device is available; it places a flash drive memory device alongside a knife blade, screwdriver, and scissors.[3] Auburn University has an industrial design department that teaches creativity through various exercises. One exercise used years ago concerned combining various household items with animals. One student combined a flashlight with a giraffe. Coincidentally, a few months later, the snake light was introduced to U.S. markets. As we look to the future, we know that our imagination is our only limitation. The science fiction of our childhood becomes our adult reality.

Radio frequency identification (RFID) chips are receiving fairly good uptake in health care. Systems to prevent infant abduction in hospital nurseries are becoming fairly commonplace. Wristbands containing an RFID chip are placed on wounded soldiers to facilitate triage when an airplane full of injured servicemen and servicewomen arrive in Germany for additional treatment. It is anticipated that an RFID will be placed inside of jewelry and could broadcast access number information for medical records in emergency situations even when the injured person is taken unconscious to the emergency department.

Expensive equipment can be located through the use of RFID chips, and barriers can be placed to sound alarms if this equipment is moved by unauthorized personnel. Patient and staff movement can be similarly tracked in a large hospital setting. There is even speculation that individual doses of medicine may someday contain an RFID identifier.

The ability to shop intelligently for devices and compare the best price on the planet to the item on the sale rack in front of you should become commonplace. These features are even being built into shopping carts in some stores. Other predicted capabilities are personal remote monitoring of a sick relative and viewing an individual broadcast of a child's soccer game during business travel. Combining GPS connectivity wherever it is appropriate brings even more power to these gadgets.

Informatics as a Discipline

The ability to systematically process data in health care should rapidly improve as health care becomes a complete digital industry. This digital world, however, will never be a perfect world. Both the benefits and constraints of using information and communication technology must be considered. Information quality for successful patient management and organizational analysis will be mission critical. A strategy to continually improve the management of this information is necessary. Constantly monitoring the tools of informatics will also be required. Students who are equipped with foundational informatics knowledge and skills when they graduate from Doctor of Pharmacy programs will be well positioned to utilize informatics tools in practice.

We believe informatics training in any health care organization should be a part of routine operations. The byproduct of daily transactions should be the structure, design, and analysis opportunities to improve information systems along critical paths. There is no question that, as bioinformatics and genomics develop and merge, our future will be impacted by these technologies far beyond anything we can imagine today. Change-management principles will need to be utilized to track and implement system improvements. Continuing education and lifelong learning will need to be employed to maintain a sufficient knowledge base in this discipline. Increasingly, education will become just-in-time applications to support decision making and will be integrated into normal work systems.

In medicine, continuing medical education (CME) credits are already being given to physicians who have learned about medical issues and news. Physicians log onto a Web site and are given 15 minutes of CME following their experience. Once this new approach to continuing education is moved into pharmacy practice, imagine receiving a referral for a patient whose diagnosis is a rather rare disease or simply the disease about which you are unfamiliar. For example, if Wegener's granulomatosis is the diagnosis, a provider might take 3 or 4 minutes to brush up on the condition. The time in which the provider accessed the electronic references would be logged into an educational activity database. Whenever 1 hour of time was accumulated, the provider would be asked to take a posttest on the material that he or she had used with patients. Scoring 75 percentile or higher would result in the awarding of one continuing education unit.

How to Prepare for New Technology

We recommend that a strategic schematic be developed for the information flow and data repositories that exist in your organization. We suggest that you attempt to identify technologies that will impact your current operations prior to their introduction into the market. Remember that the Internet can be mined for technology innovations. Key technology meetings will have exhibitions of new products. Certain publications and reports will prepare you for this aspect of potentially disruptive technologies.

Look at new technology from more than the potential changes in access, quality, and cost. Examine how a fourth factor of brand promotion will be facilitated or hindered by the adoption of disruptive technologies. Monitor competitors from the standpoint of their technology mix. Remember that technology that was designed for improving processes and safety may actually diminish the effectiveness and accuracy of your work processes. This occurs when the change is either poorly designed or poorly implemented, or the personnel using the system rely too heavily on a potentially error-producing technology.

Finally, we suggest that administrative approval be in place from the highest level of your organization. Many projects will fail from a lack of coherent policy and determination on the part of administration to weather the pain of implementation. Involvement of clinicians who will be affected by technology adoption is another critical success factor. Avoiding cookie-cutter approaches is desirable as well. Be prepared to adjust your strategy to ensure success.[4]

LEARNING ACTIVITIES

1. Perform an advanced Google search on the phrase "disruptive technologies," but specify that the file format be limited to PowerPoint presentations on current technology considered to be disrupted.
2. Sign up for various "push" notification services on technology, and activate a Google Alert (www.Google.com/alerts) on a type of technology about which you are interested. Make sure you allow Google to send you both Web site postings and news releases on your technology of choice.
3. Use the Google blog search feature (blogsearch.Google.com) to set up a subscription for notification of new blog postings by people who describe themselves as health care futurists.

References

1. HealthTech. Available at: http://www.healthtechcenter.org. Accessed October 1, 2009.
2. OpenClinical. Artificial intelligence in medicine: an introduction Available at: http://www.open clinical.org/aiinmedicine.html. Accessed March 26, 2010.
3. ThinkGeek. Swiss flash USB knife. Available at: http://www.thinkgeek.com/gadgets/tools/ad41/. Accessed October 1, 2009.
4. Bauer J. Technology and the future of healthcare: guidelines for making unaffordable investments you can't afford not to make. Available at: http://www.superiorconsultant.com/ Pressroom/Articles/TGI_Bauer_TechnologyFuturePaper.pdf. Accessed October 1, 2009.

Glossary

Note: *Boldface terms that are part of a definition are also defined in this glossary.*

A

Active clinical surveillance: Surveillance system that processes data through a **knowledge base** and alerts a health care practitioner when criteria for clinical intervention are met. (See also **Passive surveillance system**.)

Acute care enterprise clinical systems: See **Computerized patient record systems.**

Admissions/discharge/transfer database: A database in an integrated health information system or module-based system that contains patient-specific demographic information and the patient's current location within the health system.

Application Service Provider (ASP): An Internet-based organization (the provider) that provides and hosts software for pharmacy data, manages the server, and maintains the software.

Arithmetic and logic unit (ALU): A subcomponent of the central processing unit that performs arithmetic and logical operations on integers.

Asynchronous communication: Communication that does not occur in real time; the message is sent and received at a later time. (e.g., e-mail, postal mail).

Attenuation: In telecommunication systems, a weakening of an electrical signal over time or distance.

Attribute: A characteristic of an entity in a database (e.g., patient attri-butes such as drug allergies, date of birth, etc.).

Automated dispensing cabinets: Devices that maintain medication inventory via an audit trail of receiving and dispersal activity, automate charging of medication products as they are released for use by a patient, and prompt for inventory replacements according to usage and par levels.

B

Backward chaining: A reasoning process used in rule-based systems in which the conclusion is known but the path to that conclusion is unknown; therefore, the direction of reasoning is in the "backward" direction going from the conclusion through the rules or conditions to see if the conclusion is supported. (See also **Forward chaining**.)

Bandwidth: A measure of the ability to carry increasing data (bits) over time (a second).

Best available external clinical evidence: In evidence-based medicine, clinically relevant research into the accuracy and precision of diagnostic tests (including the clinical examination); the power of prognostic markers; and the efficacy and safety of therapeutic, rehabilitative, and preventive regimens.

Bioinformatics: Application of informatics to cellular and molecular biology.

Biomedical and health informatics: Optimal use of information, often aided by the use of technology, to improve individual health, health care, public health, and biomedical research.

BIOS (basic input/output system): Firmware that performs the first phases of the start-up (booting) processes and serves as the interface between the **operating system** and other computer components (e.g., monitor, keyboard, etc.).

Bit: The smallest parcel of datum stored or used in a computer (also called "binary digit"). A bit is represented by a "0" or "1."

Bootstrap (boot): A computer process that starts up and initializes hardware, and monitors and controls input/output.

Broadcast media: Telecommunication media that include infrared, radio, microwave, cellular, and satellite.

Bus: Collection of communication wires in a computer.

Byte: A computer storage unit that comprises 8 consecutive **bits**. Data made up of 8 bits can represent a single character and can be a number, letter, or symbol. Bytes are grouped consecutively to form one or more words.

C

Cable media: Telecommunication media that include twisted-pair cable, coaxial cable, and fiber-optic cable.

Cache: Special purpose memory that is much faster than main memory and permanent memory and that, compared with other types of slower solid state and magnetic memory, can speed up processing and read/write operations.

Carousel cabinet: A type of automated dispensing cabinet in which medications are stored in shelves that are attached to a carousel; the carousel can cycle through the shelving and deliver the appropriate shelve(s) to the user.

Case-control study: A medical research study that evaluates patients with a specific condition and compares them with people who do not have the condition (controls).

Case report/case series: Descriptive reports on the treatment of individual patients. Case reports/series do not use control groups.

Central processing unit (CPU): The controlling executor of the computer, which executes program instructions.

Chaining: The process of connecting a set of if-then rules generated in a rule-based expert system either to arrive at a conclusion (see **Forward chaining**) or to take a conclusion and reason back to the source (see **Backward chaining**).

Channel: In telecommunications, the path of communication between the source and destination.

Clinical data repository (CDR): A large database that houses clinical data from multiple information systems within an organization and serves as a foundational component of **electronic medical records**.

Clinical decision support (CDS): Provision of basic clinical knowledge and appropriate patient-specific information to aid health care providers in making the appropriate clinical decision for a given patient.

Clinical decision support systems (CDSS): Computer programs that are equipped with a knowledge base of clinical and patient information, and that can analyze items of patient data to generate case-specific advice to aid health care providers in clinical decision making.

Clinical informatician: Clinically trained individuals whose expertise is applied at the intersection of information technology and health care, and whose focus is on successful adoption and use of health information technology.

Clinical surveillance: In health care, active surveillance or a "watchful waiting" that includes collection and/or analysis of specific patient or disease information that can then be used to drive decisions.

Codification standards: Standards for electronic prescribing systems that exist to support accurate interpretation of the individual data elements between systems. The primary codification standards are **RxNorm** and structured/codified SIG.

Cohort study: A medical research study that evaluates, over a period of time, a large number of patients who have a specific condition or receive a particular treatment and compares them with another group that have all the baseline characteristics but not the condition being studied.

Communication mechanism: The component of a **clinical decision support system** that allows the user to enter patient information into the application, and that is responsible for communicating the relevant information (e.g., possible drug interaction alerts, preventive care reminders) back to the clinician. (See also **User interface**.)

Communication protocol or **standard:** A set of rules that each networked device or computer follows so that data can be communicated between systems without error or communication-sharing conflicts over a computer network. Network connectivity and control hardware provide the physical connectivity and utilize network control logic to enforce sharing of the network medium in a reliable and safe manner.

Communication standard: See **Communication protocol**.

Computer networking: Interchange or intercommunication for sharing data, applications, or computerized clinical services between computer systems.

Computerized patient record systems (CPRS): Clinical enterprise systems comprising software applications that are used in acute patient care (hospital, surgery center, etc.) to manage clinical data in databases. The applications contain online functions that support inpatient workflow and online views of patient information.

Computerized provider order entry (CPOE): A process of electronic entry of medical provider instructions for the treatment of patients (primarily hospitalized patients) under a provider's care.

Consumer health informatics: Application of informatics to support the patient's health activities.

Continuity of care record (CCR): A subset of data intended to be easily shared between health care organizations across state and international borders.

Corollary orders: Tests and treatments that are ordered to ameliorate the effects of a therapeutic intervention or as a consequence of other orders.

Counting systems: Automated dispensing systems used to fill prescriptions, including countertop devices and stand-alone cabinets.

Current state functional validation: In project management, an analysis conducted during the planning stage of a project to determine potential problems. End users who will be most affected by project implementation are asked predetermined questions about staffing roles, automated systems, technologies, staff knowledge base, and possible pain points (problems).

D

Data: Discrete facts, often in the form of numbers, descriptions, or measurements.

Data communications: Electronic management and transmission of data through the use of electronic systems that supply, manage, transmit, and store data.

Data definition language (DDL): A component of a relational database management system that defines the data and relationships of the data elements stored in the database files/tables.

Data manipulation language (DML): A component of a relational database management system that allows the user to access, query, update, and delete data.

Data mining: A technique used to examine large databases for trends or patterns in the data.

Data warehouse: A large database that is designed to support organizational decision making; the database contains data from numerous organizational and external systems in a manner that provides drilldown functionality.

Database: A grouping of related files.

Database management system (DBMS): A category of software that can serve two functions: as the interface between a database and application programs, or as the interface between a database and the user.

Database model: The logical structure (i.e., how the data are related) between the data within separate files of a database.

Decoder: In telecommunications, a device that converts the received, transmitted signal into the appropriate form for receipt, which is usually the original form (e.g., fax machine).

Demodulation: The process of converting an analog signal into digital form.

Denial of service attack: An attack on a Web site carried out by infecting hundreds or thousands of computers with a virus programmed to continuously access a target site, thereby disabling the Web site.

Destination: In telecommunications, the device that is intended to receive data, usually a computing system.

Diagnosis: In an evidence-based clinical question, establishing the power of a test to differentiate between those with and without a target condition or disease.

Differential diagnosis: In an evidence-based clinical question, establishing the frequency of the underlying disorders in patients with a particular clinical presentation.

Dispensable: Term used in **pharmacy information management systems** to denote an available drug product.

Dispenser: Term used by the Centers for Medicare and Medicaid Services to specify the pharmacy and pharmacist.

E

Electronic health record (EHR): An aggregation of all data generated by individual **electronic medical records** and computerized patient records. The EHR is intended to receive patient data from multiple sources and to share patient data nationally and internationally.

Electronic medical record (EMR): An electronic record of health-related information on an individual that can be created, gathered, managed, and consulted by authorized clinicians and staff within one health care organization.

Electronic protected health information (ePHI): Protected health information stored in an electronic form, including any transmission media used to exchange stored PHI, such as the Internet, intranets, or any network. (See also **Protected health information**.)

Electronic prescribing: See **e-Prescribing**.

Electronic signature: An electronic sound, symbol, or process that is attached to or logically associated with a contract or other record and executed or adopted by a person with the intent to sign the record.

Encoder: A device that modifies a signal into a form suitable for transmission; a modem is an encoder in data communications.

Enterprise clinical system: A system engineered to be highly reliable and to handle large volumes of data while supporting many concurrent clinician users throughout a large health care enterprise.

e-Pedigree: An auditable electronic record of every step taken by a retail package of prescription drugs as it moves from the manufacturer to the final point of sale.

e-Prescribing: The electronic processing of a prescription that begins with the prescriber entering the prescription directly into an electronic format, followed by all required parties verifying and processing the e-prescription in an electronic format. The final result is a labeled medication product, supportive documentation, and updated sharable patient electronic medication profile.

Evidence threshold: In clinical decision support systems, the minimum amount of evidence that should exist to substantiate presenting a drug-related problem to a pharmacist.

Evidence-based medicine: The conscientious, explicit, and judicious use of current best evidence in making decisions about the care of individual patients.

F

Failure mode effects analysis (FMEA): A method of assessing risk of occurrence of an error by identifying problems that involve products or processes. The process involves a systematic analysis of possible problems and factors associated with them before the errors occur.

Field: In databases, a grouping of characters into a word, small group of words, or a number.

File: In databases, a compilation of related records.

Filler: A component of a **computerized provider order entry** application that can respond to or perform a request for orders or services, produce an observation, originate requests for new orders or services, add additional services to existing orders, replace existing orders, put an order on hold, discontinue an order, release a held order, or cancel existing orders.

Firewall: A set of security-related computer hardware and/or software programs that prevents unauthorized users from accessing an individual computer or a computer network.

Firmware: Software installed in the various components of a computer network.

Floating-point unit (FPU): A sub-component of the computer processing unit that processes decimal numbers, but not integers.

Forward chaining: A chaining process that begins from a set of conditions and moves toward arriving at a conclusion. (See also **Backward chaining**.)

Functionality criteria: Criteria for assessing the ability of a health information application to perform certain features and functions to support clinical and administrative activities.

Future state functional validation: In project management, an analysis conducted after completion of the project design to identify and resolve the pain points (problems) identified in the **current state functional evaluation**, to plan for integrated testing, and to project the future staffing roles and technology functionality.

G

Geosynchronous: The condition of orbiting in the same direction and speed as the earth.

H

Harm: In an evidence-based clinical question, ascertainment of the effects of potentially harmful agents on patient-important outcomes.

Health 2.0: A health care concept that uses a specific set of Web tools to provide better health education, promote collaboration between patients and providers, and help providers deliver desired health outcomes.

Health information exchange: The electronic movement of health-related information among organizations according to nationally recognized standards.

Health information management (HIM): Discipline historically focusing on medical record management (in a paper environment); as medical records transition to digital, HIM has begun to overlap with informatics.

Health information technology (HIT): Use of information and communication technology in health care settings.

Health Level 7 (HL7) standard: A human-readable messaging standard that exists to move patient information between disparate information systems. "Level Seven" refers to the seventh level (i.e., application level) of the Open Systems Interconnection model developed by the International Organization for Standardization.

Hierarchical database: Database model that uses a parent-child relationship in which a parent record may have multiple child records, but each child record has a single parent. This model is organized in an inverted tree manner, in which data access starts at the top and moves down "limbs" of the tree.

Hierarchy of evidence: In evidence-based medicine, a system of classifying and organizing types of evidence, typically for questions about treatment and prevention.

I

Imaging informatics: A broad term that indicates the application of informatics to the management of images in health care.

Individual clinical expertise: In evidence-based medicine, the proficiency and judgment that individual clinicians acquire through clinical experience and practice.

Inference engine: The component of a **clinical decision support system** that forms the brain of the system and works to link patient-specific information with the information in the **knowledge base**.

Informatician (informaticist): Practitioners of **informatics**; they focus more on information than technology.

Informatics: Use of computers to manage data and information.

Information: In the context of data management, a collection of data that has been interpreted into a relevant form and has meaning. Specifically, data have been processed through relational connections into descriptions to answer questions beginning with words such as *who, what, when, where,* and *how many.*

Information technology (IT): Activities and tools used to locate, manipulate, store, and disseminate information.

Information and communication technology (ICT): Term often used to indicate information technology with a focus on communication and networking.

Infrared communication: In telecommunications, a medium that uses light waves to transfer data. This medium has a short range, usually less than a few meters, and is used in television remotes and to connect computer peripherals such as printers.

Interactive voice response (IVR): A system that allows patients to use their telephone, keypad, and voice to communicate with the pharmacy's computer system to request refills, determine the status of prescriptions being filled, leave messages for the pharmacy staff, and perform a host of other activities.

Interface: In information systems, hardware and associated software that allow two or more disparate systems to share information in a standardized manner.

Interface standards: Standards that define how data elements are organized into an electronic transaction that flows between disparate information systems.

Interoperability: The ability of different information technology systems and software applications to communicate; to exchange data accurately, effectively, and consistently; and to use the information that has been exchanged.

Interoperability criteria: Criteria for assessing an application's ability to exchange information using agreed-upon standards.

K

Knowledge base: In a **clinical decision support system**, the component that contains clinical knowledge, such as drug interactions, diagnoses, or treatment guidelines.

L

Laboratory database: A database in an integrated health information system or module-based laboratory information system that contains current and historical patient-specific laboratory information.

Latent needs: Needs that are present but have not been consciously realized. In **clinical decision support systems**, an example is notifying a clinician when a patient's medication dose needs to be adjusted for worsening renal function.

Line of sight: In telecommunications, the condition in which an unobstructed view is required between stations; this requirement makes a medium susceptible to disruption by weather.

Local area network (LAN): The smallest collection of networked computers sharing the same range of Internet Protocol (IP) addresses.

Longevity: In telecommunications, the operating life of the medium, which impacts maintenance costs.

M

Main memory controller (MMC): The computer subsystem that manages and controls the read/writes to and from main memory.

Main memory unit (MMU): A computer's primary solid state storage unit for executing operating system routines, programs in use, and data required by executing programs, including data used by the operating system.

Malware: Malicious software designed to infiltrate or damage a computer system without the owner's informed consent.

Meaningful use: In the context of the American Recovery and Reinvestment Act of 2009, demonstration of meaningful use of electronic patient records by eligible providers (institutions and physicians) to be eligible for financial incentives and to avoid financial penalties.

Medical home recognition: A process that objectively measures the degree to which a primary care practice meets the operational principles of a patient-centered medical home.

Medical informatics: The field of information science concerned with the analysis, use, and dissemination of medical data and information through the application of computers to various aspects of health care and medicine.

Medication database: A database in an integrated health information system or module-based **pharmacy information management system** that contains current, and in some cases historical, patient-specific medication information.

Medication reconciliation: The process of comparing a patient's historical and current medications to determine the accurate, current medication list.

Medium: A substance or device that carries a communication signal (e.g., air, fiber-optic cable).

Memory control unit (MCU): A specialized computer subsystem that handles writing data to and reading data from memory.

Meta-analysis: A medical research study that uses statistical techniques to combine the results of several studies as if they were one large study.

Microbiology database: A database in an integrated health information system or module-based laboratory information system that contains current and historical patient-specific microbiology information, such as culture source (sputum, blood, etc.), organism type (cocci), and sensitivity analysis.

Modulation: The process of converting a digital sound wave into analog form.

N

National Drug Code (NDC) Directory: A directory of unique codes assigned to drug products that are distributed by manufacturers and their agents, such as re-labelers; the codes are used for FDA registration and listing. The NDC comprises three segments and includes the labeler code, the formulation code, and the trade package size information.

National Patient Safety Goals (NPSGs): Requirements developed by the Joint Commission to promote and enforce major changes in patient safety in participating health care organizations. The goals highlight problematic areas in health, describe evidence and expert-based solutions for these problems, and focus on system-wide solutions, wherever possible.

Near miss: A situation in which a medication error was detected before it affected and/or reached the patient.

Network database: A database model in which a member record is linked to an owner (parent) field, while simultaneously the member (child) record can function as the owner of multiple other members. For example, in the real world, a pharmacist has many patients and patients often have more than one pharmacist.

Network switching services: Services that route claims for the pharmacy and can be used to perform pre-edits and postedits as well as an increasing number of other services.

Noise: Any unwanted signal introduced into a communication system (also known as interference).

O

Operating system: A computer's software system that acts as the interface between programs, hardware, and systems resources such as the system bus, computer processing unit bus, main memory, and hard disk. A user utilizes the operating system to interact with a computer.

Order: A request for service generated by a **computerized provider order entry** (CPOE) application that can be sent to another CPOE application for fulfillment or can be fulfilled by the requesting CPOE application.

Order detail segment: A component of a **computerized provider order entry** (CPOE) application that can carry order information. Each CPOE application has several order detail segments.

Orderable: Term used in **pharmacy information management systems** to denote an ordered drug item.

P

Passive surveillance system: A surveillance system that requires the end user to recognize that the information presented in the clinical surveillance system warrants action. (See also **Active clinical surveillance**.)

Patient-centered medical home: An approach to providing comprehensive primary care in which a personal clinician takes responsibility for ongoing care of a patient and coordinates patient care across the continuum of the health care system.

Permanent storage/memory: Data stored permanently in a computer (even when the power is turned off) so that the data can be used at some time in the future. Storage devices include hard disks, digital video disks, compact disks, and Universal Serial Bus (USB) flash drives.

Personal health record (PHR): A subset of data managed together by patients and caregivers.

Pharmaceutical supply chain: The means through which prescription medications are delivered to patients. The major players are pharmaceutical manufacturers, wholesale distributors, pharmacies, and pharmacy benefit managers.

Pharmacy informatics: Use and integration of data, information, knowledge, technology, and automation in the medication use process for the purpose of improving health outcomes.

Pharmacy information management system (PIMS): A computer system that is found in virtually all pharmacies (acute and ambulatory) and that supports pharmacy administrative, clinical, financial, and distributive functions.

Pharming: A form of identity theft in which scammers (pharmers) attack the servers on the Internet that direct network traffic and instruct the servers to redirect the computer user's request for a Web site to another site set up by the pharmer.

Phishing: A form of identity theft in which a scammer uses an authentic-looking e-mail to trick recipients into giving out sensitive personal information.

Placer: A component of a **computerized provider order entry** (CPOE) application that can originate a request for an order or services. The originator can be the CPOE application or a user of the application.

Placer order group: A list of associated orders for a single patient sent from a single location to a **computerized provider order entry** application.

Post-edit: A report of all prescriptions that were paid under circumstances that negatively impact pharmacy operations and reimbursement rates.

Potential adverse drug event: An event in which an error occurred but did not cause injury (e.g., the error was detected before it reached the patient, or the patient received a wrong dose but was not harmed).

Pre-edit: A review of claims for payment of prescriptions before their transmittal to the payer.

Prescriber: The health practitioner who has the legal authority for ordering ambulatory medications. Physicians, dentists, nurse practitioners, physician assistants, and pharmacist practitioners are examples.

Primary key: A unique identifier for a database record that allows one or more applications to access, organize, and retrieve data. For example, a medical record number is a likely primary key in a patient table.

Privacy: An individual's ability to control how and what personal information is shared with others.

Prognosis: In an evidence-based clinical question, the estimation of a patient's future course.

Protected health information (PHI): Any information that can identify the patient, including information related to past, present, and future physical or mental conditions, and to any health service or treatment.

Q

Quality: In health care, the degree to which health services for individuals and populations increase the likelihood of desired health outcomes and are consistent with current professional knowledge.

Query: A database search function that allows the user to search across multiple tables and extract data that meet predefined, desired parameters.

R

Randomized controlled trial (RCT): A medical research study in which subjects are randomly assigned to a treatment, no treatment, or placebo group. An RCT is usually blinded (i.e., neither the researcher nor the subject knows which intervention the subject received).

Receiver: In telecommunications, a device that accepts the encoded message from the transmitter and passes it along to the decoder.

Records: In databases, a grouping of related data fields.

Redundant data storage: Off-site storage of **data** by a service provider who backs up regularly and houses the data in geographically dispersed computer data storage facilities for additional security.

Registers: A type of temporary computer memory that stores data to be used immediately (e.g., instructions to direct processing of register data, the current executing instruction, and the next instruction).

Relation: A table within a relational database.

Relational database model: A database model that uses relationships within existing, separate data sets (tables) to store, manage, and retrieve **data**. In each table (file), each row is a **record** and each column is an **attribute**.

Repeater: A device that receives a signal and resends it at a stronger power.

Research informatics: A broad term that indicates the application of informatics to health and biomedical research.

Robotic cart filling system: An automated dispensing device that uses bar coding to locate, obtain, package, label, and deliver medications for specific patients by filling unit-dose carts.

Root cause analysis (RCA): An investigation technique that systematically seeks to understand the underlying (root) causes of an error by looking at all the systems involved.

RxNorm: A clinical drug nomenclature standard produced by the National Library of Medicine, which provides standard names, strengths, and dosage forms for clinical drugs and cross-links these three identifiers, as well as other modifiers such as flavor, salt, or diluents, to all branded products represented by National Drug Codes.

S

SCRIPT: A data transmission standard developed to support the communication of prescription information between prescribers and pharmacists, including transmission of electronic prescriptions, refill requests, prescription change requests or clarifications, fill status notifications, and prescription cancellations.

Secondary key: An identifier in a database record that is not unique but can be used to identify database records (e.g., birth date, address).

Security: In telecommunications, the condition of being free from unwanted or unauthorized access.

Security and reliability criteria: Criteria to assess a software application's ability to maintain the **privacy** of patient data and ensure robustness to prevent data loss.

Security incident: Unauthorized access, use, disclosure, modification, or destruction of **electronic protected health information** (ePHI), including interference with the health information system, improper network activity, and misuse of PHI data.

Semantic interoperability: The ability of two (or more) information technology systems to exchange data on the basis of an agreed-upon vocabulary, thereby guaranteeing same interpretation (semantics) of notions for the users of the interoperating systems.

Severity threshold: In **clinical decision support systems**, the minimum severity that a drug-related problem must achieve prior to being presented to the pharmacist.

Signal: The message sent in a telecommunication system.

Smart pump: A device that administers medications and contains drug libraries and dosing parameters for commonly used medications.

Social bookmarking: See **Social tagging**.

Social tagging: A method by which individuals who have a common interest can denote (tag) Web resources that they deem to be valuable assets within their focus area.

Software as a service (SaaS): Software that is based on an **Application Service Provider** model.

Source: In data communications, the source, or origin, of data signals is most frequently some type of computing system.

Spyware: Malware that secretly tracks computer users' activities, key strokes, log-in names, passwords, and Internet usage.

Structured Query Language (SQL): A unique language that is used to perform actions on data within a database and is the standard query language in relational database management systems.

System: An independent but interrelated group of parts working toward a common goal. Telecommunication systems can include people and are composed of a group of core components, including the signal, source, encoder, transmitter, medium, decoder, and destination.

Systematic reviews: A medical research study in which multiple randomized controlled trials (with sound methodology) are identified through extensive literature searches and then evaluated to answer a specific question.

Synchronous communication: Two-way communication that occurs in real time (simultaneously). Examples include the telephone, instant messaging, and text messages.

T

Telecommunications: Electronic communication over distance.

Telecommunication medium: Anything that can carry an electronic signal from its source to a destination.

Telehealth: Use of electronic information and telecommunication technologies to support long-distance clinical health care, patient professional health-related education, public health, and health administration.

Telepharmacy: A subset of telehealth activities focused on medication management, including education, patient care, and administration.

Therapy: In an evidence-based clinical question, determination of the effect of interventions on patient-important outcomes (symptoms, function, morbidity, mortality, costs).

Total parenteral nutrition (TPN) compounder: Automated dispensing device that performs the complex admixture processes of computing a TPN formulation from clinical requirements, and then drives a machine to deliver the ingredients in the correct amounts and in the correct sequence.

Transmitter: A device that sends an encoded signal over the medium.

Treatment, payment, or operations (TPO): These processes include general health care operational use, such as quality improvement, infection control, credentialing, peer review, case management, clinical training, customer service, and some fund-raising activities.

Trojan horse: A special type of computer virus that performs malicious acts while seemingly running as an innocent program.

U

Unified Medical Language System (UMLS): A collection of "knowledge sources," including the Metathesaurus, that are available from the National Library of Medicine and can be implemented to facilitate the development of computer applications that behave as if they understand medical terminologies. This functionality allows users to search and query across terms that are synonymous or have other relationships with each other.

User interface: The mechanism used by the health care practitioner to access information in an information system.

V

Viral marketing: An Internet marketing method that uses primarily social networks to increase awareness of a Web site, blog, or other Internet feature.

Virtual private networking (VPN): Secure logon procedures and authentication certificates that allow remote access to private networks that have firewalls.

Virus [computer]: Malware that is capable of reproducing and infecting computer files and programs: executables, documents, or the boot sectors on disks.

W

Web 2.0: Interactive and social media applications that comprise the second generation of the Internet, which developed after the 2001 collapse of the dot.com bubble.

Wholesale acquisition cost (WAC): The baseline price at which wholesale distributors purchase drug products.

Workflow management: In pharmacy, the application of computer systems, software, bar code scanning, photography, and other automatic identification methods to streamline and systematize work processes, and to improve visibility of the current state of those processes for individual work items.

Workflow system: In pharmacy, a **pharmacy information management system** that has multiple workstations with assigned specific tasks.

Worm: Malware that automatically copies itself and distributes the copies to other computer systems via e-mail attachments or direct connections. Worms do not necessarily infect other executables; instead they proactively spread themselves over a network (possibly by mass e-mailing).

Index